The Dark Pocket of Time

War, Medicine and the Australian State 1914–1935

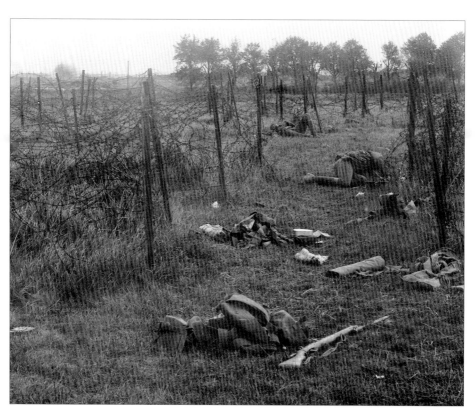

Barbed wire entanglement, Anvil Wood, 2 September 1918 (*detail*)
[Australian War Memorial neg. no. E03149]

The Dark Pocket of Time

War, Medicine and the Australian State, 1914–1935

Kate Blackmore

LYTHRUM PRESS
ADELAIDE
2008

Lythrum Press
PO Box 243 Rundle Mall, Adelaide
South Australia 5000

www.lythrumpress.com.au

First published in 2008

National Library of Australia Cataloguing-in-Publication entry:

Author:	Blackmore, Kate, 1949 -
Title:	The Dark Pocket of Time: War, medicine and the Australian state, 1914–1935 / Kate Blackmore.
Publisher:	Adelaide: Lythrum Press, 2008.
ISBN:	978 1 921013 19 5 (pbk.)
Notes:	Includes index.
	Bibliography.
Subjects:	Australia. Repatriation Commission.
	World War, 1914-1918 – Health aspects – Australia.
	World War, 1914-1918 – Veterans – Australia.
	Veterans – Medical care – Australia.
	Military pensions – Australia.
	Australia – Politics and government – 1914-1918.
	Australia – Politics and government – 1918-1922.
Dewey Number:	362.8680994

Cover design: Stacey Zass, Colorperception
Text design and typesetting: Michael Deves, Lythrum Press
Printed and bound by Everbest Printing Co. Ltd, China

Front cover illustration: Otto Dix, *Der Krieg*, XIX, Totentanz Anno 17 (Höhe Toter Mann),
  Dance of Death 1917 (Dead Man's Hill)
Back cover illustration: Otto Dix, *Der Krieg*, IV, Trichterfeld bei Dontrien von Leuchtkugeln
  erheltt, *Crater field Near Dontrien Lit by Flares*

Images courtesy National Gallery of Australia; © Otto Dix, licensed by VISCOPY, Australia 2008

TABLE OF CONTENTS

Acknowledgements   vii

Abbreviations   viii

Note on Sources   x

List of Illustrations   xi

Preface   xii

CHAPTER 1   Introduction   1

CHAPTER 2   The Great Ordeal   10

CHAPTER 3   'The Old Lie': The Soldier's War on the Western Front   29

CHAPTER 4   Setting up a Department   59

CHAPTER 5   Doctors and Soldiers: New Chapters in the History of Medicine   77

CHAPTER 6   Demobilisation, Repatriation and Australian Productivity   101

CHAPTER 7   War, Medicine and Responsibility for Illness   128

CHAPTER 8   War Pensions: The 'Clinical toss up' and the 'National purse'   150

CHAPTER 9   What an Australian is Worth by Cut and by Kilogram: a leg, an eye and other case studies in the war pensioning process   172

CHAPTER 10   Epilogue   194

Notes on the Chapters   214

Appendix 1   Fortnightly differential rates of war pensions paid 1920 for 100% incapacity   245

Appendix 2   Categories of invalids used by the AAMC in 1918   246

Bibliography   247

Index   273

... they were a sea of mud into which everything was in danger of sinking without trace and which stank of what it had already swallowed, corpses, the bloated carcasses of mules, horses, men ... It would go on forever. The war, or something like it with a different name, would go on growing out from here till the whole earth was involved ... They had fallen, he and his contemporaries, into a dark pocket of time from which there was no escape.

David Malouf

Fly Away Peter

Penguin, Ringwood 1982, pp.102-3

Acknowledgements

This book has a long history of debts. At Macquarie University, Professor Duncan Waterson and Dr George Parsons were wonderful mentors and friends. Dr Bill Edmonds was a partner in ideas and more.

The research entailed very lengthy periods in a few key archival repositories: the Australian War Memorial; Australian Archives New South Wales; and Australian Archives Canberra. My sincere thanks to the personnel who made the time productive and rewarding.

Obtaining access to veterans' records was not easy; indeed it took nearly two years of negotiation with the Department of Veterans' Affairs. My thanks go to those involved.

The research entailed significant financial outlays. This was immeasurably helped by funding from the Australian War Memorial's John Treloar Research Grants and the Australian Army History Unit. To these funding bodies I owe a debt of thanks.

The Australian War Memorial, the National Library of Australia, and the National Gallery of Australia kindly allowed reproduction of the images.

Special personal thanks are due to Brendan O'Keefe whose unstinting intellectual support, advice, collegiality, and warm accommodation in Queanbeyan was a pleasure and benefited the work immeasurably.

Finally, my thanks to Robbie Johnson for his moral support in the final editing, support given with concern, generosity and great humour.

Kate Blackmore

Acknowledgement and Disclaimer

The author expressly wishes to acknowledge the support of the Australian Government Department of Veterans' Affairs, which provided a grant to assist publication under the Government's commemorations program, *Saluting Their Service.*

The Department has not participated in the research or production or exercised editorial control over the work's contents, and the views expressed and conclusions reached herein do not necessarily represent those of the Commonwealth, which expressly disclaims any responsibility for the content or accuracy of the work.

Abbreviations

AA	Australian Archives
AAH	Australian Auxiliary Hospital
AAMC	Australian Army Medical Corps
ACT	Australian Capital Territory
ADGMS	Assistant Director-General Medical Services
ADH	Australian Dermatological Hospital
ADMS	Assistant Director of Medical Services
AGH	Australian General Hospital
AIC	Australian Intelligence Corps
AIF	Australian Imperial Force
AMA	Australian Medical Association
ASR	Australian Soldiers' Repatriation (Fund/Bill/Act)
AWM	Australian War Memorial
BEF	British Expeditionary Force
BMA	British Medical Association
CO	Commanding Officer
CCS	Casualty Clearing Station
CMG	Companion of the Order of St Michael and St George
CMR	Commonwealth Medical Referee
CPD	Commonwealth Parliamentary Debates
CPP	Commonwealth Parliamentary Papers
DAH	Disordered Action of the Heart
DC	Deputy Comptroller or Commissioner
DDMS	Deputy Director of Medical Services
DGMS	Director General Medical Services
DMO	Departmental Medical Officer
DMS	Director of Medical Services
DSO	Distinguished Service Order
DWS	Due to war service
EEF	Egyptian Expeditionary Force
FPWC	Federal Parliamentary War Committee
FRCP	Fellow of the Royal College of Physicians
FRCS	Fellow of the Royal College of Surgeons
GOC	General Officer Commanding
GSW	Gun shot wound

ICT	Inflammation of Connective Tissue
LMO	Local Medical Officer
MC	Military Cross
MO	Medical Officer
MRC	Medical Research Committee
MU	Medically Unfit
NDWS	Not due to war service
NSW	New South Wales
NYD	Not yet diagnosed
NYDN	Not yet diagnosed – nervous
OBE	Order of the British Empire
OIC	Officer in Command
PDMO	Principal Departmental Medical Officer
PU/PB	Permanently Unfit
PUO	Pyrexia of Unknown Origin
RMO	Regimental Medical Officer
RSSILA/RSL	Returned Soldiers and Sailors Imperial League of Australia
SMO	Senior Medical Officer
SNPP	Soldiers National Political Party
VC	Victoria Cross
VD	Venereal disease
VVAA	Vietnam Veterans Association
WS	War Service

Note on Sources

The bulk of the empirical data on war pensions was found in Departmental files held at Australian Archives (AA) Canberra and Sydney. The vast majority of the files were classified as 'open'. However, in order to obtain detail of the pensioning *process*, analysis of individual case files was necessary. The Department of Veterans Affairs ultimately granted conditional access to personal Pension, Hospital and Medical files of World War One veterans. This required entering into a binding legal agreement with the Department to safeguard the identity of the veterans. Consequently, no names or file numbers are used here; the references in the text are to Box numbers only; names are fictitious.

The personal files themselves provided another methodological problem, given their number. Considering the broad scope of the work, the files were used to indicate procedures and practice instead of attempting a quantitative study. As argued throughout the work, bureaucratic procedures were followed with rigorous consistency throughout the period under study. Files which revealed continuous processes of review and re-assessment over many decades provide the strongest evidence of how decisions on eligibility were reached. Only New South Wales files were used for this purpose. (There were 138 073 First AIF files held in the New South Wales branch of AA). A random sample was generated from the Box numbers within the 12 AA series in New South Wales. Each Box held between one and twenty files; the 'Table of random numbers' was then used to select files within each box. Over 1000 files were examined and approximately 200 finally used.

List of Illustrations

Front cover   Otto Dix, *Der Krieg*, XIX, Totentanz Anno 17
(Höhe Toter Mann), *Dance of Death 1917 (Dead Man's Hill)*

Frontispiece   Barbed wire entanglement, Anvil Wood, 2 September 1918
[AWM E03149 - *detail*]   page ii

Figure 1   Otto Dix, *Der Krieg*, XII, Sturmtruppe geht unter Gas vor,
Shock Troops Advance Under Gas   page 34

Figure 2   Soldiers of the 45th Battalion wearing gas respirators in a trench
at Garter Point, in the Ypres Sector, 27 September 1917
[AWM E00825]   page 35

Figure 3   A set of 180 gas projectors alongside the Albert-Amiens railway
in front of the Casualty Clearing Station at Dernancourt,
14 June 1918 [AWM E04897]   page 36

Figure 4   Australian soldiers gassed at Villers-Bretonneux 27 May 1918.
[AWM E04851]   page 41

Figure 5   Swollen face of a soldier affected by mustard gas at a Casualty
Clearing Station on the Amiens-Corbie road, 27 May 1918
[AWM E04853]   page 42

Figure 6   PH Helmet gas respirator, c 1916 [AWM RELAWM04043.001]   page 44

Figure 7   Small Box Respirator, c 1918 [AWM RELAWM12424.001]   page 44

Figure 8   Otto Dix, *Der Krieg*, XXIII, Toter in Schlamm,
Dead Man in the Mud   page 50

Figure 9   Dead German soldier in water filled crater, near Zonnebeke
in the Ypres Sector, 17 October 1917 [AWM E00927]   page 51

Figure 10   Australian troops at Chateau Wood walking over duckboards
in the waterlogged fields to Zonnebeke, October 1917
[NLA, nla.pic-an23478230]   page 52

Figure 11   Mule team bogged in thigh deep mud near Potijze Farm in
the Ypres Sector, 19 October 1917 [AWM E00962]   page 53

Figure 12   Otto Dix, *Der Krieg*, IX, Zerfallender Kampfgraben,
Disintegrating Trench   page 54

Figure 13   Captured German trenches strewn with dead after the
battle of 20 September 1917, Menin Road area [AWM E00766]   page 55

Figure 14.   Australian ambulance men at Bernafay conveying soldiers
               suffering from trench foot to a transport, December 1916
               [AWM E00081]   page 56

Figure 15.   The cost of living and the basic wage, 1919-1920   page 111

Figure 16.   Comparative rates for war pensions by country 1920:
               totally (temporarily) incapacitated Privates   page 112

Figure 17.   Comparative rates for war pensions by country 1920:
               totally (temporarily) incapacitated Privates with dependants page 113

Figure 18.   War pensions in relation to cost of living 1920   page 115

Figure 19.   Attendance of Commissioners at Meetings of the Repatriation
               Commission, July to November 1918 (30 meetings)   page 122

Figure 20.   History of assessment of incapacity, Private William O,
               1917-1935   page 190

Figure 21.   Commonwealth benefits and war pensions: liability June 1919   page 205

Figure 22.   Commonwealth benefits and war pensions:
               number of recipients June 1919   page 205

Figure 23.   Average fortnightly pension rates for incapacitated soldiers,
               1919 and 1920   page 206

Figure 24.   Number of pensions paid for incapacitated soldiers,
               1919 and 1920   page 206

Figure 25.   Total number of war pension claims 1924-1934   page 212

Figure 26.   Percentage of total war pension claims rejected 1924-1934   page 212

Figure 27.   The village of Pozières some months after the battle, April 1917
               [AWM E00532]   page 213

Back cover   Otto Dix, *Der Krieg*, IV, Trichterfeld bei Dontrien von
               Leuchtkugeln erheltt, *Crater field Near Dontrien Lit by Flares*

Preface

This book is a history of the *relationship* between war, medicine and the Australian state between c1914 and c1935. The book thus traverses a number of historical areas. There is a vast literature on the relationship between war and medicine which, until fairly recently, has been dominated by positivist or populist accounts or hagiography. Similarly, there is a significant body of literature on the relationship between war and modernity. Only in the last decade or so has a small body of work emerged that addresses all three entities. As Cooter has noted, the relationship is 'remarkable for the silence that surrounds it'.[1]

Part, if not the whole, of the problem of writing about this history is the length, breadth and depth of the topic. To do it justice it can't be the 'epiphenomenal' approach that has characterized so much of the literature, an approach equally decried by Cooter, but rather it needs embedding within the political, social and economic history of each conflict period. How many historians, then, would it take to write this history? Any wonder the subject remains barely visible, as too does the relationship between law, medicine and the state as problematized in the workers compensation process. And in an age of revived classical liberal values (economic rationalism), what resonance does such history create in a reading public?

The history databases are relatively silent on global approaches to the subject in the past few years. Ahistorical, atheoretical, populist or post-modern cultural histories are even declining in number. So perhaps, if nothing else, this work is an attempt to be *agent provocateur*. To engage in controversy, debate, or dialogue, would be infinitely preferable to continuing silence.

Finally, there are a small number of illustrations in this book. Some explanation for their choice is warranted. The five prints are all the work of Otto Dix (1891-1969) and all are from the 1924 *Der Krieg* (War) series of 50 etchings. Dix enlisted with enthusiasm in 1914 and served as a machine-gunner for four years with the German army witnessing the Somme, Pozières and Bapaume. He painted and drew obsessively during this time. He has been described as 'guilty of turning from model soldier into sacrilegious artist … of showing what he should have refrained from depicting: carnage, decay and horror'.[2]

The images in *Der Krieg* have parallels with the subject matter of some Australian wartime photography; indeed a number of comparisons are drawn in this work. However, what Dix, as artist, does is distill the experience of the front. He concentrates on death and decaying bodies, on trenches filled with such carnage and putrefaction. These are frequently brutal, shocking images; no doubt, given Dix's German social and political context in 1923-4, intentionally so. But they are nevertheless real. Dix portrays what soldiers have described: the images of the real war on the Western Front that haunted so many survivors; images rarely used in publications on the Great War.

Dix's (living) soldiers are often ugly and sometimes portrayed as indifferent to their surroundings; whether corpses or French civilian life. His wounded are terrified. On the whole, Australian artist-soldiers and official artists during the Great War produced a very different corpus. Heroism, bravery, epic tragedy, pride, stoicism, sacrifice and larrikinism are the hallmarks of Australian artist-participants from George Lambert to Ellis Silas. Death and wounding are ennobled. Beautiful young men populate the images. These are not depictions of the reality of war so have little value for this work despite their unquestioned artistic merit. Chapter 3, 'The Old Lie', attempts to portray some of this reality using available documentary sources and Dix's etchings have a resonance not found elsewhere. One of Dix's prints from *Der Krieg* has been reproduced many times (not here).[3] Unlike the majority of the images in *Der Krieg*, this is an image of a living soldier after the war. It is a disturbing image of a man with facial injuries who has undergone a skin graft.[4] The Australian War Memorial has many thousands of images of World War One. Tucked away in the vast documentary archive of the Official Medical Historian of the Great War, A.G. Butler, are a very small number of images of severe facial injuries and reconstructive surgery carried out on Australian soldiers during and immediately after the war.[5] Within these images there is one image which could have been the subject for Dix's image. Comparing the images, the veracity of Dix's work is undeniable.

Yet this image is, in one way, unique. While there are indeed many images in Australian collections of the war's horrors[6] – bodies decaying in trenches, skulls in trenches, individual young bodies with almost recognizable faces – *all* of these images are of 'the enemy'; of decaying German dead in trenches, of German skeletal remains. There are a small number of images of dead Australian soldiers but those examined were photographed immediately after the particular engagement and undoubtedly the bodies were properly buried by their units.[7]

Two questions arise here. How does one explain the sanitized nature of the Australian collections? And, are the Australian collections typical of the collections in other participating nations, that is, did all nations only photograph, collect and keep celebratory images of their own soldiers while documenting the death, decay and destruction of the enemy? These are big questions indeed and, while fascinating in themselves and deserving of further research, they are beyond the scope of this particular work. A few very tentative explanations are offered as follows.

Given the emphasis on gassing, trench foot and trench fever in this book, particular attention was given to finding accurate and graphic representations of precisely what soldiers suffered. There are few surviving images in Australia, more particularly surviving graphic images. This may be partly (or wholly) explained by wartime censorship. In August 1916, Private James Agnew wrote to his mother that 'cameras are unfortunately prohibited in France although the papers are still full of war pictures I suppose'.[8] This sentence says a lot. Images of death, decay and destruction were indeed appearing in the press around the world but, in Australia at least, such images were censored. Individual soldiers did (illegally) take photographs – but of what? Despite the massive number of privately owned photographs donated to the Australian War Memorial in the 90 odd years since the Great War, there are still no graphic or disturbing images of 'our' dead or their decay in the trenches of the Western Front. Self-censorship, it seems, may be just as powerful as official censorship – precisely what makes Dix's work 'sacrilegious'.

Censorship of images of wartime trauma, injury and atrocity is a big subject and not pursued here. Arguably the Vietnam war, the first 'TV' war, changed the nature of that censorship forever: the Eddie Adams, Nick Ut and Ronald Haeberle photos of atrocities did that. Such photographs of World War One do not exist in Australia, or, if they do, they are held in private collections. Of the private donations to public collections, from veterans, their families or friends, it is understandable, perhaps, that soldiers serving on the Western Front who witnessed the unearthing of trenches filled with the rotting remains of their comrades were unwilling, or unable, to document such a nightmare. But that is pure speculation. It doesn't fully explain the existence of many photographs of the rotting bodies of others, German dead in particular.

Brief searches of the World War One online photographic holdings of both the Imperial War Memorial and Canadian War Memorial reveal a similar story. There are a very small number of photographs of dead allied soldiers. However, all but one are of soldiers awaiting burial or being buried. The images of the long-dead are almost uniformly of German dead. We await further research on the role of nationalism, on national censorship (both official and unofficial) with regard to photography, and on (perhaps) the policies and directives that dictate the nature of collections over time.

In the end, the images included here were chosen because they give some indication of the reality of trench warfare on the Western Front from the general (trenches, entanglements, landscapes, conditions) to the particular (faces, feet). They are not intended to shock but, rather, to inform.

In memory of

W.D. (Bill) Edmonds, 1945–1994

CHAPTER 1

Introduction

In David Malouf's *Fly Away Peter*, the central character, Jim, and two of his friends were out of the lines at Armentières, about to have a cup of tea when they were shelled. Jim, when conscious enough to recognise what had happened, realised that Eric had lost both legs, one just above the knee, the other 'not far above the boot'.

Some days later Jim visited Eric in hospital. The boy was apprehensive:

> Listen, Jim, who's gunna look after me? …When I get outa here. At home'n all. I got no one. Just the fellers in the company, and none of 'em 'ave come to see me except you. I got nobody, not even an auntie. I'm an orfing. Who's gunna look after me, back there?
>
> The question was monstrous … He didn't know the answer any more than Eric did and the question scared him. Faced with his losses, Eric had hit upon something fundamental. It was a question about the structure of the world they lived in and where they belonged in it, about who had power over them and what responsibility those agencies could be expected to assume.[1]

There were 2200 amputees like Eric back home in Australia by 1919.[2] There were nearly 100 soldiers who were totally blinded.[3] Then there were the 59 000 who died: to the Australian public in the immediate post-war years, these men were icons symbolising the supreme sacrifice for the nation and the imperial cause. Sydney's Anzac Memorial proclaims '*Pro Patria Mori Dulce et Decorum est*'. Blinded soldiers and amputees likewise were used in propaganda of the period to symbolise sacrifice and, after the war, to celebrate their rehabilitation by a grateful nation.

By 1920, the 264 000 surviving members of the First AIF were home. It is estimated that around 160 000 were sick or wounded. In the same year, over 90 000 were receiving a war pension. A further 135 000 pensions were paid to widows, wives and other 'dependants' of incapacitated or dead soldiers.[4] As well as the war pension, there were re-training schemes, land settlement schemes, 'sustenance' payments, schemes for the education of soldiers' children and other forms of assistance. During the war years, returned soldier organisations had formed to act as political advocates in securing benefits. The largest, the Returned Soldiers and Sailors Imperial League of Australia (RSSILA), had a membership of 150 000 in 1919. Politically, the sheer numbers of soldiers and their families constituted a powerful electoral bloc guaranteeing some form of patronage: on the eve of the 1919 election, a war gratuity payment was promised and later realised in the War

1

Gratuity Act of 1920. This list of 'benefits' is what is usually understood in Australia as 'repatriation'. It is often described as 'an exceedingly generous system' for a 'privileged class of welfare recipients'.[5] Yet such interpretations conceal more than they reveal.

Considered historically, these measures must be understood as responses to a social and economic crisis of a scale hitherto unexperienced in Australian history. The period from August 1914 to 1920 saw immense political upheavals leading to the defeat of a federal Labor government in favour of a coalition of Labor deserters and Liberals – the Nationalist 'Win-the-War' Party – which became the 'economy government' of the period 1917 to 1922. With the passing of the War Precautions Act in 1914, government by fiat became commonplace, the 'soldiers' friend', W.M. Hughes, taking control. This period also witnessed the enormous social divisiveness of two unsuccessful conscription referenda and a re-invigoration of xenophobia which outlived the war years. As well, the financial cost of the war was beyond the wildest expectations of Commonwealth Treasury: Commonwealth debt prior to the war was less than £10 million; by June 1922 the war debt alone had risen to nearly £370 million.[6] With the cost of living rising sharply and real wages falling, industrial disputes were frequent and militant, and the reaction of the state ruthless. The AIF returned to Australia amidst this chaos.

Yet, the political, economic and social factors mentioned here leave much about the Great War and its aftermath unexplained. Malouf's character, Jim, incisively and insightfully pierces the heart of the problem: what was the structure of the world they returned to? Who would have power over them? And what responsibility would those agencies assume? To answer these questions the starting point must be France and the end point Australia in the 1930s. To answer them demands an understanding of the nature of warfare in the Great War – the Australian soldier's war in particular. It also requires a context of Australian welfare history to locate service benefits within a broader historiographical and historical framework. It requires an understanding of the character of the Australian state both during and after the war, its administrative arms in particular. And, finally and most importantly, it necessitates an understanding of the role and function of medicine both during and after the war.

The places where these diverse strands of history intersect are the war-pensioning process, and its predecessor, the medical boarding process. Both processes involved the interplay of state authority (Defence and Repatriation Departments) with professionalism (both military and medical). Both processes used evaluation of a soldier's documented war history as an instrument to express either personal or group values and belief systems (ideologies). Both were driven by 'economy' – either maximising the number of 'effective' troops, or reducing the pension 'burden' and, in the period under study, both processes were characterised by a pervasive militarism.

These themes form the substantive focus of this study. Each is problematic historically in Australia due largely to a lack of historical attention, but also to a lack of critical analysis in what history has emerged.

Welfare benefits and compensation payments[7]

Prior to the outbreak of war, the Australian welfare system consisted of maternity allowances and old age and invalid pensions. Maternity allowances (1912) were inspired by gender based notions of women's role in the reproduction of the population and in the labour force. Federal responsibility for the aged poor (1908), on the other hand, was seen by contemporaries as a state debt. The invalid pension (1910) was quite different. It was always considered a charitable handout, or a gift to the indigent sick; eligibility criteria were considerably restricted when compared to the old-age pension. Central to an application for the invalid pension was the earning capacity and health of the individual, that is, the person had to prove 'permanent incapacity for any work'. Such 'proof' was established or denied by a variety of investigative processes, including assessment by the police and examination by at least two doctors, one a Commonwealth Medical Referee.[8] The control of these pensioning procedures was firmly vested in Treasury. Examination of Treasury rulings on pensions between 1911 and 1920, an archive previously unused in histories of the welfare process in the period, reveals a distinct change in philosophy after 1913, that is prior to the outbreak of war.

The reformist liberalism that characterised the previous decade and witnessed the introduction of these benefits came to an abrupt end when the Secretary of Treasury, George Allen, went into semi-retirement and was replaced by James Collins. Collins, the son of a miner, together with his old friend C.J. Cerutty and another associate, C.J. Cornell, controlled Treasury from 1914 until 1920. In the latter year, Collins left Treasury and Cornell moved to Repatriation as Officer in Charge of Pensions. Cerutty went on to become Auditor General in 1926. Together they reformulated the nineteenth century distinction between the deserving and undeserving poor into that of the deserving and undeserving sick. This poor law mentality along with a constant mindfulness of public spending ensured an ideological conformity in decisions on pension eligibility and pension policy throughout the period under study.

Yet it was not simply Treasury bureaucrats who controlled the cost of pensioning. An important distinction must be made here between the social wage benefits like the old age and invalid pensions or even the later service pension, and a war pension. Indeed the latter is a misnomer; it was not a pension. The war pension was paid as compensation, not as a benefit. Like workers compensation it was designed with cost-containment in mind. In this instance the employer, the Australian state, compensated the worker/soldier for incapacity suffered in the course of employment at war. The compensation payment (war pension) was based on the medical assessment of a degree of incapacity expressed as a percentage. That percentage became a percentage of the monetary value of a full pension. The vast majority of war pensions paid in Australia in the 1920s were for partial incapacity. In New South Wales, for example, 44% of war pensions in 1925 were paid at less than 25% of a full pension; another 30% were paid between 25% and 50%.[9] One of the central arguments here will be that medicine and medical practitioners played an instrumental role in controlling the cost of these pensions through the assessment process.

The Australian state

Macintyre has provided a succinct definition of the state as 'the authority that constitutes the members of a society as citizens in conjunction with the formal apparatus that includes legislature, courts, administration and police'.[10] How that authority and its political, judicial and executive wings are understood is a thornier problem. There is a tacit assumption in this work that the nature and function of the state is always historically specific. A theme which arises intermittently in this work, particularly in relation to the crisis of 1914-1918, is the extent of the state's autonomy from the economically dominant class. In the specific circumstances of the First World War and its aftermath, the level of practical autonomy attained by one section of the Australian state (Repatriation) was possible only because of the dominance within its bureaucracy of values which matched those of the ruling economic elite. That is, in a situation such as that of 1918, where a new state bureaucracy was staffed by men hand-picked for the compatibility of their interests and values with a conservative political regime, and when the crisis of war granted enormous power to a central government, a high degree of autonomy was achieved by the administrative agencies of the state. In other words, to maintain a liberal-democratic society, the state was required to intervene on a scale far beyond that envisaged by classical liberalism. This is perhaps nowhere clearer than in the relative autonomy allowed to the senior Repatriation bureaucrats during the period under study, an autonomy which posed no threat to the conservative government because a pervasive ideology ensured unity of purpose.

Ideology was the glue that created cohesion in the Repatriation department. Clay Ramsay describes ideology as 'not so much a coherent set of ideas that can be ascribed to one side in a conflict, as it is a basic conceptual frame indistinguishable from the grand lines of the society to which it belongs'.[11] In the period under study, this 'frame' was characterised by rationality (efficiency) – what Gellner describes as 'the cool rational selection of the best available means to given, clearly formulated and isolated ends'[12]; control of public expenditure ('economy'); notions of self-help and self-improvement, both of which assisted in ensuring an 'economy' of government; and a grudging recognition of the need to assist the helpless, the sick and the poor. In other words, an ideology grounded in classical liberalism.

In classical liberal democratic theory (Bentham, James Mill), 'government was needed for the protection of individuals and the promotion of Gross National Product, and for nothing more'.[13] But in the late nineteenth century the ethical or developmental liberalism characteristic of J.S. Mill became influential, promoting policies of social amelioration. The result was what Macpherson calls the development of models of liberal democracy (here called reformist liberalism) which included an enhanced role for the state in improving society, notably by creating the necessary conditions for the self-improvement of the poor. The repatriation scheme at its inception was a mixture of both forms of liberalism. The breadth of the schemes of self-help, such as land settlement and vocational training, satisfied the ameliorist tendencies that survived the Deakinite years, while the intense concentration on 'economy', productivity and the selection of 'suitable men' to implement these imperatives reflect the way war revived the values of classical liberalism. During the post war years these values came to dominate.

One final aspect of the state apparatus requires comment. Max Weber's model bureaucracy was characterised by 'precision, speed, lack of equivocation, knowledge of the documentary record, continuity, sense of discretion, uniformity of operation, system of subordination, and reduction of frictions'.[14] It was also a 'paid, full-time administration by professionals, regardless of their social and economic position' and one that rejected 'decision-making from case to case'[15] in favour of 'coherence or consistency, the like treatment of like cases'.[16]

With regard to the first set of characteristics, the Repatriation bureaucrats rapidly acquired these administrative virtues. Many of the senior bureaucrats had been co-opted from other departments: Nicholas Lockyer from the Interstate Commission, James Semmens from the Victorian Fisheries and Game Department, L.T. East from Customs, and there were others. From 1920, when Semmens effectively ran the Department, any departure from such model behaviour was quickly and effectively dealt with. In one notable instance, a Deputy Commissioner, under investigation for mismanagement, was transferred interstate from where he chose a self-imposed exile in South Africa, committing suicide some years later. Yet the bureaucracy was also something of an anomaly in Weberian terms. The paid Commission of three men who sat at the top of the bureaucratic tree consisted of a storekeeper (Barrett), a chaplain (Teece) and a career public servant (Semmens). Two of the three had little administrative experience and even less experience in the public service.

This apparent anomaly can only be explained if we look at other qualifications that were common to these three and to many other senior bureaucrats in the Department. The most fascinating of these is a widespread association with the Australian Intelligence Corps, the creature of J.W. McCay established in Melbourne in 1908. The other more obvious, and possibly more important, common factor was their military backgrounds. Among the key players, this experience went back to the militia, well before the war, and in some cases persisted after the war was over. So, in addition to possessing a common set of liberal values, these men also placed emphasis on military principles such as discipline, self-discipline, obedience and punishment. The strength of this ideological uniformity created an enormously powerful organisation within the executive arm of the state, a situation which apparently defies the principles of liberalism.

The role of medicine

Coherence, consistency and the like treatment of like cases, are also of fundamental importance to the smooth functioning of a bureaucracy. In the treatment of soldiers, this became a mammoth and insoluble problem. Medical knowledge, by its very nature, is indeterminate: no two cases are alike and, its practitioners would argue, only an expert can utilise that knowledge to assess an individual's health. Yet doctors were vital to the process: they ministered to the sick and wounded of the First AIF and they performed the assessment of incapacity for tens of thousands of war pensions. During the war years the problem was partly overcome by massive increases in codification and regulation of practice, and by insistence on consistency of treatment, in other words by the imposition of Army regulations and Army discipline on the work of doctors. In the post-war years, the dilemma was partly resolved by reducing the power of doctors who were external to the Department and by increasing the power of medical bureaucrats. This was only possible because, by the late 1920s, the senior medical staff of the Department clearly and consistently placed the interests of the state above other considerations. In the words of one senior Departmental medical officer, they were not 'nice kind doctors', they were the 'careful custodian[s] of the public exchequer'.[17]

In the post war years these doctors were primarily bureaucrats. Like the other bureaucrats, they had been hand-picked for their jobs, they had all served in the AIF, some purely as combatants not as doctors, and most had long associations with pre-war military formations. One worked closely with Monash. For these men, discipline had a therapeutic value. But as doctors, they also played an instrumental role in cost-containment. Pensioning was and continues to be an immensely complex process. What might at first glance seem a simple clinical assessment by a qualified professional, was contaminated by the incompleteness of the crucial army medical records, by the importance non-medical factors such as moral 'failing' or disciplinary infringement assumed in the assessment process, by the powerlessness of the veteran in the face of the bureaucracy, and by legislative amendments to the Australian Soldiers' Repatriation Act which complicated the assessment even further.

Delving into this morass raises more questions than can be answered here. While the practice of medicine on the Western Front may have added to doctors' clinical skills and maintained army 'strength', this was frequently at the cost of soldiers' health. The well-documented system of re-classifying invalids as fit for active service as much as the poorly documented poisoning of soldiers through wearing a particular gas mask, only hints at the health problems veterans endured after the war. This entire field of history demands attention.

Militarism, modernity and ideology

Militarism was a defining characteristic of the senior doctors of the Australian Army Medical Corps (AAMC) during World War One and also of many doctors on the staff of the Repatriation Department in the period under study. This begs a definition of militarism as used here.

Militarism is a contested concept and it trails a very long bibliography. Interpretations are roughly split into those who concentrate on the civilian-military interplay of power, particularly in pre-industrial and industrialising states, in current Third World military or paramilitary states, and in the military-industrial complex; those who seek to ground militarism in particular social and economic formations; and those who see militarism as ideology or as a value system permeating particular social formations. Put another way, most of the seminal literature on militarism looks at the relationship between professional armies (rather than volunteer armies) and the state, at the nature of that state at a particular point in history, at the historical specificity of particular wars, and at the impact of a militaristic ideology on the civilian-military nexus.[18]

In Western historiography, these various approaches necessarily invoke discussions of the relationship between liberalism and militarism, between Weberian modernity and militarism, and about scientific industrial capitalism and militarism. It is a dense theoretical area which has not been resolved to the satisfaction of any particular group of analysts. Yet militarism remains, in one commentator's words, 'a protean concept'.[19] Perhaps the seminal work on militarism to date is by Alfred Vagts, *A History of Militarism: Civilian and Military*.[20] First published in 1937 but somewhat revised in 1959, Vagts teases us in the Preface to the work with some piercing insights into the nature of militarism but fails, in general, to follow up on all but his remarkable analysis of modern mass (conscript) armies, their relationship to the state, and the power of their ideology (chiefly in relationship to Germany and Japan).

However, there are two issues raised in the Preface that have relevance for this work before, during and particularly after the Great War. The first is Vagts' contention that militarism 'displays the qualities of caste and cult, authority and belief'; that it is 'more, and sometimes less, than the love of war.'

> It covers every system of thinking and valuing and every complex of feelings which rank military institutions and ways above the ways of civilian life, carrying military mentality and modes of acting and decision into the civilian sphere.[21]

In other words, militarism as ideology, what Townshend has described as the 'spillage of military values into society at large'.[22] According to one historian, in the period between Federation and the outbreak of war, a 'romantic, bellicose patriotism' and 'nascent nationalism' was evident in Australia and continued to flourish in the post-war era.[23] This is probably a fair description of, amongst other things, the creation of the Australian Intelligence Corps in 1907 – drawn from the ranks of the militia, the introduction of compulsory military training in 1911 at Kitchener's direction and in the same year the establishment of the Royal Military College, Duntroon, and the relative ease of raising a volunteer army in the first two years of the war.[24] Beyond that it is seriously misleading. As will be shown, the 'romantic' liberalism so evident in the pre-war years, completely disappeared from Australia during the war and was replaced by an ultra conservative classical liberalism which had no difficulty accommodating militarism within its values and structures, in spite of liberal rhetoric to the contrary. Vagts points out that armies are always conservative, officers in particular.[25] In post-war Australia, the preponderance of former officers in the Repatriation Department and elsewhere represents, in Vagts' words, 'an assimilation of military thought to previously cherished social and economic thought'.[26] This theme is explored at length within this work.

The second key issue raised by Vagts is the relationship between militarism and socio-economic formations and conditions. According to Vagts, 'armies and war cannot be considered aside from their relation to society'.[27] One important and recent work on the historical relationship between war and medicine has insisted on the importance of *modernity* as a key explanatory device in modern wars.[28] Once again this requires a definition. A Weberian model of modernity, one which stresses bureaucracy, organisational and managerial systems, standardisation, rationality, efficiency, and uniformity, has become a commonplace in the limited literature on the topic. These systems and forms are extremely valuable heuristic devices, as Cooter and Sturdy point out.[29] For the purposes of this work, however, modernity signifies what Lawrence describes as a 'structural organisation of state, economy, society and culture; a power-complex and a mode of consciousness'.[30] In early 20th century Australia this translates as burgeoning industrial capitalism, a modern state and, during and after the war, a permeating ideology within some public and private sectors underpinned by classical liberal values and militarism.

In broad terms, the defining features of militarism as understood here are practically difficult to differentiate from the concrete social, economic and political reality of early 20th century industrial capitalism, with all its ideological underpinnings, even if the industrial conditions did not necessarily apply to Australia in the very early 20th century. Hierarchy, instrumentality, economy, technological and scientific positivism, planning, efficiency and order, were hallmarks of many areas in Australian politics and policy, scientific, social and economic thought, in the war and post-war years. But these characteristics were not necessarily militaristic or defining of militarism. What differentiated the ideology of militarism was its excesses. This is particularly evident in the areas of command, hierarchy, discipline, obedience, punishment and the use of brutal means to achieve ends. The ruthless extermination, oppression and dispossession of Aboriginal people in Australia in the 19th and early 20th centuries, not to mention Australian imperialist tendencies in the Pacific, and support of Britain's imperialist policies, bears witness to imperialism at home, the same imperialism that Lawrence correctly defines as one of the key hallmarks of a militarised modernism. Indeed Lawrence argues that in the 19th and early 20th centuries, 'modernity had taken charge of Western Europe and was now pointing the beam of reason at Africa and Asia'.[31] The general thesis here, of militarism being concealed beneath a mantle of colonialism and imperialism, is equally apposite in Australian history. While Gellner may have been correct in saying that the preoccupation of imperialism was industry and trade 'not by a militaristic machine', Lawrence's analysis makes it abundantly clear that the means were both militaristic and devastating.[32] In the AAMC, a rigidly hierarchical command, its demand for obedience, for medical and military discipline, and the sometimes brutal means employed for desirable ends, all resonate with the ideology of militarism.[33]

One other characteristic of militarism, a characteristic not necessarily related to modern social or economic formations, is a uniform. In all wars, including the Great War, the uniform was the creator of the anonymous 'cog' in the war machine and, in its more theatrical resplendent form, the bestower of rank and command, or authority. Outside the armed forces and the police at the outbreak of war in Australia, uniforms belonged largely within hospitals: doctors had that enduring symbol of science-as-healer, the quasi-uniform of the white coat; nurses had institutional uniforms. Inside hospitals doctors perched at the top of a rigid hierarchy: they had command and authority as medical and institutional administrators as well as being the supreme authorities on human ills and their treatment. These uniforms were superficial indicators of a hierarchical and militaristic structure. Indeed there was a natural affinity between the army and the hospital, something Foucault explored at length in his works on micro-sources of power.[34] In Australia in 1910, approximately 25% of all doctors in practice were participating in military activities. In September 1914, all but eight doctors in the Australian Army Medical Corps had previous military experience. Although the exact number of doctors who served in the AAMC overseas is unknown, the example of South Australia is telling. In that state over 90% of doctors joined the AAMC Reserve.[35] In Germany, 24,000 out of 33,000 (73%) male doctors served.[36]

During the war and, markedly, in post-war Australia, military values together with those of classical liberalism dominated the workings of the Repatriation Department and its medical process of pensioning. A vast majority of the medical staff had pre-war experience in the militia, university regiments, or the Reserve AAMC and all had served in the AAMC during the war. The service records of most of the key senior medical administrators are not those of frontline doctors; rather they were administrators or pure combatants. Many continued their active involvement in military life after the war. This militaristic 'caste' within Australian society was to have an exceedingly long legacy.

CHAPTER 2

The Great Ordeal

Voluntarism: August 1914 to May 1916

> Not until news was received of the shiploads of casualties following upon the historic landing of the first divisions at Gallipoli did the public mind begin seriously to exercise itself with the civilian fate of those who would be returning scarred and worn by the Great Ordeal.[1]
>
> D.J. Gilbert in 1920

Much has been written on the meaning of Gallipoli to Australian history, culture and national identity.[2] It is not proposed to enter this debate here, yet Gallipoli had a functional importance for this work. In December 1914, Assistant Minister for Defence, J.A. Jensen, had anticipated an invalidity rate of around 1600 soldiers per annum.[3] This figure quadrupled in the six days from the 25th to the 30th of April 1915.[4] By the latter date, 25% of casualties were killed and of 5 235 evacuated, 180 died at sea of wounds. In June and July, diarrhoea, typhoid, enteritis and other gastro-intestinal afflictions became 'quite out of control' and the Assistant Director of Medical Services (ADMS) of 1st Division reported that 30% of the soldiers were unfit.[5]

In Egypt, which had become the base for the AIF, there were 11 000 sick and wounded Australians by the end of June. The first group transported to Australia consisted of 269 invalids, of whom only 49 had been wounded, and 54 soldiers sent home for a 'change'. This last group were not for discharge as Medically Unfit but were to convalesce and then be returned to duty. There was no principle to guide the boarding officers in their selection of individuals for transfer to Australia at this date other than a directive that 'all venereals were to be got rid of'.[6] The arrival of the *Kyarra* in Melbourne on July 18 therefore presented families as much as civil institutions with a range of complex problems that were to grow worse. Institutions were required for the sick and wounded, for those labelled 'mentals' and for those requiring convalescence. But in the first shipload, like all subsequent shiploads, there were also those soldiers and, later, other personnel, whose physical or mental breakdown was not so visible or severe to warrant institutionalisation, but which was sufficient to make the transformation from soldier to civilian exceedingly difficult, if not impossible.

The federal government responded to the situation by forming the Federal Parliamentary War Committee (FPWC), a body consisting of six members from each Party 'to whom questions affecting the war and Australia's participation in it can be referred by the Government'.[7] In August the Committee recommended an organisational structure for delivering voluntary services and voluntary funds to soldiers and their families in need. The federal body was to supervise and coordinate. At the next tier, State War Councils composed of up to 12 members representing the Federal government, State government, Local government and business interests were to keep records of all discharged personnel, raise and disburse funds, ascertain land available for settlement and act as de facto employment bureaux. The third tier, the War Service Committees or Local Committees, were based on Local government areas and were intended to facilitate local employment and relief.[8] The work of these Councils and Committees, however, relied entirely on voluntary funds.

On 3 May 1915, the 'First Casualty List' was promulgated.[9] From this date until mid 1916, the bleak reality of death, wounding and disease spurred what one commentator called 'the first great emotional impulse' towards returning soldiers: the establishment of patriotic funds.[10] These private funds had been responsible for the repatriation of Australian soldiers and care of their families after the South African War. From the outbreak of war in 1914, such funds again appeared, initially directing energy, gifts and money to relief of invaded allies. However, from mid 1915 the larger organisations, especially the Red Cross and the Australian Comforts Fund, recognised the need for something more than spontaneous donations. On July 30 an appeal 'day' modelled on the successful Belgian Day appeal of the previous May was planned.[11] While the organisation of the appeal day may have been successful – some £800 000 raised in New South Wales alone – the disbursement of the collected funds was not. Ernest Scott, the author of the homefront volume of the Official history of the war, celebrates a 'noble devoted service', but his student, L.J. Pryor, describes a process full of 'confusion and duplication':

> Lack of co-ordination meant waste; absence of responsible control gave the unscru-pulous an opportunity to make money out of their more patriotic and humane fellow citizens.[12]

It was also clearly recognised that these funds when distributed locally were simply supplementing an inadequate pension.[13] In this respect the experience of Australia was similar to Britain where it was assumed that private charity would supplement pensions.[14] At the same time Australia had volunteered every available recruit to the British government. While the patriotic press reported the success of fund-raising drives it was simultaneously reporting the outcome of recruitment drives. Indeed the two were considered part of the same effort. When Andrew Fisher agreed to the recommendations of the FPWC that State War Councils control recruiting, he also agreed to the principle that 'some control' of the funds should be initiated.[15]

The July recruiting figure, however, turned out to be the highest of the war and, without evidence to the contrary, it seems the Australia Day appeal in July was the apogee of private subscription.[16] As a result, at the same time that the states undertook various forms of regulation and supervision of voluntary funds, the funds began to shrink. As these ameliorative funds diminished, more and more soldiers returned to Australia needing help and more recruits were required. Not surprisingly other forms of 'benefit' were introduced to attract new recruits and substitute for cash amelioration.

Land settlement was mentioned in the Victorian Legislative Assembly in May. Across the Tasman the New Zealand Prime Minister simultaneously announced the setting aside of 'suitable blocks of land' for members of the New Zealand Expeditionary Force.[17] Land settlement, however, was only one part of a state policy fundamentally concerned with the potentially explosive issue of the employment of returned soldiers. The effects of the disruption of trade were felt immediately. The number of unemployed trade unionists jumped from around 6% to nearly 11% between the second and third quarters of 1914. Unemployment and under-employment grew in 1915 and at the same time prices rose rapidly and wages were frozen to pre-war levels in all states.[18]

In 1915, in a measure designed both to provide some employment for soldiers and bolster recruitment, the Commonwealth Public Service Act was amended to give preference to returned soldiers, to raise the maximum Public Service recruitment age to 25 and to severely limit recruitment of males otherwise eligible to enlist in the AIF.[19] Returned soldier preference was to become an increasingly valuable political tool during the war years. Marilyn Lake draws attention to the equally political use W.M. Hughes made of land settlement: for Hughes, who had succeeded Andrew Fisher as Prime Minister in October, land for British soldiers was an important part of his bartering stock for British war loans.[20]

The idea of land settlement grew like a weed. It also became a powerful piece of propaganda – like returned soldier preference – both in recruiting drives and in pre-empting dissatisfaction amongst former soldiers.[21] For the Commonwealth government, on whom the principal burden of war debt fell, this combination of preference to ex-soldiers, which cost the government nothing, and land settlement, which was to be financed through loans to the states, had an obvious appeal. The only direct cost to the federal Treasury was war pensions.

On 3 September 1914, Senator Millen, then Liberal Minister for Defence, announced a pension scheme for Australian soldiers, one that was welcomed by the the *Argus* as 'not unduly generous, but reasonable and fair'.[22] This announcement, part of a final flourish by the doomed Cook government, probably represents the earliest indication at Federal level of recognition of the need for state intervention. Until May 1916 it was the only intervention.

The Fisher Labor government, which took office in September, delayed some two months before introducing a Pension Bill. It is clear that ascertaining the cost of the new pension to the Commonwealth was one factor in the delay. On 15 October Senator Pearce, Minister for Defence, referred to the 'pensions scheme' as 'still under consideration of Cabinet'. He was prepared to guarantee a minimum annual pension for a widow of £52 – £2 more than Millen's proposed scheme – but also proposed a drastically reduced rate for incapacitated soldiers.[23] By the date of the introduction of the Bill on 28 November, this latter rate had been adjusted so that a totally incapacitated soldier received £52, his wife receiving 50% of that.

Meantime, the question of who would control pensioning, Defence or Treasury, had arisen in the corridors of the Treasury Department. It is clear from the files that Treasury was determined to gain the same control over War Pensions that it exercised over Invalid and Old Age Pensions. The political culture of Treasury was one of economy, represented as economy 'in the public interest'.[24] By July 1914, Treasury had a centralised permanent staff of more than 200.[25] Treasury officials saw themselves as custodians of Commonwealth capital and this custodial mentality allied to an obsession with fiscal restraint generated an unashamed hostility towards the seeming profligacy of other Departments, notably Defence. Given that the cost of war to the Commonwealth was more than £15 million by June 1915 and over £56 million by June 1916, and that around 93% of this money was raised by loan, Treasury's obsession is understandable.[26]

On 17 October F.J. Ross, Chief Clerk of Treasury, wrote to the Secretary, George Allen, as follows:

> At present all payments of compensation, pensions and gratuities, which are granted under the Constitution … are approved by the Governor General on the recommendation of the Treasurer.
>
> It would appear that the Treasury which will provide the money should have a voice in the granting of the military and naval pensions. Many of such pensions will be payable years after the war is over, and the fact that the Treasury will have an oversight in these matters will not only be a guarantee of uniformity, but will doubtless be of advantage both to the Departments concerned as well as to the recipients.[27]

Once the Bill was circulated, Ross became more adamant, pointing out in another Memorandum to the Secretary on 30 November that there were intrinsic weaknesses in the Bill, chief of which was the authority given to the Minister for Defence. Allen promptly submitted the matter to Andrew Fisher, then Treasurer as well as Prime Minister, and an amending clause was drafted within days by the Attorney General's Department providing the Treasurer with full authority to administer the Act.

The Act provided for the constitution of a Pensions Board of three members, one of whom was a medical officer. In December, Allen wrote to the Minister for Customs asking for the nomination of a medical officer to the Board, and to the Minister for Defence also asking for a nomination. On 7 January the Board was appointed, consisting in the end of two Defence representatives, Lt Col Dodds and Surgeon General Fetherston, and F.J. Ross from Treasury.

One month later the Board wrote to the Treasurer complaining that although several members of the Forces had died and others had become incapacitated, none of the chief functions prescribed under Section 4 of the Act had been placed before them for consideration. These clauses were critical to the functioning of the Act, incorporating as they did all the investigative and assessment activities that by this date had become part of the repertoire of Treasury officials in their assessment of claims for other pensions.[28]

The response from Treasury was predictable. James Collins, Assistant Secretary, considered that the administration of the Act generally needed review.

> The Board's decisions have no effect without the approval of the Treasurer. Thus the final responsibility for all the action rests upon the Treasurer, who will not be guided by the Board's recommendations alone, but who will insist upon a review of the evidence. Just as the Treasurer must take the responsibility for determining a claim, so it would seem he must be satisfied with the method of collecting the evidence. I submit, therefore, that the proper course is to take up the whole business of the pensions as one of the ordinary functions of the Department.

Collins went on to criticise the Board's inactivity and its failure to show how it was going to carry out these functions. He also pointed out that the machinery already existed within Treasury to investigate claims throughout the Commonwealth. Treasury could

> get police reports; can check statements made in relation to marriages, ages of children and means of livelihood or claimants. Our Commonwealth Medical Referees also can be employed in the examination of incapacitated soldiers. In addition to all this, the system of payment of and accounting for invalid and old-age pensions would naturally extend to payments under the War Pensions Act.[29]

In effect, the Board as constituted could only make a recommendation regarding a War Pension if Treasury officials concurred with the recommendation. The Board was also forced to use Treasury investigations and assessments as its source of information, there being no facility provided within the Act for the Board to gather information itself. At the same time the Act directed the Board to make determinations and recommendations. This ineffectiveness led to the abolition of the Board in an amending Bill of July 1915 when War Pensions became the sole province of Treasury until pensioning was transferred to the Repatriation Department in 1920. The enormous ramifications of this transfer to Treasury are fully explored in Chapter 8. What needs to be made clear at this point is that the administrative and organisational models established during Treasury's period of direct control remain largely unaltered to the present.

At the end of June 1916 there were only 8754 pensions being paid with a total expenditure for the financial year of £138 000.[30] Further, the proposed loans to the states, which were primarily intended to be used as advances to soldier settlers, were controlled by the federal government fixing a maximum advance to ex-soldiers of £500, despite the seeming inadequacy of this sum.[31]

The outcome of these piecemeal measures was a de-centralised organisation of voluntary

State Councils whose only reliable income was to be via limited Commonwealth loans earmarked largely for advances to soldier settlers. The Councils' systems of appointment varied from state to state, as did their control of voluntary funds.[32] Yet the demands made on the Councils and Local Committees was rising. Medical supplies, payment of debts, allowances to wives and widows designed to supplement pensions were just some of the increasingly urgent needs of returning soldiers and their families. In the words of D.J. Gilbert, 'while they [the Councils] were given much work to do, they were supplied with no funds to do it with'.[33]

In February 1916, the FPWC proposed a state-controlled Repatriation Fund 'from which advances might be made to returned soldiers or their dependants'. Administrative control of the Fund was to be vested in a Board of Trustees consisting of fourteen members, six being members of the Committee and another eight nominated by the federal government.[34] In the same month, this proposal was put to a conference of federal and state Ministers who endorsed the idea. The Fund, still voluntary in nature, was to be used solely for the 're-establishment' of soldiers as opposed to more immediate ameliorative activities.

> Soldiers returning to good positions are not likely to require assistance; but all soldiers or dependants of soldiers in need of financial support towards re-establishment will participate in the benefits of the Fund. Ex-soldiers who are mechanics and artisans may be helped in the purchase of tools to enable them to resume work at their trades. Others who may desire to set up in a small business for which they are fitted may be advanced the necessary capital. Those who take up land can be helped, where necessary, to maintain themselves until their land becomes productive … In short, assistance of a general kind will be afforded to returned soldiers and their families, as distinct from ameliorative aid dispensed by other funds.[35]

The State War Councils were to organise, collect and distribute the Fund while all services in connection with the Fund were intended to be gratuitous. In March, J.C. Watson, former Labor Prime Minister and then Honorary Organiser of the FPWC travelled to Sydney to interview potential Trustees. In a confidential letter to Acting Prime Minister G.F. Pearce, he reported that the prosperous merchant Samuel (later Sir Samuel) Hordern was 'quite sympathetic' although concerned that any contributions he made would be tax deductible. Hordern was also 'doubtful whether voluntary effort would bring in some of the wealthier people who so far have kept aloof from such movements'. Watson also recommended Edward Grayndler, then Secretary of the Australian Workers Union (AWU), to Pearce as a 'clear-headed chap' representing 'a body with branches right through Australia'.[36]

However, not all the potential Trustees were consulted in this fashion. Sir John Forrest, at that time a Western Australian representative on the FPWC, was appointed a Trustee without his knowledge. There is also evidence that Pearce undertook no consultation with the states, other than Queensland, over the nomination of representatives.[37] Despite these anomalies, on 18 April the Fund was launched with a joint federal and state appeal and at the end of May the Commonwealth government passed the Australian Soldiers' Repatriation Fund Act.

Conscription: May 1916 to January 1917

The new Board of Trustees met provisionally on 5 May. At that date the membership consisted of the Prime Minister, as ex-officio Chairman, and E. Millen (NSW), Sir William Irvine (Vic), James Page (Qld), A. Poynton (SA), Sir John Forrest (WA) and J.J. Long (Tas) all from the FPWC. Commonwealth government nominations, stated to be representative of the general public, were A.S. Baillieu (Vic), Sir Langdon Bonython (SA), J.J. Garvan, E. Grayndler, Samuel Hordern, Denison Miller (NSW), J.M. Hunter (Qld) and O. Morrice Williams (Vic).[38] An Executive comprising the Chairman plus Bonython, Baillieu, Grayndler and Williams was appointed later. Given the seminal role this Executive played in shaping the organisational structure of the Repatriation Department it is worth noting its membership in more detail.

One member of the Executive was amongst the wealthiest men in Australia. Sir John Langdon Bonython, a man of 'unswerving ambition', was owner and editor of the Adelaide *Advertiser*. A stern Methodist, his political and philanthropic interests, outside his business enterprise, seem to have focused on technical education for working-class men, something he had in common with other so-called progressive liberals and a prominent feature of the later Repatriation scheme.[39] It is also suggested that he had some influence with W.M. Hughes.[40]

In contrast to Bonython, Edward (Ted) Grayndler was the Sydney-based Secretary of the Australian Workers Union (AWU). Grayndler was an avid anti-conscriptionist but in other respects a conservative unionist, which probably explains his choice by Watson.[41] Described by one biographer as 'a keen sports fan and a convivial drinker', Grayndler's attendance at full meetings of the Board of Trustees – let alone the Executive – was scant. His later attendance as nominal representative of labour interests on the Repatriation Commission was equally unimpressive.[42] Yet these two members of the Executive, Bonython and Grayndler, survived the subsequent dismantling of the Fund and the constitution of a Repatriation Department. The remaining two members of the Executive did not.

Arthur Baillieu was the brother of W.L. Baillieu, the founder of the Collins House empire. Although little has been published on Arthur, the relationship between W.L. Baillieu, W.L.'s intimate friend W.S. Robinson and W.M. Hughes would suggest that by 1916 the connection to the Collins House group was of unequivocal political value, notably in the trade of base metals.[43]

Similarly, given the anticipated size of the ASR Fund, it is perhaps not surprising to find a banker appointed to the Executive. Oliver Morrice Williams, Inspector and General Manager of the London Bank of Australasia Ltd, and President of the Bankers

Institute, was elected Deputy Chairman of the Executive.[44] In effect, Williams and Baillieu together ran the Fund. Of the 68 meetings of the Executive, these two attended 65 each. The next closest attendance was Bonython at 16 meetings.[45]

One other figure intimately associated with the Board and with the formation of the Department deserves attention. David John Gilbert was appointed Secretary to the Board in early May 1916.[16]Gilbert had worked as a journalist and editor on the *Bulletin*, the Brisbane *Courier* and the *Daily Telegraph* prior to becoming leader-writer on the *Sydney Morning Herald* in 1907. In 1911 he founded the *Land* but then left journalism for two years, returning in early 1914 to accept J.C. Watson's offer of editorship of a proposed new Labor paper, the *World*. With the outbreak of war, however, and Watson's move to the FPWC, the paper did not materialise and Gilbert became Watson's assistant and Secretary of the New South Wales State War Council.[47] It will be seen in the following sections that for one who was to later describe himself as 'the framer of the Repatriation scheme', this association with Watson, a Labor man subsequently cast as one of the 'rats' of the labour movement, is of particular interest.[48]

The Fund of the Board of Trustees was established by one large donation and the promises of two more: the Commonwealth government donated £250 000; Messrs Baillieu promised £25 000 and the Hordern family and firm promised £20 000.[49] The first task of the Trustees was to frame regulations for the administration of the Act. The key provision was the instruction to the State War Councils to form special sub-committees which should conduct appeals and determine applications for assistance. In general, such assistance was designed for any person who was, or had been, a member of the Commonwealth Forces on active service outside Australia, or their dependants.[50] The Regulations also carefully prescribed conditions of eligibility. Anyone with 'adequate means', anyone 'adequately provided for in any scheme promoted by any Governmental or private agency' – a clear reference to both War Pensions and the Patriotic Funds – or anyone 'not in receipt of an honorable discharge' was deemed ineligible. It would seem that only the indigent and honorable soldier or his dependants could apply.[51]

By December 1917 more than 40 000 soldiers had been discharged, of whom more than one quarter applied for assistance from the Fund. Of this number, more than one third were refused. In terms of cost, the greatest outlay by the Councils was on loans. A total of £158 000 was loaned to ex-soldiers or their dependants, the major purposes being for 'Small Businesses and Plant', 'Farming, Plant, Seed, Livestock' and 'Homes'. In contrast, only £73 000 was approved as 'Gifts'. At least £16 000 of this represents 'Sustenance' payments made 'to those in need of assistance during the initial period of re-establishment'. A further £4500 went to 'special instruction' where the states could not provide free appropriate technical or other training, and small amounts went to 'Tools of Trade' and the 'Renewal of Artificial Limbs'. By far the greatest proportion, however, went to 'Furniture'. Indeed, some 2253 claims for furniture were approved by the Councils.[52]

Furniture was just one commodity that the 'Anzac Work' scheme, a somewhat utopian idea where manufacturers donated plant and workers their labour, was supposed to produce as 'goods' which could be allotted to soldiers in lieu of cash.[53] However, the launch of the scheme – the brainchild of Gerald Mussen, an intimate business associate of the Collins House group[54] – was delayed. The Executive of the Fund therefore directed the States to 'regard them [the applications] conservatively'. They also cautioned the Councils that these applications were the 'subject of abuse'.[55] In January 1917, the Board circularised the Councils proposing that the grant (the gift of furniture) should remain the property of the Trustees for a period of twelve months and then be given to the applicant. The Secretary of the Victorian State War Council objected:

> We have frequently been told by returned soldiers that if we are not prepared to make a gift of what they regard as a paltry amount for furniture, we can keep it. If your proposition were carried out, I am afraid that it would give rise to very serious complaint, against the War Council, which we are desirous of avoiding.[56]

Undeterred, Gilbert wrote to the Secretary directing the 'policy' be put into effect. The Board's reasoning was clear:

> It is realised that in the case of many soldiers furniture is used to raise sufficient to get them out of a tight corner; with the bona-fide applicant there should be no objection whatever, and if not bona-fide, the man is not deserving of consideration.[57]

The parsimony of the Board may be partly explained by what has been described as 'the traditions of charitable action' in Victoria.[58] This tradition, which according to welfare historians was still flourishing in the early twentieth century, relied on tests of eligibility – both work tests and moral tests of 'character' – in the same way that the English Poor Law had relied on the deterrent effects of the workhouse. One member of the Board, Sir William Irvine, while Premier of Victoria in 1902, had vigorously opposed aged pensions, reduced the budget allocation for pensions by one third and tried to 'ensure the administrators assessed moral worth before dispensing what he regarded as state charity'.[59] Yet even attempts at economy, such as we have seen in the Regulations and advice to the states, required a fund to regulate.

The promises of moneys to the Fund were slow in realisation: Hordern's earlier concern over tax deductibility was not without foundation. While the Board recommended such a principle to the government, no formal reply was forthcoming, although Hughes did indicate that it was likely in a speech in Sydney in August. The Trustees complained in their final Report of how this delay and indeterminacy had 'militated against the appeal for funds'.[60] According to the Report, many donations in cash or kind were promised but on this condition of tax deductibility. The Trustees pointed out that they 'could not accept contributions to which a condition was attached'. Furthermore, they had 'evidence of misapprehension on the part of several who are disposed to be large contributors' that they would be just as liable as others who had not yielded to this 'sacrificial impulse'.[61]

The Board's worst fears were indeed realised. At the end of December 1917, after 19 months of operation, such sacrificial impulses totalled less than £110 000, that is, only £65 000 after the Baillieu and Hordern donations. Pryor considered the response to the appeal 'strangely disappointing'.[62] It seems even more 'disappointing' when account is taken of the estimated total of Patriotic Funds raised by public subscription up to the end of June 1919 which was over £14 million.[63]

The reasons seem clear. To begin, the State War Councils were responsible for raising voluntary funds which were seen to be controlled by the Commonwealth government, but, as noted above, there were no formal tax exemptions. Moneyed donors were thus discouraged. Second, the fund-raising efforts, along with the 'Anzac Work' scheme, were organised for launching in October 1916 which, as it transpired, was at the height of the conscription debacle. As a result, they were both postponed – indefinitely as it turned out.[64] Third, during September, while attempts to control other funds and fund-raising activities were introduced through the use of the War Precautions Act – largely by control or prohibition of the use of words such as 'Anzac', 'Repatriation' and 'AIF' – there was simultaneously a clear message from the federal government that it intended to finance repatriation through taxation – specifically through a wealth tax.[65] So again those with capital to contribute had cause to re-assess the necessity. Indeed, state intervention in the whole question of repatriation seemed imminent. Finally, and most importantly, there was the devastating reality of the war itself.

Events on the Western Front reverberated throughout Australian society. The first Battle of the Somme saw 1 Anzac Corps suffer 23 000 casualties at Pozières with another 5500 casualties at Fromelles from the 5th Australian Division. During August Generals Birdwood and White drew up a plan for reinforcements – 20 000 initially plus 16 500 per month – which was cabled by the Secretary of State for the Colonies to the Prime Minister. On 30 August Hughes put the proposal to Parliament as one that was impossible without conscription.[66]

The background to the conscription referendum requires brief description. On 5 January 1916, British Prime Minister Asquith introduced the first Military Service Act which provided for compulsory military service for single men.[67] In early March, the Australian Prime Minister arrived in London, and between that date and 29 June when he left London for Australia, Hughes, together with his two associates, W.S. Robinson and Melbourne journalist Keith Murdoch, strutted the British 'corridors of power', dealing and negotiating over the purchase of Australian primary produce – notably wheat, wool, meat and zinc.[68] Hughes's frequent companions during this period were Lloyd George and a coterie surrounding Lord Milner, the founder of the Round Table society and a government adviser on trade.[69] Hughes's other abiding interest on this visit was obtaining clarification of Britain's position on the question of Australian sovereignty in the south Pacific as against alleged Japanese interests in the region.[70] Hughes had limited success on both accounts. He required the co-operation and patronage of the British government in both the purchase of Australian produce and in British dealings with Japan. Yet his bargaining power in the climate of 1916 was extremely limited. One of the few 'commodities' he could bargain with – and one that was expressly requested by London – was troops. On his return to Australia, in the face of militant Labor opposition, Hughes was forced to a referendum on the issue. The effects of the subsequent referendum resulted in what one historian has labelled 'a Nation Divided'.[71]

In addition to the socially divisive effects of conscription, some glimmer of the deaths, maiming, sicknesses, the exhaustion and despair that was daily life in France began to touch ever-increasing numbers of families and friends in Australia. The gloss was lost, the euphoria dead. In late 1916 only the conscriptionists could produce copy saturated with the language of loyalism that had intoxicated so many in 1914. It is worth noting that pre-eminent amongst the pro-conscription propagandists was the General Secretary of the National Referendum Council, a body responsible for producing 'a torrent of conscription material'. From September 1916, that Secretary was D.J. Gilbert.[72]

With hindsight it is easy to interpret Hughes's September announcement of a wealth tax to finance repatriation as just one of many ploys invented as a result of the seeming necessity of conscription.[73] With the labour movement in open revolt against the proposal, Hughes, in alliance with political conservatives, created bogeys that relied on the power of racist ideas, sectarianism and fear of bolshevism.[74] Peter Love's analysis of 'Fat', radical labour's depiction of the usurer capitalist profiting from war, provides a succinct description of part of the opposition Hughes faced and a ready explanation for the touted wealth tax, one designed to pay for the human legacy of 'Fat's' profits.[75] The referendum failed and the wealth tax did not eventuate. Instead, income tax was increased by 25%.[76]

Thus, by November 1916, just as 1 Anzac Corps went back to the Somme, Hughes faced political chaos, a divided society and no conscription of either men or wealth. The £10 000 000 loan he intended to raise in London to finance land settlement loans to the states did not materialise.[77] Repatriation was sustained by voluntary donations, was run by an honorary Board and consisted largely of loans. So far, state commitment to the returned soldier was rhetorical only. Yet this manifest voluntarism was to have a profound affect on the organisation of the Repatriation Department.

In 1916 it is clear that the ideology of the Board of Trustees was pre-eminent in the organisation, regulation and administration of the Fund, within the limits of the Act. Individualism and commitment to the status quo characterise the Board's dealings. The Executive of the Board, as noted above, were drawn from the business elite. Robert Cuff has described a similar phenomenon in the United States, notably in the career of Herbert Hoover as director of the Food Administration department. According to Cuff, the ideology of voluntarism was used to justify the movement of private men into public places and therefore counter charges of conflict of interest – a charge that might easily have been levelled against Baillieu and Robinson.[78] Such voluntarism placed emphasis on 'public service, character, and probity' – Pryor's 'men of sympathy and vision'.[79]

In one other important respect, there is a parallel between the state response to war in the US and Australia. Weinstein and Wiebe have described the way the liberal state in the US fashioned its bureaucracies on a corporate model in the first two decades of the twentieth centuries.[80] The model emerged from the increased co-operation of the federal state with key industries, a symbiotic co-operation where federal regulation could provide what Kolko describes as a 'bulwark against democratic ferment nascent in the states'.[81] One key feature of this model was centralised control. Such control was noticeably absent from the administration of the ASR Fund. As constituted by the Act, the states controlled the real disbursement of the Fund and this lack of control over the money was the target of serious and loud complaint by the Executive.

In late 1916 the Board forwarded a memorandum to Hughes wanting 'definition of the functions of the States in relation to the administration of the [Fund]'. Hughes's response was an 'intimation' that land settlement finance as well as general repatriation would need to be met by the Fund and a statement that 'the repatriation question as a whole, must be considered as a Commonwealth responsibility'. The Board was instructed to prepare recommendations as to how the 'problem' could be dealt with. The recommendations that resulted, both those of the Board and the minority report of Baillieu and Williams, were for an organisation very clearly modelled on a corporate structure with highly centralised control. In little more than a year these recommendations formed the basis of a new state organisation: the Repatriation Department.[82]

Intervention: January to September 1917

This period is one of the most bleak and perhaps the most critical of the war both on the Western Front and in Australia. In France, 'Shell Shock' was being re-defined. From late 1916 there were two classes of diagnosis: 'Shell Concussion', cases where there were visible signs and symptoms of concussion caused by a shell or other explosion, and 'Nervous Shock'. In this latter category were 'all other cases which may be grouped under the term "Inability to Stand Shell Fire" from whatever cause arising'.[83] The former were 'wounded', the latter suffered a 'trivial ailment', were neurasthenic or lacked 'nerve stability'. The Adjutant General, G.H. Fowke, circulated all Armies in October 1916 with a secret command on disciplinary methods of dealing with such 'offenders':

> It should be for a Court Martial to decide whether the evidence as to the existence of actual disease is such as to justify absolving an offender from penal consequences.[84]

In August the Assistant Director of Medical Services (ADMS) had circulated members of the AAMC in charge of various Field Ambulances requesting accounts of the manner in which 'Shell Shock' was handled. Major D.W. Carmalt Jones of the No 4 Stationary Hospital reported that it was made clear to soldiers that 'they will return to the front as soon as fit, without alternative, and that evacuation to England or transfer to a Base will not be considered'.[85] Some doctors used more practical solutions. Major Woollard of 48th Battalion wrote that 'with our reduced numbers we had the same extent of ground to defend and the question of evacuating for Shell shock became of paramount importance'. Woollard's solution was a substantial dose of morphine: 'At about the end of ¾ an hour I was able to rouse them and the men would volunteer they felt better and would return to the line'.[86] Others denied there was a problem. Lt Col Huxtable, commanding the 7th Field Ambulance noted that 'a large number of cases were not suffering from Shell shock at all, on arrival, but were merely bruised by trenches being blown in, and by burying'.[87]

There were other problems harder to deny. During the 1916-17 winter on the Somme, units were losing up to 80 men per week with Trench Foot. Then there were the diseases such as Trench Fever, pneumonia and bronchitis brought about by exhaustion, malnutrition and exposure. Graham Butler witnessed the Somme winter and compared the effects of battle with this slow torture:

> The men of the 1st Division had come out of the Battle of Pozières as from the Valley of the Shadow of Death; but the troops of the 2nd Division who dragged themselves step by step through the mud from Flers seemed to reach a further degree of reaction – being almost past caring.[88]

But there was worse to come. Australian casualties from July to November 1916 were well over 38 000, the battle of Bullecourt in April/May 1917 claimed another 14 000, the three days, 7-9 June, at Messines another 18 000 of a total of over 27 000.[89] Ypres and Passchendaele were still ahead.

The significance of these figures to the higher command of the British Expeditionary Force (BEF) and the AIF was the need for replacements. At home the referendum had failed and, worse, it adversely affected voluntary recruiting. From 11 520 in October recruits were down to 2617 in December.[90] The 'urgent need for men' that was continually being cabled to Australia in order to maintain five infantry divisions translated into a minimum of 5500 men per month. By May 1917 the Chief of General Staff cabled that 7000 would need to enlist each month to meet requirements. In August fewer than 3000 volunteered.[91]

There was another complicating factor. Many of the recruits were described as being 'of quite a different type'. 'Elderly and weakly men', 'useless' men, 'deformed' men, men blind in one eye, 'mental cases', not to mention those suffering from rheumatism, bronchitis, shortness of breath, cardiac insufficiency, hand or foot deformities, hernias, epilepsy, asthma and septic teeth, started to make up an ever increasing percentage of the new recruits. The report of the ADMS at Tidworth to the Director of Medical Services (DMS) on these 'Senile' volunteers was damning:

> With regard to Senility, the majority are weak old men, not only permanently unfit for General Service, but quite unfit for employment on any Military duties whatsoever in England, and who require to be returned to Australia before the winter commences.

As the results of statements made to me by these soldiers, I have ascertained that the following appear to be the chief reasons for the inclusion of such a large number of soldiers over Military age in these drafts:

1. In very many cases they have very much under-stated their real age on enlistment.

2. Many of the men state that they have been encouraged to so under state their correct age by Recruiting Sergeants and Recruiting Officials, although these Recruiting Sergeants and Officials know well that the men concerned are far over Military age.

3. In one instance a soldier states that he gave his correct age as 49 and that this was knowingly entered up as 44 at the Recruiting Office.

4. Another soldier states that the Recruiting Committees are encouraging these under-statements of age and that the idea has therefore grown up among the public that old men should state their 'Military' age as opposed to their Real Age in order to enlist.[92]

These suggestions are borne out by the experience of Harvey Blackburn, a veteran of the South African war, who desired to go to Officers School in 1914. In 1915 he was 'sent for' but on the way had an accident. Eighteen months and six operations later he lost one foot, but with the formation of Railway Units he volunteered again. Having been accepted by the doctor at the recruiting depot 'after a bit of parlava', he went to camp. The medical examination at camp was somewhat more difficult. The examining doctor did not notice the artificial leg either on the Attestation papers or in the 'flesh' but his colleague did; Blackburn was told to 'get around the room' without his artificial leg. The second opinion was that 'he [the doctor] would pass 1,000 men like [Blackburn] tomorrow if they came along'. Blackburn went on to serve over three years in France and England.[93]

In 1930 Dr Kenneth Smith, then Senior Medical Officer (SMO) in Sydney and later Principal Departmental Medical Officer (PDMO), wrote about the 'influence and pressure of higher authorities' during the recruiting campaigns of this period.[94] Butler describes the problem from the vantage point of the Director General of Medical Services (DGMS), Fetherston:

> From the beginning of 1917 … General Fetherston found himself more and more compelled to submit to a policy of dilution, which he was ultimately induced to support, but which General Howse [DMS overseas] resolutely refused to accept.[95]

Fetherston was even clearer in a letter to Howse: 'The Prime Minister, Mr Hughes, is very angry because we are rejecting so many'.[96]

Hughes's seamy tactics in relation to recruiting and the second referendum have been well documented. Pearce, as Minister for Defence, was no less guilty of the anti-German 'scapegoating' so vividly described by Raymond Evans.[97] In March of 1917 Pearce announced to the press that the Department of Defence possessed damning evidence that Germany was preparing to seize Australia. Charles Bean later recalled the 'wide currency' this statement had in the AIF and asked Scott to look into it during his research of *Australia During the War*. Scott found the 'evidence' in question in four files relating to the activities of Dr Eugen Hirschfeld. According to Scott, Pearce placed 'a certain interpretation upon the documents in the four files'. He went on to assure Bean that 'they do not bear that interpretation, if read without a desire to strain their meaning'.[98]

It would appear that under the extreme circumstances any tactic was legitimate if it held an answer to the Imperial imperative. The federal body politic meanwhile mirrored the chaos and divisiveness of society at large. The stalwarts of the National Referendum Council – Watt, Hume-Cook and Irvine – proceeded to form the core of a 'Win-the-War' party, a coalition of Liberals and Labor defectors, ultimately headed by Hughes.[99] Negotiations over the make-up of the new party ministry lasted from December to 17 February when the powerful coalition of conservatives, liberals and conservative labor was sworn in only two months after a similar coalition took office under Lloyd George.[100] The newly created Nationalist Party not only won the May 1917 election decisively but held government in Australia until 1929.

While the battle for power in Cabinet raged, another war of position was being lost. In January Hughes circulated the recommendations of the Executive of the Board of Trustees at the Premiers' Conference. In brief, these recommendations were for a Commonwealth authority which controlled all aspects of repatriation. This authority, the Board suggested, could be the Board itself. The authority would devise uniform policies for administration by state-based Commonwealth bodies (the former State War Councils).[101] Hughes introduced the matter to the Conference on 5 January commenting 'I think there must be some central control. What form that control is to take, and the extent of it will be determined later'.[102] With the states' control of land settlement assured, the Conference agreed to the principle of Commonwealth control.

On 11 January, the Board met and discussed the nature of the new organisation. Hughes's preference was for authority to be vested in 'a capable man whose sole business was to deal with Repatriation matters'. Irvine, Cook, Forrest and Morrice Williams argued that authority should lie with a trustee body, with administration the responsibility of a 'well paid experienced man, immune from political influence'.[103] The arguments put forward by Williams and his coterie against Hughes's suggestion seem unconvincing: there would be 'divided control'; it would be difficult to determine where the Board's activities should cease and the Commissioner's began; and

> with the Commissioner an independent authority, the Board's position would be no more satisfactory than it is now. It would merely hand over money without having the power to see that it was effectively spent.[104]

The antagonism of the three Liberals to Hughes's proposal can perhaps be better understood when it is recognised that in the week preceding this meeting, Irvine, Cook and the 'dinosaur' Forrest were manoeuvring in the lead-up to the establishment of the coalition party to displace Hughes as Prime Minister, each believing the position theirs.[105] In the end, however, the Board recommended the appointment of a Repatriation Commissioner for Australia, the Commissioner's relationship to the Board being that of a Chief Executive Officer to a Board of Directors.[106]

Hughes, for his part, publicly repeated his belief in the need for a 'responsible central authority'.[107] As for the Board, Williams and Baillieu submitted their personal views to Hughes suggesting that there was no one man who could possibly possess all the qualities required by the job of Commissioner:

> The area of criticism is so wide, and the feelings of the public in this regard are so tender, that even the best individual performance is likely to fall short of expectations; and to expose an individual to the full brunt of the criticism which is inevitable, would be to jeopardise his health if he should be a sensitive man, and if he be not a sensitive man, he, most probably, would lack the fundamental qualification for the position.[108]

Instead they proposed a paid Commission of three men, one being a returned soldier, who would also be members of the Repatriation Board and act as its Executive.

No indication of the outcome of these recommendations was made public until after the Cabinet battle was fought out. For Hughes the outcome of that encounter was the loss of 6 National Labor Cabinet places to Liberals. The new Cabinet, sworn in on 17 February, brought in Forrest as Treasurer, Cook as Minister for Navy, Watt as Minister for Works and Rail and Millen as Vice-President of the Executive Council.[109] Five days later, George Parkes, a member of the Repatriation Special Committee of the New South Wales State War Council, wrote to Morrice Williams complaining that his Committee was 'somewhat in a quandary'. The morning papers had announced the appointment of Senator Millen as Minister in charge of a Repatriation Department and the appointment of two Commissioners, Nicholas Lockyer and Brigadier-General Williams.[110] That this was Morrice Williams's first intimation of such an arrangement is made clear in his own letter to Hughes on 26 February where he abruptly pointed out that

> the procedure followed is scarcely in keeping with the understanding reached at the last meeting of the Repatriation Board, viz: that before making any public announcement you would discuss the Government's proposals with the Executive of the Board. This, you will remember, was your own suggestion … I will be glad if you will make this known to Senator Millen, and suggest to him that he might find it advantageous to utilise the resources of the Board's office until such time as he has made his permanent arrangements.[111]

The following day Williams instructed Gilbert not to provide Millen with copies of either his and Baillieu's letter to Hughes, or the Executive's recommendations.[112]

Meanwhile the character of federal politics deteriorated even further. Late in February the House of Representatives carried a motion by Hughes that the Imperial Parliament be requested to legislate for the extension of the duration of Parliament for the duration of the war.[113] However, Labor then held a majority in the Senate. In the weeks following the Bill's passage through Representatives, Hughes and Pearce allegedly brought 'considerable persuasion' to bear on a number of wavering Labor Senators to achieve its passage through the upper house.[114] The melee which followed forced an election and the House was dissolved on 5 March.

During March, the Board of Trustees appeared more conciliatory, observing that by making repatriation the business of one minister the Commonwealth government had 'taken the first step towards placing this extensive and intricate and pressing business upon a broad Australian basis'.[115] In the same month the Board furnished a detailed report of its activities and expenditure and that of the New South Wales organisation.[116] Whether these were provided to Millen or Hughes is unclear, but on 20 April, at the height of the election campaign, Millen announced a new repatriation scheme to the press. In accepting 'full responsibility for the care of its returned soldiers and sailors', Millen argued that the government needed control of the executive and administrative agencies. The new organisation, as described by Millen, retained the Board of Trustees as 'a guarantee that the scheme would be administered without political influence on one hand, or red tape on the other', but also provided that a Minister of Cabinet be Chairman of the Board. The Board's powers were to be enlarged and an executive of three men was to be appointed and made responsible to them. Millen went on to refer to certain activities to be incorporated into the scheme and the need to rationalise the Patriotic Funds.[117]

Superficially the scheme and its organisation appeared scarcely different from the existing organisation with the exception that the Prime Minister's role was replaced by a Minister and that an executive along lines suggested by Baillieu and Williams was introduced. Indeed Pryor considered Millen had not done 'much constructive thinking since his appointment'.[118] In May, however, after a landslide victory in the election, a far more detailed document, based on the April press release, was submitted by Millen to Cabinet. In this instance Millen left no doubt in the minds of his colleagues as to his aims:

> When the Cabinet entrusted me with the duty of proposing a Repatriation Scheme it gave no indication either of the policy it proposed to adopt or of the type of organisation it desired to see created. I have therefore felt free to consider the question quite apart from anything that has been said or done in the past and to ignore the existence of the present machinery except where it appears desirable to incorporate part of it in the proposal now submitted ... Repatriation, as I understand it, implied setting a man to work, but amelioration when indiscriminately administered may become an inducement to him to remain idle.

As to the administrative machinery, Millen's proposal bears quoting at length:

> The certainty that the problems arising out of the re-establishment of the returning army will induce emotional conditions with a powerful political reflection suggests

the prudence of interposing a buffer between claimants and their sympathisers and the Government. A non-political Board would supply this buffer …

The Repatriation Board of Trustees is already in existence. I propose the abolition of this Board, but the creation of a similar one limited to … members, consisting of the more active members of the existing Board, and two representatives of the Returned Soldiers League, and eliminating all Parliamentarians other than the Chairman …

The Minister will be the nexus between the Board and the Government and Parliament and I propose that he shall have a power of veto in respect of any decision of the Board whatsoever.[119]

During the next two weeks Millen's proposal for an executive of three was reduced to one.

It can be seen that while the appearance of the new organisation closely resembled the existing one, the Board had been emasculated. On learning of the proposals, Williams reaction was swift and blunt:

Instead of the Board being, as you wish it to be, a 'buttress' do you not think that political enemies will soon learn the extent of the powers of the Board and of the Minister's power of veto, also that the Board meets say once a month only, and is, in brief, really an Advisory Board?

… Under your proposal the Minister would become, almost of necessity, the active administrative head, and the permanent officer, no matter how capable he may be, merely the executant of the Minister. In these circumstances I can see little essential difference between the organisation of the Board and that of an ordinary Government Department, open to all the influences to which the ordinary Government Department is exposed.[120]

The following month Millen's proposal, largely unaltered, was elaborated into the Australian Soldiers' Repatriation Bill and introduced into the lower house. In August a Bill was passed abolishing the ASR Fund and in September, after lengthy and heated debate[121], the government majority passed the ASR Act, an Act to be administered by the new Minister for Repatriation, E.D. Millen.

In this complex situation of crisis and flux, no one factor or agency was or could have been responsible for the passing of the Act and for the Department it generated. There was no grand scheme but rather great expediency. The political and administrative history of repatriation from the outbreak of war to September 1917 is very much a reflection of the history of federal politics in that period, a history of reflex manoeuvres and piecemeal controls aimed at preventing the total rupture of the status quo.

During late 1916 and early 1917, however, Australian conservative forces coalesced into an organisation with one clear aim: to participate fully in an Imperial conflict at all cost. The progressive marginalisation or suppression of any political opposition worked with massive propaganda campaigns to assure political and ideological hegemony. While Williams's complaint about Ministerial autocracy was quite valid, the interests served by that Minister and his Party were, in essence, identical with those of Williams.

In 1928 Charles Bean, the official historian of World War One, identified this process as revolutionary:

> One of the most striking results [of the war] seems to have been the almost complete attainment of unification, partly through the War Precautions Act and the Defence Act. It seems to me extraordinary how smoothly this revolution was effected under the constitution of the Commonwealth, which of course, I suppose, was designed largely to meet this contingency.[122]

The same constitution that was designed to protect state rights could, in a situation perceived as a national emergency, allow the exercise of untrammelled central power provided there was a clear majority of politically and ideologically united members in both houses – a situation which came about in May of 1917. Yet this political history, that of the rich or powerful in Australian society, provides only one story of the war years thus far. The mammoth Department that was established at this time was purportedly designed to manage and provide assistance to returned soldiers. However, a vast majority of those directing its establishment at this date were not soldiers and had no experience of trench warfare. Theirs was a second-hand, a vicarious experience of war, with all the gloss that entails. These men saw the statistics of deaths, injuries and illness and they saw the fiscal and administrative problems that that produced. The other crucial story comes from the Western Front; from the lived experience of the volunteer 1st AIF.

CHAPTER 3

'The Old Lie': The Soldier's War on the Western Front

Bent double, like old beggars under sacks,
Knock-kneed, coughing like hags, we cursed through sludge,
Till on the haunting flares we turned our backs
And towards our distant rest began to trudge.
Men marched asleep. Many had lost their boots
But limped on, blood-shod. All went lame; all blind;
Drunk with fatigue; deaf even to the hoots
Of gas shells dropping softly behind.

Gas! Gas! Quick, boys! – an ecstasy of fumbling,
Fitting the clumsy helmets just in time;
But someone still was yelling out and stumbling,
And flound'ring like a man in fire or lime…
Dim, through the misty panes and thick green light,
As under a green sea, I saw him drowning.

In all my dreams, before my helpless sight,
He plunges at me, guttering, choking, drowning.[1] (1917)

How do we understand the soldier's war within the context of this work? For most of us, as remote observers, there is the vicarious experience of valour, bravery, endurance, suffering, pain and horror. We experience this via books, poems, film, television, memoirs and many other media. The fascination of the front line soldier, of trench warfare, is generally not an intellectual one but a powerful emotional one. The soldier is in a foreign place, isolated from his own social and cultural milieu, fighting (with real and lethal weapons) a dangerous enemy. His 'story' is better than any Boy's Own adventure. Yet, just as unreal.

Wilfred Owen's poem is frequently quoted in part or full in works dealing with gassing in World War One. And this is for a very good reason. Unlike so much other war poetry, the poem provides us with a glimpse of the real war. Not a glamorised or romanticised or censored artifice, or a propaganda piece, but a vile and sickening image of drowning lungs and a powerful indictment of wartime propaganda and of war itself. Similarly, for any serious historian of the war, Otto Dix's cycle of prints, *Der Krieg*, with its images of the Somme in the winter of 1916/1917 are an enduring reminder of the modern soldier's war. As one curator of his work has recently written, 'Dix's war is a modern war – the scale is vast. Not only are men killed in an arbitrary, anonymous and indiscriminate way, the landscape itself is torn apart, desecrated and ravaged'.[2]

In the (nearly) 100 years since the Great War, the number of publications depicting the war defies the bibliographer. Yet few dwell on this gruesome detail. Even historians of the War and its aftermath have only recently engaged in a critical fashion with disease, illness and trauma during the war.[3] A smaller number have looked at their post-war consequences. To date most of this history has come from Canada, Britain and Europe. A serious engagement by Australian historians is sadly lacking.[4]

So how do we approach an understanding of illness and injury amongst the 1st AIF? The war at the front for the Australian soldier started in 1914 and ended at the Armistice. Gallipoli has attracted inordinate attention yet the Middle East war almost none – perhaps a cultural artefact of Australian historiography. Yet there are good reasons to look to France for the soldier's war. France provided the longest period of service and a vast majority of soldiers served there. Medical record-keeping was better in France while records at Gallipoli were poor. Also, most post-war problems dealt with by the Repatriation Department, the post-war adjudicator of service-related health problems, arose in France. This is not to disdain illness or injury at Gallipoli, rather this choice of battlefield reflects pragmatic decisions on the value of the records available for historical analysis as well as the volume of empirical evidence.

Illness and injury in France

According to Butler, the official medical historian of the First AIF, the medical problems experienced by Australian soldiers on the Western Front in the period 1916-1918 consisted, in gross terms, of approximately 54 000 soldiers who died in battle or of battle wounds, approximately 202 000 soldiers who were sick, approximately 114 000 who were wounded, and approximately 16 500 who were gassed.[5] Putting aside for now those categorised as 'wounded' or 'gassed', Butler also provides a very rough breakdown of illness and disease (the 'sick') on the Western Front. His figures possess many serious shortcomings and of particular significance here is the fact that he regarded AIF figures on cardiac disease 'useless' and believed that all medical officers, 'from front line to base', had 'failed in their duty' in relation to documentation in this respect.[6] Heart conditions – 'soldier's heart', 'disordered action of the heart' (DAH), or 'effort syndrome' – were to become the third leading cause of discharge from the British Army.[7] It is also worth highlighting the fact that figures for Trench Fever and Trench Feet were significantly under-reported. Taking cognisance of those facts, Butler's gross figures indicate that the most significant causes of sickness in order of sheer numbers admitted to Base Hospitals (total admissions 157,547) were[8]:

- Venereal disease (29,610 or 19%)
- Respiratory tract infections (23,289 or 15%)
- Inflammation of connective tissue ('ICT') (8960 or 6%)
- Pyrexia of unknown origin ('PUO') (7280 or 5%)
- Trench fever (5525 or 3.5%),
- Trench feet (4648 or 3%), and
- Scabies (4893 or 3%).[9]

'PUO' and 'ICT' are problematic diagnoses. The first simply indicates a high temperature of unknown aetiology (cause). The second ('ICT') is somewhat akin to 'chlorosis', that is, a disease that no longer exists, one that no longer populates medical nosology. Whilst these were the diagnoses recorded at the time of the soldier's admission to hospital, it became clear later in the war, and indeed after the war, that 'ICT' was a 'camouflage' (Butler's term) for Trench Foot, while 'PUO' was most commonly Trench Fever.[10] Thus, a revised list of illness rates appears rather different:

- Venereal disease (29,610 or 19%)
- Respiratory tract infections (23,289 or 15%)
- Trench feet (13,608 or 8.5%)
- Trench fever (12,805 or 8%).

Moreover, these are figures for admissions to Base Hospitals, not to Casualty Clearing Stations or Field Ambulances. That is, they reflect illness that required evacuation from the vicinity of the front for treatment. If we look at sheer numbers of admissions to Field Ambulances in France another picture emerges. Between April 1916 and March 1919, Butler records approximately 212,000 admissions. In descending numerical order, the most common causes for admission were as follows:

- Respiratory tract infections (41,300 or 19.5%)
- Trench Fever (including PUO) (approx 28,593 or 13.5%)
- Scabies (19,920 or 9%)
- Trench Feet (including ICT) (13,780 or 6.5%)
- Venereal disease (13,105 or 6%).

Between them, Butler's figures for respiratory tract infections, scabies-borne illness and trench feet account for nearly half all admissions to Field Ambulances in France during these three years.

Further down the scale of illnesses were the various 'mental' disorders and within this category was 'NYDN': 'Not yet diagnosed – nervous' (n = 3351 at Base Hospitals and n = 4293 at Field Ambulances). Within this group was Shell Shock.

By contrast with disease and illness statistics, battle casualty statistics for the AIF do not exist. Butler lamented the destruction and/or non-existence of these figures throughout his three volumes and ultimately decided to present the figures of the BEF on the basis that they were not dissimilar to those experienced by the AIF. Butler extrapolated the percentages of injuries to various parts of the body contained in the British figures to the AIF and included these in Volume 3 of his work. According to his hypothesis, over 38% (n = 51 812) of all injuries were to the lower extremities of the body, some 29% (n = 39 801) to the upper extremities, and over 16% (n = 22 453) to the head, face and neck. An additional 1.5% (n = 2 018) of injuries to the lower extremity resulted in amputation.[11] This latter figure is consistent with other sources.[12]

Ignoring the distinctions made between the nature and causes of illness and injury on the Western Front, and concentrating instead on the question of army 'wastage', in other words on the *most important* causes of incapacity or disability amongst the AIF, Butler's statistics present the following picture.

Major causes of incapacity in the AIF

Nature of illness or injury	Estimated number*
Wounds to the lower extremity	51,812
Wounds to the upper extremity	39,801
Venereal disease	29,610
Respiratory tract infections	23,289
Wounds to the head, face and neck	22,453
Gassing	16,500
Trench feet	13,608
Trench fever	12,805

* Figures for wounds include all theatres of war and all years. Figures for illness are for the Western Front only in the years 1916-1919. Figures for illness are those reported as admitted to Base Hospitals.

The reality of the soldier's war can now be more readily appreciated. First, of the total of 330 714 soldiers who embarked for duty overseas, around 59 000 died overseas (a ratio of 5:1). Second, whilst wounding constituted an immense loss of manpower, 'sickness' was the cause of even greater losses. On the Western Front, the major sicknesses experienced by the AIF were almost certainly venereal disease, respiratory tract infections, the effects of gassing, trench fever and trench feet.

There are four problematic issues embedded in these figures that demand further exploration. First there is the distinction made between wounds/injury and disease that permeates the contemporaneous (and current) medical nosology. Second, there is the problem of 'diagnosis' – the now well documented social constitution of disease entities.[13] Third, and of significance here, there is the question as to whether the disability that ensued from illness was 'war-related', and thus pensionable. And, finally there is the illnesses themselves. These issues are examined throughout the work.[14] The last – the nature of the illnesses themselves – tells us more about the soldier's war.

Three illnesses are examined here: gassing, trench fever and trench foot. The rationale behind the choice is relatively straightforward. Venereal disease has had significant critical attention in the past two or more decades from social historians.[15] Respiratory infections deserve a work of their own. These are an exceedingly complex set of diagnoses given that they incorporate diagnoses of influenza, bronchitis, pneumonia, pleurisy and many other contemporaneous diagnostic tags, and all of varying aetiology, including the after-effects of gas. As a disease group it almost defies historical or medical analysis due to contemporaneous understandings as much as war-time record-keeping. Its importance as a cause of 'wastage' is nonetheless recognised and its significance in post-war pensioning noted elsewhere.

The three remaining key illnesses of the AIF in France are examined here wherever possible in the light of medical and scientific research in ensuing decades. A key principle of war pensioning in Australia from the introduction of the 1920-22 Act was giving soldiers the *benefit of the doubt* when decisions were made on the attribution to war service of then current signs and symptoms.[16] While this Pandora's Box of ideology, politics and bureaucratic imperative is dealt with at length in Chapter 8, it is instructive to compare contemporaneous understandings of the nature and aetiology of these conditions with current understandings. All three were 'new' to medical officers during the war and the aetiology unknown for some time. Even when there was a crude understanding of obvious signs and symptoms, and aetiology (cause), the sequelae are still imperfectly understood.

Gassing

> If in some smothering dreams you too could pace
> Behind the wagon that we flung him in,
> And watch the white eyes writhing in his face,
> His hanging face, like a devil's sick of sin;
> If you could hear, at every jolt, the blood
> Come gargling from the froth-corrupted lungs,
> Obscene as cancer, bitter as the cud
> Of vile, incurable sores on innocent tongues, –
> My friend, you would not tell with such high zest
> To children ardent for some desperate glory,
> The old Lie: Dulce et decorum est
> Pro patria mori.[17]

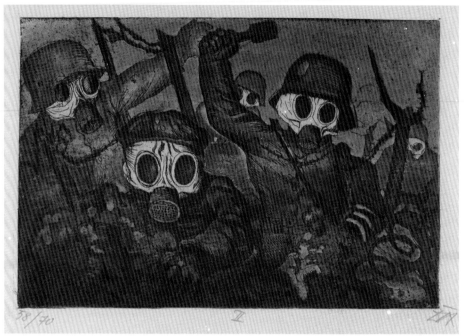

Figure 1. Otto Dix, *Der Krieg*, XII, *Sturmtruppe geht unter Gas vor*, Shock Troops Advance Under Gas

[Courtesy National Gallery of Australia; © Otto Dix, licensed by VISCOPY, Australia 2008]

On 22 April 1915, Canadian doctors near Ypres observed 'a long cloud of dense yellowish-green smoke'. This was the first successful and well documented use of *lethal* chemical gassing in the Great War.[18] The gas was chlorine. According to Butler, during the ensuing four years and seven months, over 30 chemical substances were used as weapons.[19]

For the purposes of this work chemical warfare is defined as the purposeful employment of chemicals, based on a contemporary scientific understanding of their action, in a military engagement. As such, chemical warfare is not old. It is a modern idea, one coterminous with the 'chemical revolution' at the end of the eighteenth and beginning of the nineteenth centuries. Sulphur dioxide, cacodyl cyanide, chlorine, ammonia, hydrogen chloride and other less lethal compounds were put forward by the military, by chemists and by lay people as potential military weapons for nearly 100 years prior to the Great War.[20] Indeed according to one historian, if Germany had not taken the initiative, 'some other combatant would soon have attempted something similar'.[21]

The arsenal of chemical substances used during the war was delivered by both sides of the conflict. The extent of both tactical and strategic use was determined by a host of factors such as the state of chemical industries in a nation, political will, capacity for production of exploding shells to deliver the gas, contemporary military strategic

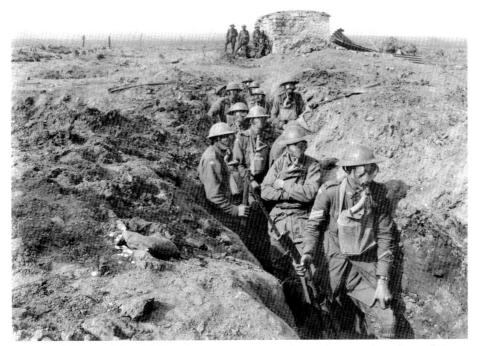

Figure 2. Soldiers of the 45th Battalion wearing gas respirators in a trench at Garter Point, in the Ypres Sector, 27 September 1917. (Photo Frank Hurley)

[Australian War Memorial neg. no. E00825]

thinking, and three key environmental factors: prevailing winds, temperature and rain/moisture.[22]

Gas use started early in the war – allegedly a tear gas was used by France (ethylbromo-acetate) late in 1914 or early 1915 and by Germany (dianisidine chlororsulphonate) in late 1914.[23] Tear gases used throughout the war also included benzyl bromide, xylyl bromide, bromacetone, brom ketones, and brombenzylcyanide.[24] They were primarily used as 'lachrymators', that is they were a strategic device used with the same intent as current tear gases: to temporarily incapacitate an opponent. The chemicals attacked the eyes, the skin and the respiratory and gastro-intestinal tracts (the latter if ingested). The eyes became red, painful and tearful very quickly and inhaling the gas resulted in a cough and sore throat. Benzyl bromide is currently described as a 'severe skin, respiratory and eye irritant'; as 'corrosive' and 'lachrymatory'.[25] On combustion benzyl bromide forms toxic fumes including hydrogen bromide. It also 'attacks' many metals, especially in the presence of moisture. Thus, for the purposes outlined here, it had a twofold usage: rendering soldiers blind and incapacitated and rendering their weapons useless. A similar substance, benzyl chloride, is an established carcinogen but in 2002 there was insufficient data available on the long term effects of benzyl bromide to determine its carcinogenicity.[26]

Although the effects of the tear gases were painful and debilitating, and the long term

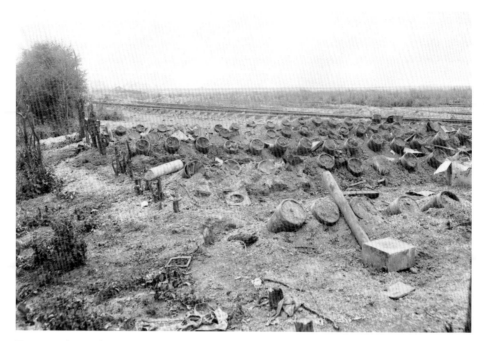

Figure 3. A set of 180 gas projectors alongside the Albert-Amiens railway in front of the Casualty Clearing Station at Dernancourt, 14 June 1918

[Australian War Memorial neg. no. E04897]

sequelae not properly understood, even now, the introduction of chlorine in 1915 was a moral and ethical seismic shift. Chlorine was discovered by a Swedish pharmacist, Carl Wilhelm Scheele, in 1774, and health problems and deaths following exposure to the gas were known by the late eighteenth century.[27] Thus, unlike tear gases, the use of chlorine in gas cloud attacks by Germany, and soon after by Britain in the disastrous attack near Loos, was with the intention of lethality or, at best, serious physical damage to the respiratory tract of soldiers.

There were, however, problems with chlorine as a cloud gas from a purely military standpoint. Chlorine was first used by Germany on the Eastern front against Russia in January 1915 but the gas did not vaporise at subzero temperatures and had no effect.[28] As a cloud gas it was part of a 'cumbersome immobile system' of cylinders, each weighing up to 100 pounds and up to 12 000 cylinders were used in any one gas operation.[29] The cloud also relied on wind direction and with prevailing winds travelling from west to east on the front the last use of cloud gas by Germany was on 8 August 1916. Britain, on the other hand, with prevailing winds generally favouring its position on the front, and a chronic shortage of shells until around 1918, continued to use cloud attacks to the end of the war.[30]

The effects of chlorine on soldiers, like that on humans generally from other airborne chemical exposures, depended upon the concentration of the chemical in the air, the length of exposure, the susceptibility of the individual, and the efficacy of personal protective devices – in this case gas masks. No *effective* masks were available to the AIF or other allied soldiers until the Small Box Respirator was in common use by late 1917.[31] Smoking was common amongst the AIF, as was tuberculosis at this time, making many soldiers more susceptible to respiratory gases. The concentration of the gas has been assessed as being very high and, given the nature of trench warfare, the duration of exposure was long enough for thousands of casualties to be recorded on all sides.[32]

The AIF had little exposure to chlorine gas clouds in the period from April 1915 to around July 1916 (the despatch of Australian Infantry to France began in March 1916). For those who were exposed, as toxicologist Chris Winder explains,

> The most obvious effect of chlorine in high enough concentrations is to displace oxygen from air by dilution sufficient to cause asphyxia ... While chlorine is sparingly soluble in water, it will begin hydrolysing in the moist linings of the airways, forming a solution of hypochlorous and hydrochloric acids ... Continuing exposure will produce effects further and further into the respiratory system ... These changes will be manifested as loss of respiratory function ... the development of inflammation of the lungs, or pneumonitis. Pneumonia develops as consolidation (where the air spaces fill with exudate) proceeds. Hemorrhagic pneumonia is a severe form, with loss of blood and lung structure.
>
> While some of these reactions will cease as exposure ceases, others are part of the inflammatory response and will continue.

The other effects of chlorine include chest pain, dyspnoea (difficulty breathing), production of white or pink sputum, sore and reddened eyes, and coarse wheezes and crackles when breathing. Pulmonary oedema (lungs filled with fluid) will occur either immediately or be delayed by several hours.[33] Butler describes the symptoms as 'choking, coughing, gasping for breath ... retching, sternal pain and thirst followed by the phenomena of anoxaemia, weakness and lassitude'.[34]

Current scientific knowledge on the long-term effects of acute chlorine exposure is based on 'conflicting data'.[35] Residual effects of exposure in occupational settings over the past 35 years have been 'inconsistently observed'. Das and Blanc's 1993 review of such research concluded that 'airway obstruction ... may persist following acute inhalational injury due to chlorine gas'. They also draw attention to the dearth of research that examines the effects of pre-existing conditions (for example, asthma) or the role of risk factors (for example, smoking) on the duration and severity of long-term effects.

Despite its toxicity, on the Western Front chlorine was soon superseded by a far more insidious and sinister chemical: phosgene. Phosgene was introduced by Germany in December 1915 as a cloud gas.[36] It was first used by France in February 1916. It was used throughout the war due to its toxic and lethal efficacy. In November 1917, an Australian soldier, Lance Corporal Serjeant of 'B' Company 14th Battalion, wrote in his 'Gas Notes' that phosgene was the 'most dangerous' gas used by the enemy. He also noted that 'Our gas' was 'mainly Phosgene'.[37] In practice, phosgene (carbonyl chloride) was commonly mixed with other chemicals within shells. The most common blends were with chlorine, diphosgene (trichloromethyl chloforormate), diphenyl chlorarsine (chlorodiphenylarsine) and/or chloropicrin (trichloronitromethane), although these last three chemicals were also used alone or in other combinations by both sides.[38] These chemicals are highly toxic and all affect the respiratory tract.

Phosgene was used in liquid-filled shells that vaporised quickly once detonated.[39] As a gas it is colourless and is 3.5 times heavier than air so quickly settled into valleys and trenches once dispersed.[40] Reportedly it smells like newly cut hay or green maize/corn, but the odour is not always noticed.[41] While chlorine is a household commonplace and widely known and used worldwide for its bleaching action, for water purification, disinfection and in plastics manufacture, it is less widely recognised that phosgene is almost as ubiquitous in its current usage. Phosgene is currently used in the manufacture of dyes, pharmaceuticals, polycarbonates, polyurethanes and pesticides. It is considered one of the 'most potentially lethal of modern, large-volume chemicals'.[42] Historically it was reportedly used by Japan against China during World War Two, by Egypt against Yemen in the 1960s, and by Iraq and Iran during the 1980s.[43]

The smell of phosgene soon disappears and it can be readily masked by other smells,[44] notably by mixing it with chlorine. However, its most alarming feature is its insidious toxicity. Like the relatively benign lachrymators, in high concentrations it produces red, painful eyes and blurred vision *immediately* together with throat irritation and a cough. However, the delayed symptoms are more lethal. These are due to deep tissue damage within the lungs. Sufferers may be free of symptoms for many hours before developing severe pulmonary oedema and the onset of this may be precipitated by exercise.[45] In Butler's words, 'men who had passed seemingly unscathed through the gas dropped dead some time later after slight exertion'.[46]

The long term effects of phosgene poisoning are unclear, however, it is known that 'complete recovery … may require up to several years' and that for individuals with 'pre-damaged lungs' (smokers, those who suffer from asthma or bronchitis, for example) there may be continuous deterioration of lung function. Because the pulmonary oedema that can develop from acute exposure is so marked, and because the brain is deprived of oxygen when the lungs are filled with liquid, it also seems clear that some after effects are due to this anoxia (lack of oxygen). These symptoms can range from psychological disturbances, including depression, to paralysis of limbs.[47] Finally, phosgene belongs to a class of organic chemicals known as alkylating agents. These chemicals react with DNA and DNA replication and are therefore considered potentially carcinogenic.

Diphosgene is a combination of phosgene and chloroform. At the time of its use on the Western Front it was known to have a 'disagreeable suffocating' odour and to be more persistent than phosgene.[48] It seems it was developed quite specifically to penetrate the early gas mask filters used by allied soldiers, filters designed to combat phosgene. Its first recorded use is believed to be May 1916 (the German 'Green Cross' shell).[49] Like phosgene, it has low water solubility so significant amounts can be inhaled before any symptoms appear. It also has a similar action to phosgene, that is, it penetrates deeply into the airways and causes fatal pulmonary oedema. Doses of diphosgene are cumulative as it is not detoxified in the body.

Diphenylchlorarsine is a dark brown liquid that decomposes on heating producing toxic fumes, including arsenic fumes and chlorine. Used alone it was designated 'Blue Cross' by Germany, 'Sternite' by France, and 'DA' by Britain. Reportedly it has only a slight odour.[50] The gas affects the eyes, skin and entire respiratory tract. It also affects the nervous system with high exposures causing loss of consciousness. Like phosgene and diphosgene, its effects on the lungs are often delayed and are exacerbated by exercise. Pulmonary oedema results from high exposures.[51]

Butler describes the 'more severe cases' as follows:

> [they experienced] intense pain in the nose, mouth and throat, gums and jaws, tingling and smarting of the face, copious discharge from the nose, tightness in the chest, nausea and retching. The pain in the eyes and head … when severe, was agonising and accompanied by intense mental distress.

Diphenylchlorarsine degrades to diphenylarsinic acid. Little information is available on the toxicity of diphenylarsinic acid in cell reproduction, however, in high concentrations it is thought to cause chromosomal aberrations.[52]

Finally, there is *chloropicrin* (trichloronitromethane). Chloropicrin is a slightly oily, colourless liquid with a pungent odour. It was used alone by both Britain ('PS') and France ('Aquinite') or in combination with stannic chloride, phosgene or diphosgene. Britain's use of chloropicrin was specifically to penetrate German gas masks. According to Heller, chloropicrin

> seeped into the masks and created intolerable eye irritation, coughing, vomiting, and inflammation of the respiratory tract. Enemy soldiers forced to remove their fouled masks were then subjected to a shelling with lethal phosgene.[53]

Chloropicrin is widely used today in fumigants, in fungicides and insecticides. In agriculture it is widely used to sterilise soil and seeds. In quite low concentrations it causes profuse lacrimation (tears), red eyes, pain and blurred vision. Inhaled it causes abdominal pain, cough, diarrhoea, dizziness, headache, sore throat, vomiting and weakness. In higher concentrations it causes profound inflammation of the lower respiratory tract and potentially leads to fatal pulmonary oedema. At the time of its use on the Western Front chloropicrin was known to be cumulative in action and that 'repeated exposure to small concentration leads to increased susceptibility…Brief exposure to strong concentrations may cause temporary unconsciousness'.[54]

The toxicity 'profile' of chloropicrin is not well-documented; indeed the literature on its effects on humans is described as 'mostly anecdotal'.[55]

These toxic gases, known rather benignly as 'lung irritants', were used throughout the war. However, July 1917 saw something new and far more devastating – 'mustard gas' or 'yperite' (dichlorethylsulphide). In Butler's view the introduction of sulphur mustard was 'an event of outstanding military importance'. In his opinion 'the nature and action of the substance was determined in a few days; the box respirator was effective, and a line of treatment promptly evolved. But the problem set to the defence was new and in some respects insoluble – as it is to-day'.[56] Whilst his views on preparedness, on the effectiveness of the respirator and on treatment can be seriously questioned, he is correct in viewing 'defence' against the gas as insoluble, even now.

Sulphur mustard is currently regarded as one of the most important agents of chemical warfare. It is easily produced, even in underdeveloped countries, and it has no effective therapy.[57] It was synthesised around 1822 by Despretz but first developed as an agent of chemical warfare by Fritz Haber in the Great War. According to one source, over 1.2 million soldiers were exposed to the gas during the war with approximately 400 000 requiring 'prolonged' medical treatment.[58] Since the war, sulphur mustard has been used by Italy in a campaign against Ethiopia (1935-6) and extensively by Iraq against Iranian soldiers and the Iraqi Kurdish population between 1983 and 1988. Sulphur mustard was one of a number of identified chemical weapons used in the killing of 5000 Kurdish civilians in Halabja in 1988.[59]

Sulphur mustard is a colourless to yellow oily liquid with an odour of garlic, onions or mustard. It is highly soluble in oils, fats and organic solvents so quickly penetrates the skin as well as certain textiles, rubber and heavy leather. It breaks down much slower in water and forms hydrochloric acid. It is this release of hydrochloric acid in body tissues that is responsible for its characteristic delayed damage to skin, eyes, and the respiratory and gastrointestinal systems. High temperatures and increased moisture potentiate the effects and their severity.[60] As a poison it spreads throughout the body, but concentrates in the liver, lungs and kidneys.[61] Its primary role in warfare is as a powerful blistering agent. Within 12-24 hours after exposure large, thin walled, pendulous blisters develop. The burns tend to be 'partial thickness' but in warm moist areas they are deeper.[62]

Its value as a chemical weapon is its persistence and ability to incapacitate rather than its lethality. Soil, food, and any porous material become contaminated for very long periods of time, especially in cold and damp climates.[63] On the Western Front it was first used by Germany ('Yellow Cross') on 12 July 1917. In a report marked 'Very Secret', the Physiological Adviser of RAMC Gas Services, Lt Col Douglas, noted that between July 1916 and July 1917, total casualties from gassing in the British Army were 8806 and deaths were 532. But from July 1917 to July 1918, casualties were 105 910 and deaths 2973. These figures, he wrote, under-represented the true situation: they did not include deaths in the trenches or prisoners of war.[64] Similar figures, however unreliable, are not available for the AIF. The explanation for the great increase in deaths and casualties in 1917 was twofold: more gas was used from the beginning of the spring offensive and

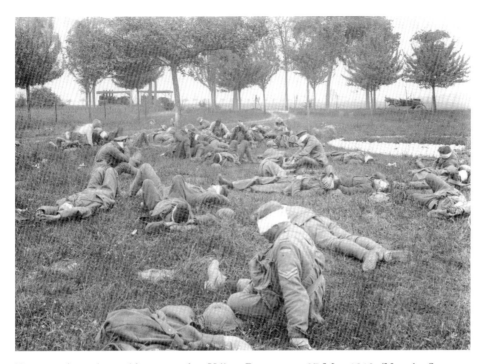

Figure 4. Australian soldiers gassed at Villers-Bretonneux 27 May 1918. (Note by Sergeant A. Brooksbank, Gas NCO, 10th Australian Infantry Brigade: 'Examples of what should not be done. Casualties should have removed contaminated garments. Lying on the ground with contaminated clothes and not wearing respirators means that they are inhaling quantities of vapour and adding to their injuries') [Australian War Memorial neg. no. E04851]

mustard gas was introduced. Sulphur mustard was also mixed with prussic acid which destroyed the sense of smell making detection extremely difficult.[65]

If the liquid in the exploded shell sprayed the skin it blistered and if the blisters were rubbed, more blistering occurred. The eyes were burned and so watered, the lids swelled and temporary blindness ensued. The nose burned, there was nausea and vomiting. The trachea and bronchi became inflamed, there was intense coughing, and tissue died, leading to bronchitis or broncho-pneumonia. Because it could penetrate all ordinary fabrics, moist protected skin, especially the scrotum and penis, became red then blistered within 24 hours. Its persistence in clothing and in the soil meant that men were 'gassed', as in the experience of the 2nd Australian Division, by 'sleeping beside men who had got some gas on clothes':

> A few men were gassed by returning to dugouts from fatigues or carrying, gas having got into their dugouts during their absence … A considerable number were affected in the eyes by taking off the upper part of the mask in order to see the duckwalk. They were members of carrying parties who were surprised by [a] barrage while going or

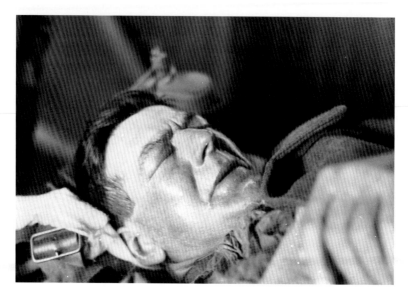

Figure 5. Swollen face of a soldier affected by mustard gas at a Casualty Clearing Station on the Amiens-Corbie road, 27 May 1918   [Australian War Memorial neg. no. E04853]

returning along [the] duckwalk. The night was very dark and it was impossible to see the duckwalk through the goggles. They had either to remain in the barrage, which was very heavy, or free the eyes in order to get out of it. They chose the latter …Men were slightly gassed when digging in ground which had been bombarded …Men were affected by going into shell holes to stool.[66]

Ever concerned with prevention, Butler noted that at Villers Bretonneux in July 1918, during an intense bombardment, Green Cross shells were 'thrown in first to make the men sneeze and deaden the sense of smell'. These were then followed by an 'overwhelming' bombardment with mustard. He went on:

With regard to the prevention of gas casualties from Yellow Cross, the matter is extremely difficult. It is almost impossible to move a battalion any distance at night if all the men are wearing gas masks as it is very hard to see trenches and wire, and, in addition, the enemy very often surrounds his gas shelling with a barrage of HE [High Explosives] …In addition, it is extremely difficult to keep on a gas helmet for more than a few hours at a time. A few of the ambulance men were gassed some by coming in contact with gas patients and others by carrying patients into and through the gassed areas.[67]

Sulphur mustard is commonly known as a 'vesicant' agent, that is, a blistering agent. Although it has been studied and produced by many countries its mechanism of action remains unknown.[68] What is known is that it is mutagenic, carcinogenic, and cytotoxic; that it is known to cause respiratory cancers, skin cancer, leukaemia, chronic respiratory disease, bone marrow suppression and eye damage.[69] It is also thought to cause cancers of the oesophagus and stomach.[70] The single greatest cause of long-term disability amongst those exposed to sulphur mustard is respiratory problems. Importantly, (see Chapter 9) chest X-ray is 'not sensitive enough for detection of respiratory complications'.[71]

Gas masks

The preceding paragraphs provide a thumbnail sketch of a vast topic. Those chemicals that are still in use today are the subject of extensive research by physicians, toxicologists and others dealing with the sequelae. Current medical and scientific knowledge is incomplete and constantly changing. In particular, the long-term effects of these chemicals are only now partially understood, and in most cases treatment and, more importantly, prevention of health effects is rudimentary.

On the Western Front, likewise, treatment was reflexive and reliant on contemporary medical and scientific understandings. Blood-letting ('venesection'), for example, was a widespread treatment for gassing. Defence – prevention – centred on the development of gas masks, that is, on protecting the respiratory tract of soldiers. Gas masks were developed by both sides of the conflict and had various mutations through the course of the war. For Australian soldiers the key developments were the British 'Hypo' helmet respirator (issued to troops in the vicinity of the Anzac area in anticipation of Turkey's use of gas which did not eventuate), the PH or PHG helmet, issued to all Australian troops on arrival in France, the Large Box Respirator and the Small Box Respirator, the latter being the first effective mask used by Britain and its allies. These masks were the equivalent of what is now known as Personal Protective Equipment in the vernacular of occupational health and safety. Masks are still used extensively in industries with toxic fumes/gases and many of the problems experienced by soldiers in the Great War persist.

The 'Hypo' helmet was introduced in May 1915 and by June all British soldiers on the Western Front had been issued with this helmet. Made of grey woollen Viyella or flannel, it was hot, stuffy and had no valve for the intake or expiration of air so filled with carbon dioxide. Visibility was impossible through the Mica, celluloid or cellulose acetate 'window'. The 'filter' in the 'Hypo' helmet was achieved by soaking it in sodium phenate. This mask was designed specifically to overcome gassing by chlorine.

As outlined above, phosgene was introduced by Germany in December 1915 and continued to be used in shell attacks to the end of the war. In January 1916 the 'PH' gas helmet was introduced as a form of protection (Figure 6).[72] The 'P' stood for a breathing valve in the helmet, itself a cloth hood tucked into the collar and impregnated with sodium phenate, and the 'H' for the addition of hexamine, the latter chemical, suggested by Russia, acting to 'take up' phosgene. This chemical combination was also used in the earliest 'respirator', the Large Box Respirator. In his draft of the chapter on 'Chemical Warfare', Butler expressed considerable reservations about the PH helmet, reservations that were not included in the final published chapter.

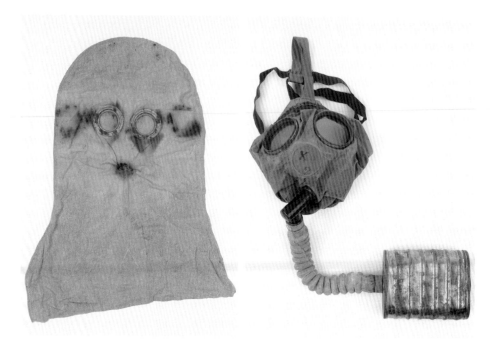

Figure 6. (*left*). PH Helmet gas respirator, c 1916

Figure 7. (*right*). Small Box Respirator, c 1918

[Australian War Memorial neg. nos. RELAWM04043.001 & RELAWM12424.001]

In the 'alert' position it had to be worn pinned to the front of the tunic and tucked inside the breast; so that in warm weather the jacket could not be removed as it carried the helmet … A further serious objection was the fact that the moisture of the brow bringing the chemicals of the fabric into solution produced irritation and burns – due to the phenyl compound – if the helmet had to be worn for any length of time.[73]

By early 1917, the better designed and more effective Small Box Respirator, which filtered breathed air through charcoal and soda lime, had been issued to British and Australian soldiers (Figure 7). According to Butler, by early 1917 'the anti-gas equipment of each of the fighting troops then consisted of a small box respirator and a reserve P.H. helmet'. The 'reserve' PH helmets, which 'afforded no protection against either the arsenical warfare gases or mustard gas' were withdrawn in February 1918. Thus, in the period from early 1916 to early 1917, soldiers subjected to gas attacks were using either a PH mask or the Large Box respirator, both of which were impregnated with hexamine. From early 1917 to February 1918 the back-up device, clearly still in use, was the PH helmet.

The affect of phosgene on the hexamine contained in the PH helmet and Large Box Respirator caused them to give off formalin fumes. Soldiers were told that formalin 'irritates the throat but is quite harmless [and the] mask [is] not to be taken off on that account'.[74] Formalin (formaldehyde) is now known to be a lethal chemical, highly toxic in vaporised form and a proven carcinogen. Exposure to the fumes over a period of time can destroy the sense of smell, so vital to gas detection for all soldiers on the Western Front. Just how many soldiers suffered both short and long-term health effects merely from wearing these masks or the early respirator in gas attacks will never be known.

Trench Fever

In December 1914 soldiers started suffering from a sickness characterised by a high temperature and little else. It came on quickly and lasted for from four to six days. The high temperature itself caused a general malaise but no other signs or symptoms were manifest. In the spring of 1915 a variation of this illness was recorded. The appearance – the signs and symptoms – were identical but the illness was characterised by 'periodicity', by relapses. Although no other symptoms were present, the recurrence of the fever was debilitating. By the end of 1915 the same illness was still present amongst soldiers but now another symptom appeared. 'Shin pains' became 'almost universal'. During 1916 a familiar pattern of illness became established. It was characterised by 'severe and often intractable pain', irregular high temperature, great debility that often required a convalescence of several months, loss of muscular strength, fine tremors, a rapid heart beat, a heart murmur, enlargement of the left side of the heart, and loss of appetite and sleep. Other variations appeared during 1917 that were characterised by muscular pain. This pain was often diagnosed as 'Myalgia' on soldier's records yet true myalgia was exceedingly uncommon.

This description is based on a retrospective appraisal by Colonel A.B. Soltau, CMG, Consulting Physician to the Second Army in August 1918.[75] On the ground, however, things were not quite so clear. According to Butler, the illness was 'missed' at Gallipoli in a 'welter' of misdiagnoses, yet the BEF reported thousands of cases between April and October 1915. An article by Major J.H.P. Graham appeared in the prestigious *Lancet* journal in September 1915 describing it as a 'Relapsing Febrile Illness of unknown origin'. Gradually through 1916 medical officers became more familiar with the illness although it still appeared on hospital returns and soldiers' medical history cards as 'PUO', or pyrexia of unknown origin. In the first Interallied Sanitary Conference of May 1916 the 'discovery' of the 'new disease' was widely discussed. Within a short period of time all belligerent nations had published reports of the same illness.[76]

For military doctors the problem was differentiating this illness from many other febrile illnesses. In April 1917 Captain Roland Beard, RMO of the 53rd Battalion of the AIF wrote to the ADMS of 5th Australian Division on cases of 'an infectious fever' which he called 'Infectious Osteomyalgia … (Syn. so called "Trench Fever")'. After treating around 30 cases in three weeks, Beard was convinced that the illness was infective since comrades of the sick soldiers, those who were 'closely associated' with them, fell prey to the same illness. He also described a 'Tibial walk': 'not unlike that of a person wearing new and tight boots'. From his perspective, the disease was 'ravaging' his Battalion: 'it is a disabling affection and men are unable to do their duty efficiently in most cases for several weeks. The pain prevents sleep'.[77]

By May 1917, AIF medical authorities started enquiring about the status of inoculations of sick soldiers, about the length of time that had elapsed since their last bath and change of underclothing, and of the 'approximate date of disinfection of blankets'.[78] By the end of the month the illness, now known as Trench Fever, was reported by the Commander of the 7th Australian Infantry Brigade to 2nd Australian Divisional Headquarters as 'becoming epidemic and a serious menace to the efficiency of the Brigade'.[79] Colonel Alfred Sutton, ADMS to the 2nd Australian Division replied that 'Investigations have been carried on for a year or more as to the causation of this disease'. He went on:

> The question is still not absolutely settled, but there is a good deal of evidence in favour of the view that the disease is transmitted by lice.[80]

Sutton went on to outline some basic steps that had been taken towards hygiene and disinfection amongst that Brigade. June saw a flurry of activity aimed at eradicating louse infestation amongst the troops. Radical cleaning, scrubbing, sterilisation, baths, disinfection, use of irons for clothes, changes of underclothes all materialised – and all of this against a background of an ever-increasing 'epidemic' that was still of uncertain cause and with no knowledge of how the disease was transmitted. But this was to change.

In the period from July to August 1917 American forces arrived in France. Perfunctory research into the cause and transmission of the disease had been undertaken in Britain but with no support from the War Office. This lack of support largely hinged on the need for human subjects for experimentation. However, the Medical Research Committee (MRC) of the American Red Cross immediately set up a Medical Investigation Committee on Trench Fever and agreement was reached with the BEF that the MRC would undertake the human experimentation in British hospitals. The War Office, now under pressure, acquiesced and, as Butler puts it, two research campaigns 'were carried out in a spirit of mutual co-operation, combined with a wholesome tang of competition – the ideal atmosphere for scientific creation'.[81]

The first report of the Australian Members of the MRC to the DMS described three forms of 'PUO': a 'relapsing type' known as Trench Fever; a fever characterised by 'a single short initial bout'; and 'those showing prolonged initial fever'.[82] By the date of the third report, later in 1917, the doctors were able to confirm that 'experiment has since shown that those three are merely variations of the same infection'.

Human experimentation began in December 1917 but with negative results. By this date the number of admissions to Field Ambulances with PUO and Trench Fever had escalated. As recorded on the soldiers' medical cards there was an approximate ratio of over 20:1 admissions for PUO as opposed to Trench Fever, yet the AAMC was well aware that over 50% of the alleged PUO cases were in fact Trench Fever.[83] As well, by December 1917 many soldiers had been in British hospitals for up to six months convalescing from the disease. These particular individuals suffered particularly from anaemia, inflammation of the heart ('myocarditis'), pain and insomnia.[84]

In February 1918, however, there was a breakthrough. The Interim Report by the War Office Committee on the Causation of Trench Fever announced that 'probably the most important method of the spread of Trench Fever' was lice.[85] By May 1918 it was recognised that the effects of long-term or severe infections included enlargement of the spleen, a distinctive rash on the chest and abdomen, heart abnormalities often referred to in diagnoses as 'Disordered Action of the Heart' or 'DAH', pain, 'pink eyes' (marked 'conjunctival injection'), frontal headache and the relapsing fever. The rapid heart beat noted by the MRC and the British Medical Investigation Committee 'disables a man for a long time from duty'.[86] By this stage, and even at the date of Butler's research in the 1940s, the illness was believed to be *viral*.

From June, when Trench Fever became a notifiable disease, to August 1918, with a causative agent known and some rudimentary understanding of the condition circulating widely, the attention of the higher command of the AAMC was twofold: prevention, and the discipline of AIF doctors who were repeatedly reprimanded for 'slackness of diagnosis' and issued with ever-changing instructions as to how to diagnose, classify and deal with soldiers presenting with a high temperature. Yet despite zealous administrative efforts, by August 1918 Trench Fever was still responsible for around 20% of admissions to Casualty Clearing Stations. When this figure is considered in the context of the massive gassing of 1918 the reality of the soldier's war becomes more palpable.

'Urban' Trench Fever: Bartonella quintana

The first clear descriptions of Trench Fever appeared during the Great War although it is now known that the disease has a very long history indeed. It has been identified in the DNA of human remains in south-eastern France dated at being greater than or equal to 4000 years and has been postulated as the cause of Napoleon's retreat from Russia, again based on DNA sampling of a mass grave in Lithuania.[87] It was described sporadically after the Great War and once again appeared in focal outbreaks during World War II. However, it was not until the 1960s that the *bacterium* was isolated and described. *Bartonella quintana* and other *Bartonella* species have received significant attention since the early 1990s due to their adverse affects on patients infected with human immunodeficiency virus (HIV). The other major worldwide population seriously affected and infected by *B. quintana* is homeless people.

Homelessness is currently recognised as a major worldwide social problem in both preindustrial and highly industrialised countries. Significant statistically verified populations exist in the United States, England, France, Japan, South Africa and elsewhere.[88] The chief characteristics of the homeless that have parallels with soldiers in World War I are poor physical condition, lack of basic hygiene, poor nutrition, lack of conventional shelter, heavy tobacco usage and use of alcohol. Males are also disproportionately represented.[89] Homeless people also have little or no access to medical care in most wealthy nations.

The human body louse (not the hair louse) is the only known vector of *B. quintana* and humans are the only proven mammal host for the bacterial organism. Lice live in clothing and are transmitted to others by contact with clothing or bedding. They multiply rapidly – by up to 11% in one day – and it is estimated that about 5-10% of lice are infected with *B. quintana*. The louse's bite causes pruritus (itchy skin) and broken skin through scratching and, since the bacteria survives in lice faeces for up to twelve months in high concentrations, infection occurs when infected faeces comes in contact with broken skin. The lice retain the infection in their gut for life.[90] Humans can retain *Bartonella* in red blood cells for very long periods, with or without any symptoms. This means that lice can come in contact with the organism by biting an infected human host. In other words, given the rate of multiplication of lice populations, newly hatched lice biting infected soldiers, even those with no symptoms, would be infected and then in turn infect other soldiers.[91]

The clinical picture of *B. quintana* infection today is similar to that described above during the Great War. The difference now is that medical technology and research has allowed much greater knowledge of the causes of the various signs and symptoms described during the war on the Western Front. Four clinical entities are described in current literature: 'urban' Trench Fever; bacillary angiomatosis; chronic bacteraemia; and endocarditis. In simple language this means that infected people present to doctors with one of four types of infection – rather like the various types described on the Western Front. The first is characterised by a relapsing fever, headache and body pain and is still known as (urban) Trench Fever. Bacillary angiomatosis translates as red lumpy lesions on the skin (with or without swollen glands), fever, weight loss and osteolysis (the breakdown of bone tissue). The third, chronic bacteraemia, simply means a long term presence of bacteria in the blood. It is characterised by fever, headache, leg pain and a reduction in red blood cells (thrombocytopenia). However, it can also be present with no symptoms whatsoever. The fourth, and for the purposes of this work perhaps the most important, is endocarditis, potentially if not probably the 'DAH' of the Great War. This is characterised by fever, difficulty breathing, a heart murmur, and vegetative 'growths' around heart valves, some of which can break off and form emboli that can occlude arteries.[92]

The severity, and thus clinical picture of the illness, has been postulated as being due to a variety of factors: the size of the 'inoculum', in other words how much bacteria was transmitted to the individual; the virulence of the particular strain of the organism; the immune status of the human; and genetic variability in *B. quintana* itself.[93] What is more certain is the difficulty of diagnosis, particularly of the nature or cause of the endocarditis or heart valve disease in presenting patients.[94]

Trench foot

During the 1916-17 winter on the Somme, units were losing up to 80 men per week with the condition which came to be known as Trench Foot. Men literally got bogged in the deep sticky mud. Sometimes they were abandoned and died.[95] Standing in mud or water, in freezing conditions, for days at a time, the soldiers' feet would initially become cold but progress to an absence of all feeling. The feet would then swell in the boots. Puttees, caked with mud, formed hard uneven rings around the calves cutting off circulation. This was exacerbated by wearing Mounted Pattern Breeches which, by their design, when the knees were flexed, also restricted circulation. The result was extremely painful, red feet, swollen two to three times their normal size and making it impossible to replace boots. If they were left untreated the feet went from bright pink to a 'dead, black gangrenous appearance'.[96] The condition could and did progress to gangrene and it is estimated that approximately 121 of the total number of amputations carried out on men who subsequently survived to return to Australia resulted from Trench Foot.[97] The condition is now known as either 'immersion foot syndrome' or as 'non-freezing cold injury'.

In order to understand the nature of this condition it is necessary to understand the nature of trench warfare on the Western Front, and to understand how such a serious cause of attrition in the field got out of control. The experience of the 5th Australian Division of 1st Anzac Corps in late 1916 provides a seminal case study of the latter and in so doing highlights the antagonisms that existed between the medical corps and senior officers, and between the various levels of higher command. The Commanding Officer of the 5th Australian Division was Major General James Whiteside McCay, former head of the Australian Intelligence Corps, close associate of John Monash, and a figure encountered elsewhere in this work.

Trench warfare and the Somme winter

It has been estimated that by the end of the war there was more than 15 000 miles (approximately 24 000 km) of trenches between the North Sea and the borders of Switzerland.[98] 'Trench' summons up a picture of a neat U-shaped tunnel lined with boards ('duckboards') on the ground and sometimes boarding on the side walls. But in the winter of 1916/17 this was not the case. Wilfred Owen was then a Lieutenant in the BEF. On 12 January 1917 he wrote to his mother as follows:

> We had a march of 3 miles over shelled road then nearly 3 along a flooded trench. After that we came to where the trenches had been blown flat out and had to go over the top. It was of course dark, too dark, and the ground was not mud, not sloppy mud, but an octopus of sucking clay, 3, 4, and 5 feet deep, relieved only by craters full of water. Men have been known to drown in them. Many stuck in the mud & only got on by leaving their waders, equipment, and some cases their clothes.
>
> High explosives were dropping all around, and machine guns spluttered every few minutes. But it was so dark that even the German flares did not reveal us.

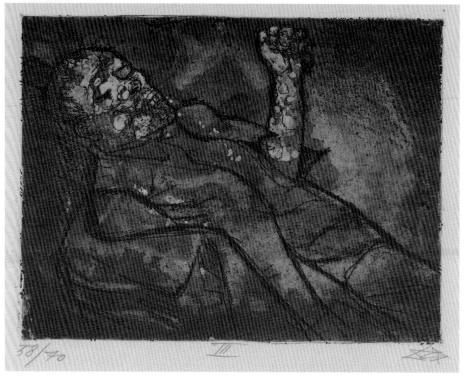

Figure 8. Otto Dix, *Der Krieg*, XXIII, *Toter in Schlamm*, Dead Man in the Mud
[Courtesy National Gallery of Australia; © Otto Dix, licensed by VISCOPY, Australia 2008]

Several days later he continued:

> No Man's Land under snow is like the face of the moon chaotic, crater-ridden, uninhabitable, awful, the abode of madness …
>   Hideous landscapes, vile noises, foul language and nothing but foul, even from one's own mouth … everything unnatural, broken, blasted; the distortion of the dead, whose unburiable bodies sit outside the dug-outs all day, all night, the most execrable sights on earth. In poetry we call them the most glorious. But we sit with them all day, all night … and a week later to come back and find them still sitting there, in motionless groups, THAT is what saps the 'soldierly spirit' …[99]

Some things even Owen didn't write about. Toilets, for example, were commonly dug behind the front line trenches. However being in full view of the enemy meant the pit had to be dug in the trench itself. When a trench was destroyed by explosives, dead bodies were incorporated into the new trench wall so the 'stench of putrefaction was added to that of urine and faeces'.[100] The harrowing images of Otto Dix's *Der Krieg* portray this reality of the Somme winter.

Over 23 000 Australians were killed or wounded in five weeks at the Somme. In October 1916 1 Anzac Corps was ordered from the Ypres salient, where they were preparing for winter quartering, to the Somme to relieve the British XV Corps in a 3600

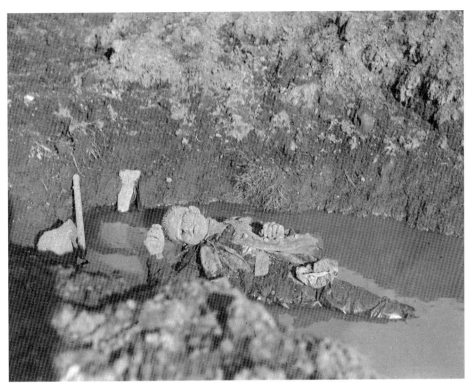

Figure 9. Dead German soldier in water-filled crater, near Zonnebeke in the Ypres Sector, 17 October 1917 [Australian War Memorial neg. no. E00927]

metre line. Michael Tyquin politely notes that the Anzac Corps 'inherited the medical evacuation scheme and routes from the previous occupant'.[101] In December, looking back on two months of warring within the Corps and within the Divisions of the Corps, the Officer Commanding 1st Anzac Corps, Lt Gen W.R. Birdwood, wrote to Headquarters of 4th Army regarding his 'heavy sick wastage' in the following terms.

> When our Divisions first took over the line the conditions were exceedingly bad …
> In the front line the trenches consisted of linked shell holes full of mud and water,
> and the men during their tour of duty, i.e. for about 48 hours, were compelled to
> crouch in cold water up to their knees. It was not possible for them to either sit
> down, lie down or move about. The trenches were in full view of the enemy and no
> movement was possible except by night, and even at night there could be no freedom
> of movement.[102]

On 9 November, 4 days after the re-commencement of hostilities, Colonel A.H. Sturdee, ADMS of 1st Australian Division wrote to Divisional Headquarters that 'a big majority of the men have never been dry since the 27th of last month, and while in the trenches are standing in mud and water, sleep being out of the question … many of them at least [have] been without hot food for the same period and longer'.[103] Unbeknownst to

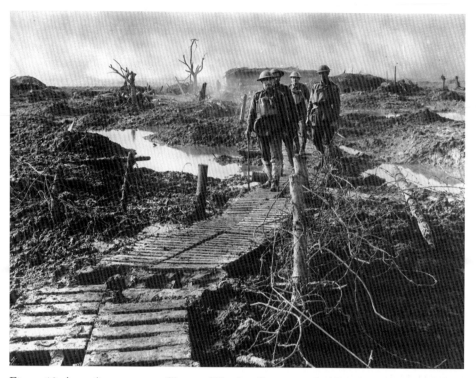

Figure 10. Australian troops at Chateau Wood walking over duckboards in the waterlogged fields to Zonnebeke, October 1917. (Photo Frank Hurley)

[National Library of Australia, an23478230]

Sturdee, the following day the Provost Marshal of 4th Army wrote to Birdwood's Anzac Corps complaining bitterly of the 'great many hundreds' of men being evacuated with a diagnosis of 'Exhaustion': 'there appear to be reason to believe that the men are in many cases not sick at all, but really aught to come under the category of stragglers'. A few days later the DDMS of 1st Anzac Corps, Colonel Manifold, a British officer, wrote to the ADMS of 2nd Australian Division complaining about the Division's sick rate, for using a diagnosis of 'Exhaustion' on evacuated men, and for the lack of hot food for men in the front line. Sturdee's Commanding Officer wrote directly to Birdwood as follows:

> As this implies lack of precautions on the part of the Division, may I point out that the trenches we took over were, without exception, full of mud and water from knee to waistdeep, and that there was no refuge for the men or possibility of cooking. Even the bomb stores in the front line had disappeared.
>
> Every effort was made, but as you know, for 24 hours we had the greatest difficulty in even getting the wounded out, and bare rations in to the front trenches.
>
> Exhaustion and trench feet were inevitable... .[104]

The following day, 14 November, the second German attack commenced. By the 17th, as Tyquin notes, 'all the approaches to, and evacuation routes from, the front had dissolved

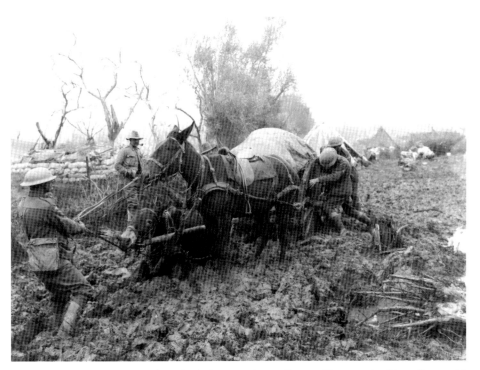

Figure 11. Mule team bogged in thigh deep mud near Potijze Farm in the Ypres Sector, 19 October 1917   [Australian War Memorial neg. no. E00962]

into the quagmire'. On 19 December the 2nd Division recorded 275 men wounded and 441 sick; on 3 December the 5th Division recorded 155 casualties and 1132 sick and much of this from Trench Foot. Needless to say the rate of attrition in 5th Division attracted the attention of those further up the command chain and various causes were floated: differences in Unit rates of sickness were put down to doctors examining soldiers without the Unit Commander first seeing the man ('cases must occur, and frequently do occur, in which the Doctor evacuates men who have little, if anything, the matter with them'); poor officer supervision ('lack of care and want of discipline on the part of Regimental Officers'); and, the soldiers' lack of attention to their health ('the men are careless of their own welfare').[105]

Senior doctors also weighed in with criticisms. Manifold wrote to Birdwood on 30 November that 'there must be something radically wrong when one Division reports 159 cases [of Trench Foot] and the other under similar conditions only three'.[106] Manifold had questioned a number of 5th Division men he found at the Corps Rest Station and was able to report that no gumboots had been issued in two Battalions, few had gumboots in another two Battalions, that 'nearly all the men were said to have had bad boots for marching up' and that 'some boots were found lying in a dump, but after some had been issued, all were recalled'. He went on:

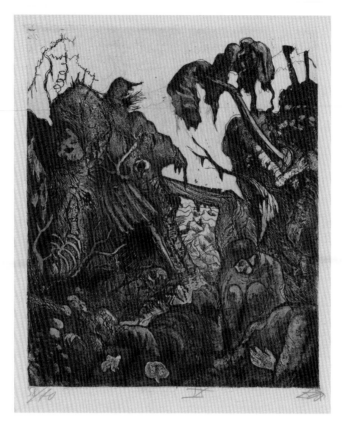

Figure 12. Otto Dix, *Der Krieg*, IX, *Zerfallender Kampfgraben*, Disintegrating Trench
[Courtesy National Gallery of Australia; © Otto Dix, licensed by VISCOPY, Australia 2008]

No inspection was apparently made to see whether men were carrying spare socks, and that in hardly any case had a man ever taken off his boots whilst in the trenches … Had a man taken off his boots in the trenches he would have done so standing half-way to his knees in water … where gum boots were worn, it is said they had been taken over wet inside; sometimes men marching up had picked them up lying in the mud of the trenches.[107]

Manifold was convinced that the problem – 'arrangements … absolutely deficient in system and organisation' – rested with Divisional officers and announced that he was going to investigate the matter 'on the spot' the next day. His lengthy and detailed 'Report' caused considerable anger and resentment amongst many senior officers and amongst other senior AAMC members. Manifold blamed the excessive rate of trench foot on four preventable factors: an inadequate supply of 'Trench boots' (gum boots); lack of 'dug-outs' and dry standing places; neglect to remove boots and socks and attend to feet hygiene; and, in Manifold's opinion the 'root of the whole matter', the 'Australian Officer' who had 'not learned to look after his men'.[108] In addition to the issues he had previously highlighted, Manifold drew attention to the bad quality of ankle boots –

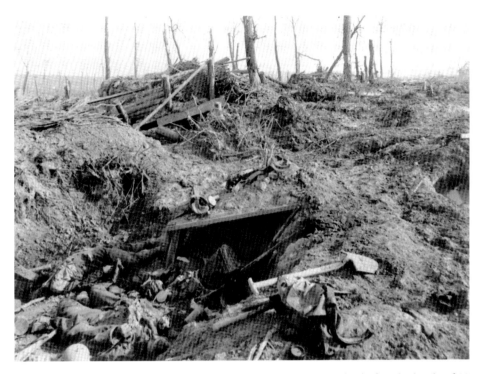

Figure 13. Frank Hurley: captured German trenches strewn with dead after the battle of 20 September 1917, Menin Road area. (Photo Frank Hurley)

[Australian War Memorial neg. no. E00766]

'I know it is quite common for men to walk back from the front line, either in their gum boots or in bare feet, not being able to get their ankle boots on their feet again'; inappropriate clothing – 'Australian Troops wear breeches, fitting very often closely and tightly constricting the knee … In consequence of the wetness of the trenches men cannot sit down with any comfort and consequently often crouch upon their hams which brings close constriction on the leg'; and food that was 'rarely warm'.

McCay had not been idle and indeed on the day of Manifold's inspection he had issued one of his many lengthy 'Special Divisional Orders' regarding trench feet. Every detail was attended to including lubrication of feet, wearing of gum boots, creation of 'shelters', availability of dry socks, slackening of bootlaces and breeches, hot drinks 'at least once during each night, and a hot meal and hot drink once a day', establishment of drying rooms and so forth. But for McCay, given the ever-increasing rate of evacuation from this illness, the solution lay in greater discipline. His Order of 1 December was intensely critical of his own officers and his remedy fairly typical: a threat of 'removal' and a charge of 'neglect of duty'.

In 1932, Butler was trying to fathom the recalcitrance of the problem and corresponded with a number of former AIF senior officers and AAMC members. Although he celebrates

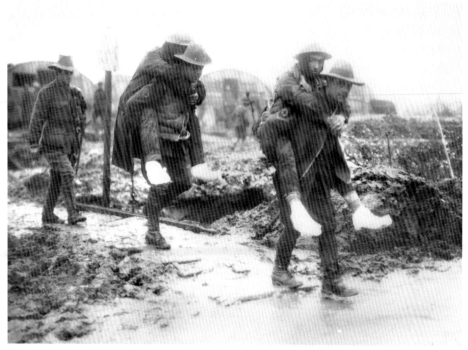

Figure 14. Australian ambulance men at Bernafay conveying soldiers suffering from trench foot to a transport, December 1916   [Australian War Memorial neg. no. E00081]

the AIF in the published version of events, some of his correspondents did not necessarily agree. General Tivey told him he had 'stood up' to Manifold about his report and believed that 'the rationing of the front line trenches was always with the Australian units an affair of honour' and that the Australian officers 'looked after their men well, even in the early winter on the Somme'. The former DADMS of the 5th Division believed that the condition of the sector taken over was so appalling that the health effects, including a high incidence of trench feet, were totally understandable and that conditions prevalent in BEF occupied trenches were far worse than in any Australian Division. However, Lt Col Crowther, an RMO in the 31st Battalion of 5th Division at this time believed the problem did indeed lie with the officers of that Division. For Crowther the Division was 'seriously demoralised': 'the Battalion officers had lost their punch and grip of the men'. And the cause of this demoralisation was 'their hatred for McCay'.[109]

In ideal conditions, dry weather and good drainage in the trenches, the problem of trench foot was eliminated. However, in winter's heavy rains and cold, and in a war environment, this was practically impossible. By 1915, miles of 'duckboards' had been placed in trenches, but, as one commentator has noted, many of these either 'floated away with the heavy rains or were trodden into the mud'.[110] The longer term solution required vigilant attention to the feet and their coverings by officers and other ranks, and a spirit of cooperation amongst all concerned – Butler's 'spirit of the game', an esprit de corps desperately missing in the 5th Division. John Monash, then commanding the 3rd Division, described his own experience in January 1917 in a letter home:

> all the men in the front lines regularly get hot food – coffee, oxo, porridge, stews. They cannot cook it themselves, for at the least sight of the smoke of a fire the spot is instantly shelled. And they must get it regularly or they would perish of cold or frostbite, or get 'trench feet', which occasionally means amputation. So I have got the pioneers to make hundreds of 'Thermos Flasks', boxes lined with straw into which the 'dixies' or cooking-pots can be packed, and these are carried on men's backs up to the forward defences, the food remaining quite hot.
>
> It is also imperative to attend to the men's boots and socks. A special organization looks after the collection of wet socks from men in the trenches, and these are taken down to the divisional baths to be washed and dried, and clean dry socks are daily sent up in sacks, by platoons. The boots I refer to are special trench boots called gum-boots, made of rubber up to the thighs. I have 6,000 on hand of which 3,000 are in use, while the other 3,000 are back out of the line, in the 'Gum-Boots Store' where there are drying rooms; this establishment being run by a special detail of men.
>
> … I have two divisional baths, one at Steenwerck, one at Pont de Nieppe, a suburb of the large town. In these are washed 2,000 men daily, with hot water in great brewery tubs. Each man hands in his old under clothes and gets in exchange a complete clean outfit. I employ over 200 girls in the laundries washing and ironing the soiled clothes.[111]

Monash's approach to the problem of trench feet emphasised systematic organisation over discipline, and it worked. The engineer was endlessly fascinated by the machine, in this case the workings of the organisation he commanded. Later in 1917, after Passchendaele, he wrote:

> Throughout every department of the work, both fighting and feeding up supplies, stores and ammunition, I strive to introduce similar systematic methods and order, so that there shall be no muddling, no overlapping, no cross purposes, and everybody has to know exactly what his job is and when and where he has to do it. To carry this into effect one has to be very firm and very strict, and anybody who does not work up to time and come up to scratch usually does not get a second chance with me.[112]

Monash's response is remarkably similar to the public health and organisational response now so familiar in global disasters and to that which was eventually commonplace on the Western Front. It required cooperation and respect between the medical corps and army officers, an understanding of fundamental public health principles, the capacity to communicate successfully with officers and all other ranks, and good leadership (in its broadest sense) from commanding officers. The fact that figures for trench foot fell dramatically over January and February to a 'trickle' bears witness to this method.

Yet the soldier's war was not all gassing, sickness, wounding and swollen feet. In France it was also long periods of utter boredom, stuck in a trench, doing nothing; the quiet times. It was also trips to local towns, prostitutes, cigarettes, long letters home, and mateship.

But for all the celebrated camaraderie and the heroism, only a small minority of the AIF were untouched by injury or illness on the Western Front. And for most it was, quite literally, an unspeakable experience.

For decades after the war, former soldiers visited their local doctors with an astonishing (then) range of signs and symptoms. Sometimes doctors admitted their lack of knowledge; more commonly they made categorical diagnoses based on their current practice and experience. But to obtain a war pension for a disability a veteran had to be examined by a different kind of doctor; one employed by the Repatriation Department. And these doctors were, in many respects, quite different from an average general practitioner. In later chapters the characters and careers of some of these doctors are examined in some detail. It will be argued that these doctors were first and foremost gatekeepers for Treasury and efficient bureaucrats rather than doctors, and that consequently the soldier's war, as recounted here, held little relevance.

CHAPTER 4

Setting Up a Department

The previous chapters have dealt with powerful social forces and with the grim reality of war. That history possesses a certain drama. By contrast, the subject matter of this chapter may appear mundane. From the broad sweep of events in Australia and overseas it shrinks to the minutiae of a nascent bureaucracy, to a group of three people: the Minister for Repatriation, the Comptroller and his Secretary. From a time frame of around three years it contracts to only six months. Yet this detail is of immense importance. There is no comparable study of a major Australian bureaucracy which provides the same intimate detail of the unfolding of an organisation, its personnel, values and powers.

The lack of such studies may partly be explained by the random survival of documents but it also derives from the nature of the subject. Departmental histories have attracted little attention from critical scholars and have frequently been subjected to some form of censorship, including self-censorship.[1] Perhaps the most eloquent expression of the problem is by the author/editor of what must be the largest official history of an institution ever published in Australia, *The Official History of Australia during the War*. Charles Bean wrote to Graham Butler in 1942 that 'one cannot take an anti-Government view (or a possibly anti-government one) in a government history. The volume would have to be censored by them and the staff'.[2]

The early history of the Repatriation Department recorded by Pryor, Gilbert and Scott, and by those who have recycled their works, suffers from precisely this problem. In addition, there has been no broad analysis of the historical process involved. The following exposition and analysis draws on an archive which reveals, first, the sources of inspiration behind the General Orders and Regulations which were to govern the nature of the Department and, second, the systematic and comprehensive procedure of making appointments, both to the staff and the voluntary State Boards, which ensured that like-minded men occupied all the key positions. This latter practice was not just the classical cronyism that saw the placement of friends in 'good' positions. It was a methodical and calculated adjudication of the available field for each position with the explicit aim of ensuring sameness of purpose, identity of interest and commonality of values from the Minister down to the Accounts Clerks. By using such appointments to establish an institutional ideology the exercise of control from the centre was greatly facilitated.

Although little is known of the small but crucially important staff gathered around the Comptroller in Melbourne in late 1917, it seems likely that similar considerations were involved in their selection. This was the staff which framed the General Orders and Regulations. In the following section, some of the documents it used to identify areas which were perceived to require regulation are analysed. Since the scope of Departmental activity was exceedingly broad, and impossible to cover in any detail here, the documents have been used to indicate attitudes or values rather than specific details of any one scheme. The selection of *what* to regulate and of the means to achieve that regulation was not a value-free process of decision-making but rather an activity consciously or unconsciously directed by the ideology of those carrying out the work. It will be seen from the next section that the final character of the Regulations, described as 'tyrannous' by their critics, was a direct reflection of the ideology of its principal authors.

Rules and Regulations

Centralised state control was the product of a deliberate policy. Those like Millen who were active in its realisation were fully aware of the process in which they participated. George Knibbs, Commonwealth Statistician, in his correspondence with Millen during the latter months of 1917, wrote in a 'Confidential and Unofficial' letter regarding the new scheme that

> The *organising* of a community trained upon individualistic methods is obviously a work of *stupendous* difficulty. We are in fact proposing to pass from pure individualism to a scheme of social organisation informally directed by the Government, and this is a fundamental change.[3] (original emphasis)

Under the new legislation, control was clearly vested in the Minister. The Act itself was merely enabling machinery. As Gilbert noted, 'it embraced no policy, embodied no scheme, and indicated no limitations of finance'.[4] This made it difficult to criticise. It was not only political prudence, or even lack of time, which precluded the elaboration of a detailed scheme, but also the Minister's determination to have control. Indeed it was for this last reason that there could not be any detailed legislation by July, only two months after Millen's appointment. That process took another nine months investigation and then another two years to fine tune.

Millen was a critical figure in the establishment phase. Working and living in north-western New South Wales in the 1880s and early 1890s, he was, like Gilbert, a journalist for many years and had a keen interest in the welfare of farmers and graziers. He entered state politics in 1894 as a free trader and supporter of George Reid, and of Federation. From 1901 to 1923 he represented New South Wales in the federal Senate, being Opposition leader or vice-president of the Executive Council in various ministries. Millen was Minister for Defence when war broke out and was initially responsible for recruiting. From late 1915 until his death in 1923 he was intimately and actively involved in the repatriation process, first as a member of a parliamentary sub-committee on repatriation and then as Minister.[5] The character that emerges from the evidence examined here is a pragmatic, tough, politically wise conservative, with little or no interest in the humanitarian or ameliorist aspects of repatriation and a talent for economising. His interviews with soldier representatives, with the original Repatriation Commissioners and others, reveal a determined and intransigent individual, whose principal aim was to personally control the entire repatriation process in the interests of economy, while maintaining a façade of generosity, a façade frequently dented by public outcries over 'his' scheme.[6]

In July 1917 there were two areas of concern to Millen: the detailed nature of the proposed scheme and its administration, hence staffing. It will be argued that these two facets of the new Department were intertwined. The process of shaping the operating ambit of a new government department by regulations provided the ideal environment for influence by powerful individuals or organisations. And once the nature of the scheme became clear, it became important to employ 'suitable' individuals to higher offices to ensure its smooth operation. What emerges from the following analysis of an extensive archive of contemporary Departmental material is the construction of a bureaucracy, and of the relationship between that process and the conservatism of the state in the period.

By late September 1917, Nicholas (later Sir Nicholas) Lockyer was acting as Comptroller, or administrative head, of the as yet unformed Department. He was the first Repatriation bureaucrat and, it seems, the first Ministerial appointment.[7] In September 1917, when appointed Comptroller, he had been a member of the Interstate Commission for four years on an annual salary of £2000. His career in the New South Wales public service had begun at age thirteen. At fifteen, he began work as a clerk in Treasury and progressed through that Department, while George Reid was a functionary, to become Inspector of public revenue, Receiver of revenue and, in 1886, Accountant to Treasury. In the previous year he had married the daughter of Geoffrey Eager, Head of Treasury from the early 1870s until his death in 1891. Allegedly with the patronage of Timothy Coghlan, New South Wales government statistician 1886-1905, Lockyer then moved to Taxation and Customs, becoming Collector of Customs and the first Commissioner of Taxation in 1896 during Reid's second Ministry – a Ministry which included Reid's ardent supporter E.D. Millen, and which faced, across the benches, W.M. Hughes.[8] In 1901, after the death of his first wife, he married the daughter of (Sir) Harry Wollaston, Comptroller of Federal Customs, and on Wollaston's retirement in 1911, Lockyer took over that position.

Coming up through the ranks during the factional period in Australian politics, Lockyer was accustomed to working within a system of patronage that ensured the 'right man' in the right place, whether from political or bureaucratic patronage.[9] Old habits die hard and despite the depression of the 1890s and the polarising affect that had on politics, and despite the emergence of a two party system, it is clear from the establishment of the Repatriation Department that such cronyism remained rampant. Indeed even prior to Lockyer formally applying in October for a Leave of Absence from the Interstate

Commission, Millen had suggested he should have a 'free hand' in making alterations to the personnel of the State War Councils 'which in his judgement he [deemed] necessary'.[10] However, the real work of staffing did not start until February 1918. In the interim the question of what precisely this staff would administer occupied the Minister, the Comptroller and his Secretary, D.J. Gilbert.

As noted in Chapter 2, Millen embarked on this project with enormous determination. In early August he instructed all State War Councils to send copies of forms and cards then in use – there was an obvious need to standardise the information that was gathered.[11] He also asked all the State War Councils and the Voluntary Funds for advice as to the extent and nature of assistance currently provided and for suggestions which might assist in formulating the Regulations.[12] There was no shortage of responses. In broad terms they were similar to the official reports of the Board in their descriptions of assistance given: sustenance, vocational training, equipment, small loans for approved purposes, tools, furniture and so forth. Yet these unofficial responses also provided an opportunity for more forthright comment and criticism, much of which was to be incorporated immediately into the General Orders and Regulations.

The State War Council of Victoria, for example, complained of the problems encountered as a result of the premature discharge of soldiers from the AIF where either a War Pension had not been finalised or the soldier's health prevented him from working. This issue of responsibility for treatment was to prove contentious until 1921 when the Department took over Department of Defence medical institutions. The Victorian Council also drew attention to the percentage of failures due to ill health amongst those returned soldiers who had been helped to start small businesses. This form of assistance was popular, it argued, because it gave an impression of independence and control that would allow a disabled soldier time to rest. Poultry farming on suburban quarter acre blocks had been especially popular and its failure rate especially high. Indeed, the Council had been forced to employ a Business Inspector to advise on the fortunes of those so placed.[13]

The New South Wales Council was rather more businesslike in its approach: 'Grantees must show that they possess the necessary aptitude, special knowledge and steadfastness of purpose to carry on the undertaking submitted'. But another factor was identified as responsible for the failure of these ventures, one which received no publicity and remained largely unrecognised by critics of the scheme for many years, although the same factor was quickly associated with failures in the area of land settlement. The Council described the problem as follows:

> It is recognised that our present limitation of assistance is in many instances too small an amount to establish a man in business. Some provision might be made that in special cases where the circumstances strongly point to success and security is good, an amount adequate for the purpose required might be granted. It is not advisable, however, that any publicity should be given to this provision, but rather that an ordinary limitation should be made known.[14]

Such suggestions did not lead to the removal of this particular kind of assistance from the benefits available from the new Department but eligibility was progressively restricted in the following two years.[15]

It can be seen that in these cases structural impediments such as conscious under-funding were just as important as the health of the individual in determining access to benefits and the outcome of that benefit. There were other less tangible tests of eligibility. As noted previously, gifts of furniture were also perceived to be a problem. The New South Wales Council saw this form of assistance as representing a most unsatisfactory principle and one to be avoided at all cost:

> In fixing definite avenues of assistance …the danger of attracting application for assistance which may not have been lodged is very real. After granting an unfortunate man a few *most* necessary articles of furniture we have been submerged with an avalanche of requests claims and demands for household articles, some of which are wilfully extravagant and not at all suited to the means and situation of the applicant.

In Victoria, on the other hand, the Council was convinced that a gift of furniture 'gives great satisfaction'. The Victorian Council was more concerned with the 'large number of soldiers [who] look lightly on their obligations' and who sold property bought from Council loans. Horses and carts in particular were a problem and the assistance of the Police was required to recover them. Two cases were being prosecuted at the time of writing but the Council urged Millen that it was 'necessary that some definite action should be taken to prevent this abuse, and also as an example to protect those who may suffer'.

The New South Wales Council's final word was the need for the new Regulations to be elastic since, they argued, in the end each case had to be treated on its merits. This theme was echoed by the Australia Day Fund Ameliorative Committee, but the 'merits' involved in their deliberations differed from those discerned by the Councils. The Victorian Council administered its funds like a Church fund. There was liberality tempered by Christian morality which frowned on simple sins like stealing (furniture) or dishonesty (Council loans). The New South Wales Council had more utilitarian notions: was the soldier fit for work, experienced, qualified? In business-like fashion, they suggested there should be no universal principle for making the grant but rather an evaluation of the merit of the proposition and the suitability of the applicant. In the case of Victoria, a nineteenth century poor law mentality guaranteed the restriction of beneficiaries. In New South Wales, economic rationalism prevailed to deter if not disqualify applicants. The Ameliorative Committee, however, brought yet another interpretation of merit and eligibility to the notice of the Minister.

The activities encompassed by the Australia Day Fund were largely concerned with cash handouts: as supplements to War Pensions or military pay; as living allowances while soldiers awaited pension decisions, employment or during vocational re-training; for purchase of civilian clothes; or to help those suffering from recurrent illnesses. The organising principle of the Fund's allocations was bodily impairment: that is, whether soldiers returned fit or unfit. The unfit, who made up the majority of applicants since the establishment of the Fund, were further subdivided into those suffering some disability due to war service and those who were not, categories closely resembling the assessment criteria for War Pensions.[16] The Committee considered that for soldiers whose war-related impairment was both partial and temporary, the supplement paid 'should be on a scale somewhat lower than the ruling rate of wage, as it has been found that there is a reluctance amongst some of the men to obtain employment and this must be guarded against'.[17] When it was permanent, they believed there should be a stable pension, commenting that 'it would be manifestly unfair to reduce or cancel the pension of a man who by his own efforts has re-established himself in civil life'.

The 'class' of men suffering from disabilities not due to war service was again subdivided into 'Men who have seen service' and – here another definition of merit appears – 'Men who have given no practical service to their Country'. With regard to the former, the Committee warned that 'there is a great risk to the Treasury in granting a pension to a man who is invalided owing to a complaint from which he suffered prior to enlistment, as in most cases it is likely to be an increasing disability with the natural corollary of an increasing pension'. As far as the latter were concerned, bearing in mind the coercive practices used in recruiting campaigns and given the importance of the issues raised, the Committee's recommendations bear quoting in full:

> It is doubtful whether it is sufficiently realised at the present time the large number of men who come under this heading, more especially those who returned in the early days when a certain amount of impersonation was practised and many men were enlisted who should never have been sent away. Included in this category are men who were epileptics, mentally deficient, physically deformed, tubercular, etc. At the present time these men are receiving the same 'discharge' and treatment as men who have done long periods of service and who in many cases have lost an arm or a leg on active service. This is manifestly unjust and should be remedied ... It is thought by some that these men should not be eligible for the benefits of repatriation or for help from the patriotic funds. There appears however to be a responsibility on the government for having passed these men into the Army as fit and subsequently discharging them as unfit. It is suggested that this might be met by the granting of gratuities by way of compensation as is done by the Imperial Authorities.[18]

There are a number of important issues here for the early history of the Department. At the outset there is reference to the enlistment of those the Committee labelled as undeserving of assistance. But there is also recognition of state responsibility for accepting these individuals into the AIF. These contradictory impulses – judgement of moral undeservedness and a grudging sense of responsibility – were to re-emerge in many of the Department's later dealings and to provide cause for some heated exchanges between the Department and its critics, particularly in the case of soldiers labelled as 'senile' – that is over forty-five years of age at enlistment – who subsequently applied for benefits.

Next is the mention of amputees in the same context as the 'undeserving'. Amputees were a highly visible group of returned solders for propaganda purposes: the plight of the soldier who had lost a limb moved even the most cynical observers to compassion. In general it was always easier to identify this kind of 'wound' as compared with the invisible effects of gassing or Trench Fever, for example. This visibility was to assume increasing importance in subsequent years.

Last there is the issue of war gratuities. The gratuity was a 1917 replacement for booty: it was a meagre sum paid to soldiers to stave off dissent. In this instance the Committee's recommendation was to use such a payment to dispose of those soldiers who had become a state 'responsibility', by virtue of their service, but whose service was not perceived to be useful. The sordid history of Australian Gratuities is described in Chapter 6.

All of these matters were important to the small group of men recruited to form the operating instructions for the Department.[19] However, the Ameliorative Committee had more advice to offer, this time on administration. In their view, there were two 'essentials' required for the satisfactory carrying out of such assistance: 'a complete system of records, and medical examination'. The records, they advised, should consist of Military History sheets, Army Medical History sheets, Pension papers, Returns from the Voluntary Funds, assistance granted by the Repatriation Fund – including land settlement matters – and Police Reports, and all this should be kept in a central bureau. As far as the Committee was concerned, it was 'impossible to have too much information in regard to each case'. In addition, they thought each man could be issued with a card on which all assistance was recorded and which would need to be compulsorily produced in order to obtain any further assistance. The second 'essential', medical examination, meant not only the weeding out of those unfit for land settlement or employment generally but an opportunity to check the health of applicants and determine whether further treatment was required or an appeal for increase in War Pension was necessary. The Committee also suggested that periodical examinations would be found to be 'the greatest check in preventing discontent'.

Both these suggestions foreshadowed with remarkable prescience the Benthamite preoccupation with surveillance and intelligence-gathering which was to underpin the administration of the Department from the outset, and to grow in extent and importance from the time War Pensions became a Departmental responsibility. As to medical examinations, an issue which will be considered extensively in later chapters, it is instructive to note the place of medicine at this early date within the voluntary system.

In late August, the Secretary of the Disablement and Training Committee of the New South Wales Council wrote to Gilbert singing the praises of their 'expert gentlemen', their doctors. But the Secretary also issued a warning on the matter of having the decisions of such experts reviewed by laymen, bearing in mind 'cures which border on the marvellous'. The Secretary continued:

> It would be worth your serious consideration and deep thought when you are fixing up the State Boards to take care that nothing interferes with this splendid work. That is to say, do not put them in the position of having their decisions reviewed by

anybody except the Minister and his Council. I mention this so that no irritation of any sort can come in. Professional men are very touchy on these matters.[20]

Certainly the review of professional opinion by a non-expert could have been viewed as a challenge to the doctors' competence. But a perusal of the Minutes of the Disablement and Training Committee in this period suggests another reason for touchiness about review. At each meeting, the Committee, which consisted of four doctors and three other 'experts', recommended further medical treatment – often private treatment – for a small number of soldiers by one of their own number or, less frequently, by another specialist.[21] Whilst it could be argued that such a professional referral system was in the best interests of the former soldier, it is also possible to see a lucrative and continuing source of business which could only be defended on professional grounds, that is, by an expert closing-of-ranks against the inquiries of a 'layman'. The delicate matter of control over medical work foreshadowed here was to be a formidable problem for the Departmental bureaucracy over the next decade. The principles involved continue to fester in the relationship between the profession and the state. However, at the end of 1917, the role of doctors within the new Department was unclear and of little importance when other staffing matters were considered.

Suitable men

While the scope of repatriation activities was being formulated by the Comptroller and the Minister, the bureaucrat's invisible hand was also manipulating the assessment and selection of staff. Just how much 'his Minister' knew is unclear, but Lockyer's career and experience must have been known to Millen, along with his (Lockyer's) public service contacts and power, before his appointment. As noted earlier, Millen was quite specific in giving Lockyer authority in this sphere. It is also clear that the Minister and the Comptroller did not always agree.

Prior to February the record of staff and the activities of Lockyer's new domain is scant since there was no official administrative entity at this date. Indeed Gilbert wrote to Lockyer in March that even then he was not a formal 'Officer' of the Department.[22] However, by September or October of 1917, a small staff was assembled at Repatriation Headquarters in Melbourne. In early October Major Lean and Lewis East, as part of that staff, were sent by Lockyer to investigate the staff of the Victorian Council then headed by Donald Mackinnon, who was appointed Commonwealth Director General of Recruiting at the end of November.[23] This proved to be an inauspicious beginning to the investigative process. East discovered that one of the temporary clerks was not a returned soldier and, worse, although of military age he had not volunteered. East reported to Lockyer that

> I took the opportunity to mention to him, in his own interests, that it was the policy of the Minister to staff the new Department, as far as possible, with returned sol-

diers, adding that I was mentioning the matter so that he might keep his eyes open for some suitable job, in order that if he were replaced by a returned man, he might not be left without employment.[24]

The following day the Council Secretary, D. Barry, called Lean and East into his office and complained that 'the whole of the men ... were beginning to feel as if a sword was being held over (*sic*) their heads'. Further, he found it inadvisable to employ returned soldiers in 'certain branches of the work':

> to employ any but men of known and undoubted integrity in the branches dealing with more particularly, records and financial assistance, was fraught with possibilities of fraud, which in the interests of the public purse it would be very unwise to risk.[25]

Lockyer wasted no time in asserting his authority. The next day he saw Barry and informed him that as there were reliable and competent returned soldiers available they would certainly be employed in the Department. The new procedure would be that pending transfer of the Councils to the Department, any returned soldier it was proposed to place in the Melbourne Office would be referred to Barry for 'an expression of opinion as to whether he is in a position to offer any objection to his employment'.[26] By about the same date Lockyer had a full list of all staff of all State War Councils and their salaries.[27]

The next period of intense activity began in mid February by which time there was a staff at Repatriation Headquarters of around thirty.[28] It is clear from the files that there was Ministerial pressure to finalise staffing and administrative arrangements generally at this time prior to the proposed proclamation of the Act in March or April. The first sign of concern by the bureaucrats is a suggested timetable drawn up by Gilbert and submitted to Lockyer on 19 February outlining a proposed itinerary for matters ranging from the printing of Account Books to Publicity over the following six weeks but also including visits by himself, Major Ryan and Lieutenant Colonel Farr – both of the latter being on the staff of Headquarters – to all states. On these visits it was intended to make appointments to the honorary State Boards (with Ministerial approval), to make staff changes or additions, to organise the Local Committees, to arrange premises, to negotiate with the State authorities over the pending transfer of responsibility and, Gilbert suggested, to arrange for the Voluntary Funds to pay sustenance under Departmental orders until the Department could take over.[29] Lockyer demurred on the role of the Voluntary Funds, commenting that he did not approve 'delegating our work to the ameliorative authorities', but in other respects agreed with Gilbert and forwarded the proposal to Millen for approval the following week.[30]

On 1 March, Gilbert arrived in Sydney on the first leg of his tour. Lockyer wrote to him that things in Melbourne were moving very slowly, it was indeed 'a heavy machine to move'.[31] One of the biggest problems facing both men was finding 'suitable' returned soldiers to fill the new positions of Deputy Comptroller in each state. In the short term, the Headquarters staff were being despatched to fill these roles or train others. Lockyer informed Gilbert that

> Mr Farr will start for Tasmania in a few days, and Major Ryan for South Australia. I have sent for Colonel Tilney ... and with the Minister's approval, will offer him Western Australia. The Premier of that State ... recommended him. I think he is very suitable'.[32]

It is also clear from Lockyer's letter that Gilbert would be taking over the job of Comptroller once the Department started operating. Gilbert's task was twofold: he needed to find suitable returned soldiers who could fill the chief staff positions but also had to finalise appointments to the new voluntary State Boards. With regard to the latter, during February lists were drawn up of possible appointments in the various states. Millen was clearly involved in this process but there may have been input from Lockyer as well. The lists were then circulated to interested parties. For example, the list of potential Brisbane appointments was sent to Groom, Assistant Minister for Defence and a Liberal colleague of Millen's, Senator Foll, a National, a returned soldier and former staff member of the Queensland Commissioner for Railways, and Thomas Givens, a National, President of the Senate and ex-member of the Queensland Labor Party. The lists were accompanied by a form letter from Millen requesting an opinion on eligibility and providing the option to add other names where preferred.[33] Givens replied that he was satisfied with the list but re-ordered the names and suggested two more. Foll replied in detail in a personal letter to Millen agreeing to Givens's number one and two but then re-ordering the rest. Gilbert, in the meantime, telegrammed Lockyer that he needed a list 'numbered by the Minister' to be posted to him care of the Council in Brisbane. This was done, with the final list reflecting Givens's order of names but with three new names added, making a total of fifteen.

Gilbert eventually proceeded to Brisbane from Sydney and late in March was sent an urgent telegram by Millen wanting the full christian names of the new Board for Gazettal on 4 April. Writing to Lockyer on this subject he reported that he hoped to be able to send the names shortly: 'two of the men I wanted to see are in Sydney, Macdonald, and Marchant. As to Macdonald the Minister seems to favour him but no one else does. I shall endeavour to suggest an alternative'.[34] Gilbert then cabled Millen that he did not recommend 'number three' on the list (Macdonald) but provided the requisite information on the others: 'William Mandeville L'Estrange, George Marchant, Dr William Nathaniel Robertson, Frederick Harris, Bootmakers Union, William McIntyre, Manager Commercial Bank, Captain Lance Allan Jones, Pubic Accountant, identified country interests, [and] Private James Hugh Gaffney'.[35] He then cabled Millen recommending L'Estrange as Chairman. All Gilbert's recommendations were accepted by Millen, were offered places on the Board, and accepted the positions.

While this clandestine process worked itself out, the Brisbane Secretary of the Returned Sailor's and Soldiers' Imperial League of Australia (RSSILA) wrote to Millen in mid March suggesting two names for the new Brisbane Board. On 2 April Lockyer wrote back to the Secretary, acknowledging receipt of his letter and apologising for the delay in reply. Simultaneously he assured the Secretary that 'Senator Millen … has had your letter before him in considering the personnel of the proposed Board'.[36] The literalness of this response together with the fact that only one of those recommended by the RSSILA appeared at all on Millen's final list (at number 11 position) and neither were selected for the final seven positions, gives some indication of the impotence of the formal returned soldier organisations at this date. There is very little evidence that such organisations had any appreciable impact on the practices of the Department throughout the period under study.

The situation in New South Wales was slightly different. Sometime prior to March, Millen approached the Chair of the New South Wales Council, W.T. Willington, for advice on suitable 'prominent citizens' to serve on the new Board. Willington approached two such men with an invitation to serve on the Board. However, by the time Gilbert arrived in Sydney the Minister's list for this Board had clearly been revised and these two were not included.[37] Always the consummate diplomat, Gilbert suggested a letter of apology to these men which was immediately forthcoming. Millen wrote to one of the offended men that

> by some mischance, probably due to my not having made myself sufficiently clear, Mr. Willington interpreted my request as authorising him to make a distinct offer. At the same time I was myself making similar enquiries and later on definitely made an offer to several citizens who signified to me their acceptance.[38]

As it transpired, the five men on Millen's list were deemed acceptable by Gilbert and accepted their positions on the Board. However, the two returned soldier positions – a quota which seems to have become unofficially accepted in this period – were not at all clear. Gilbert wrote to Lockyer that he was searching for an 'officer of a right type' but with limited success. Nevertheless, he had found a suitable 'Other Rank' in ex-private Joseph Eade. In Gilbert's view, Eade embodied the ideal returned soldier. He was a model by which others could and would be judged. For these reasons his description of Eade bears quoting in full.

> Eade, who has lost an arm, was one of the first men to return. A coal miner before enlistment and only very crudely educated, he applied himself on return to the improvement of his general education and also to acquiring some knowledge of accounts and the general routine of an office. He succeeded sufficiently well to obtain a position as a clerk in the Assets Department at the Town Hall. This suggests that he is a man of grit, and my [word omitted] concerning him personally are very satisfactory. I discussed him with Brigadier-General Jobson and also with Mr. Potter – Secretary, Returned Soldiers' Association – who is himself a very responsible type of man … I think his will be a good appointment.[39]

The image of the one-armed or amputee soldier is an enduring symbol of patriotic sacrifice, and one with international currency. In the work of George Grosz it was used in searing attacks on war-profiteers. It was also freely used in the propaganda of repatriating authorities.[40] In Australia, moving pictures of running or jumping *rehabilitated* one-legged or legless men, stirred feelings of guilt, compassion and – not least – patriotism in their audience, emotions clearly calculated to enhance recruiting. They also advertised the Department. Scenes of rehabilitation using artificial limbs and vocational re-training – a powerful duo of body and mind – were used to symbolise the work of the Department.[41]

There were 2200 amputees in the returned AIF by the end of 1919, that is, less than 1.3% of those injured or otherwise damaged by war.[42] While the problems of adapting to loss of a limb were immense and while the provision of an artificial limb – that sometimes worked – was undoubtedly of great assistance, the success of such treatment could be measured and photographed. Other treatments were not successful at all and many disabilities were invisible.

The second aspect of Eade mentioned by Gilbert is that he was a coal miner prior to enlistment with only elementary education. On his return he had 'applied' himself, 'improved' himself and acquired knowledge. This made him, according to Gilbert's view, succeed 'sufficiently well' to be employable; it also made him personally 'satisfactory'. Such a man of 'grit', succeeding against the odds, trading his miner's uniform for a respectable white-collar job, epitomised the kind of individualism that saturated the workings of the Department. This model of successful self-help, with all its fallacies, was repeatedly trotted out as a rationale for denying assistance. In the 1920s, as unemployment rose along with the cost of living and the standard of living fell for most Australian workers, and as chronic low grade war-related injuries and illnesses took their toll, such success stories were rare. Yet this icon remained, towering over the supplicants of the Department.

The final characteristic singled out by Gilbert is that Eade had the approval of the RSSILA. It has been mentioned previously that the League possessed little if any power at this date, an impotence well documented by Kristianson and evident in correspondence between the League and the Commonwealth government.[43] Gilbert's reference to their approval of Eade appears to contradict this. The explanation is twofold. In late 1917 it is clear that Millen wanted to put a stop to press notices emanating from the League that were critical of the government's policy towards returned soldiers. To this end he was prepared to 'talk' to the League about their concerns and offered them unspecified financial assistance.[44] It is possible this assistance was no more than permission to travel on trains with returning invalids to secure members.[45] Secondly, the League in this period was one of a number of competing soldier organisations of varying political persuasion. The League itself was conservative and its leaders were drawn from the same class of businessmen that Millen, Lockyer and Gilbert were combing for membership of the State Boards. (This probably explains Gilbert's remark about the Secretary of the New South Wales Branch being 'a very responsible type of man'.) It seems likely then that

Lockyer and Gilbert recognised the usefulness of the League in finding suitable men for Returned Soldier positions on the Boards and at the same time this de facto recognition invited co-operation rather than criticism. Later in 1918, in a rare if insignificant victory, a member of the New South Wales Board was pressured by Millen to resign after insulting a League deputation by referring to the 'verminous' state of soldiers applying to the Department.[46]

In the case of Eade, however, recognition of the League was purely expedient, a means of finding suitable returned soldiers. On 15 March, in a confidential letter, Gilbert wrote to Lockyer suggesting that Millen should advise Eade that accepting a position on the State Board debarred him from holding any office in any soldier organisation. Four days later an official letter was forwarded to Gilbert instructing him to 'kindly ascertain confidentially and discreetly whether [Eade] is content to sever himself from any official position in the Returned Soldiers' League'. Lockyer continued:

> Please explain to him that the reason for this is, not from any lack of sympathy with the League, but to the fact that dual positions may lead to difficulty if, in the impartial performance of his responsibilities, he is subject to a divided allegiance.[47]

Eade apparently relinquished the position with the League.[48] The officer position was filled by Major J.M. Maughan who Gilbert described as a 'solicitor of good standing', adding that there was 'an advantage in having a legal man on the Board'. Maughan, for his part, reassured Gilbert that he knew the returning AIF required very delicate handling.[49]

As for the other members of the Board, the power of the bureaucrats in the selection process is revealed in another confidential letter from Gilbert to Lockyer on 13 March where he confided to Lockyer that in his *official* letter of the same date he had sent the names of the proposed Board members in New South Wales. He continued:

> I hope the Minister will consider this list as final and that you will proceed to the appointment forthwith. If he wants to suggest any further alterations the probability is that they will all back out.

The suggested composition of the Melbourne Board also worried Gilbert.

> I am personally concerned also about his [Millen's] attitude towards the men whom I suggested in Melbourne ... When the Minister was in Sydney he said that some doubt had been raised with regard to Haynes, and suggested that he was too pernickety. Haynes is a man who is successfully running one of the biggest manufacturing concerns in the Commonwealth and I do not think that he is at all too pernickety ... Apart from this ... I would feel rather embarrassed if other names are now to be chosen.[50]

In both cases Gilbert's proposed members were offered and subsequently accepted the positions. Further evidence of the secret nature of this appointment process and of the control over the scheme exercised by the key bureaucrats is revealed in a letter to Lockyer written in March 1918. After going through some obsequious formalities, the newly appointed Chairman of the New South Wales Board, Willington, wrote that neither he nor the Deputy Chairman, Parkes, had 'any definite knowledge of the Minister's proposed scheme for Repatriation, or its regulations, neither have we any idea [or] knowledge of the composition of the new Staff ... or the conditions under which they are to carry out that portion of the work. No information has been conveyed to Mr. Parkes or myself, as to the proposed scheme'.[51]

One last aspect of the personnel of the State Boards warrants mention. It was noted in Chapter 2 that the composition of the Executive of the ASR Fund Board of Trustees included a conservative unionist, Edward Grayndler, whose participation at meetings of the Executive was minimal. Grayndler posed no threat to the ideological hegemony of the Fund's Executive, an Executive composed of ruling elites. In 1918, union representation on the State Boards appears to have been equally innocuous. Some unionists on the Boards were from craft unions – for example the Secretary of the Plasterers' Union in Victoria and the Secretary of the Boot Trades' Union in Queensland. Some were office holders like A. Vernon, Secretary of the General Labourers' Union in New South Wales, a union then in the process of amalgamating with Grayndler's AWU. In Tasmania there was no unionist on the Board.[52] Not surprisingly, none appear to have been significant in the history of the union movement or affiliated with any of the radical or socialist unions or movements of the period. In any case the Boards they joined were advisory only: they had no power in policy formulation within the Department, and membership thus had no significance other than a titular honour. The question must then be raised, what function did these Boards serve? Why were Gilbert, Lockyer and Millen so preoccupied with the selection of suitable men who had to be drawn from commerce, industry, unions and even returned soldier organisations?

The appointment of these Boards represents the tail-end of voluntarism in the treatment of returned soldiers – a view also held by Pryor.[53] As noted earlier, the fact that the Boards existed at all appears to have been nothing more than a political concession to the powerful business elites that sought control of the scheme. It was also politically necessary to ensure they appeared representative of the society from which they were drawn.[54] This had at least two purposes: to pre-empt any criticism that might adversely affect recruiting, and to assuage critics, like the Executive of the Fund, who objected to outright state control. The existence of the Boards, however, meant that there was genuine participation by those groups represented. This provides a clue as to why the selection process was so important. As Lockyer wrote to the Deputy Comptrollers in April, 'the primary function of the Board is to determine applications for various forms of assistance.[55] While the Regulations prescribed what kind of assistance could be offered and the scope of assistance, the Board could still decide on eligibility or otherwise under the Regulations. They had discretionary power over decisions such as whether or not to grant £25 to a soldier to purchase furniture; over whether a loan of £60 might be made to purchase four cows; or whether £100 could be loaned to purchase stock for a confectionery business.[56] That is to say, the Boards' decisions, within the Regulations, controlled the flow of funds.

Clearly, with men like Eade on the Boards there was a pervasive attitude that the Department would, first and foremost, help those who helped themselves. The assessment of the moral worthiness of applicants could not be regulated officially but certainly could and did form part of the decision-making process of the Boards: by placing suitable men on these Boards, Gilbert and Lockyer ensured there was no wastage of public money on malingerers, ne'er-do-wells or those lacking business sense. By carefully selecting the prospective members, there was a far greater likelihood that the rationalist conservatism of the triumvirate was mirrored in the activities of the Boards.

However, the voluntary Boards were not the most important part of the new Department. More important to the controllers and to the continuing operation of the scheme was the staff.

The Repatriation staff

Gilbert's lengthy confidential correspondence with Lockyer during his tour in March, while seriously concerned with the Boards, spends far more time on finding suitable men for the permanent staff – a process Lockyer aptly described as fishing in a well.[57] As the weeks passed and it became clear that the Act and its Regulations would be proclaimed in early April, Gilbert and Lockyer became increasingly nervous about the selection process. On 11 March Lockyer wrote 'our difficulties are great and we will certainly find unanticipated hindrances and obstructions by the dozen'.

> We simply have to overcome them as well as we can. I am unable to say when we will take over. That depends upon the Government decision, and also when our Regulation, General Orders, and Books of Account, forms, etc., are ready'.[58]

Each state had its problems. Western Australia was considered especially worrying in view of its 'distance from Head Quarters' and the 'extremely critical and touchy' nature of the state organisation.[59] Both bureaucrats bemoaned the shortage of experienced and suitable men and the lack of time to find them. In the end Lockyer was forced to use his Headquarters' staff as Deputy Comptrollers in some states, despite the reservations of Millen. This was particularly so in the case of New South Wales where Lieutenant Colonel Farr was earmarked for the job by Lockyer in February but was then sent to Tasmania to train the incoming and inexperienced Deputy Comptroller.[60] In early March Lockyer informed Gilbert that Millen was suffering a 'touch of nerves' over Farr because of Farr's quiet manner. Millen, he suggested, thought Farr did not possess the 'necessary capacity'.[61] Farr was to have a brief and troubled career as Deputy Comptroller in Sydney. In 1923 he was transferred to Perth after allegations regarding an 'indiscretion by an officer under his control' – an action he maintained was an injustice. On 10 September he disappeared and three weeks later his position was declared vacant. In 1937, having lived for fourteen years under an assumed name in South Africa, he committed suicide. Correspondence between Farr and Headquarters during his period as Deputy Comptroller (1918-1923) suggests a personal and seemingly unfounded animosity on the part of Millen combined with a vitriolic campaign by *Smith's Weekly* against the Sydney branch were key factors in Farr's ultimate demise.[62]

Yet Farr was an exception. Many of the new members of staff selected by Gilbert were of a different character. The Chief Clerk appointed in Sydney was Captain Bell – the 'most promising man' Gilbert could find and 'a good disciplinarian'. Major Shillington, suggested as the officer in charge of the Local Committee Section, was 'a man of strong personality, who, for a number of years was a Treasury official. He subsequently qualified for a Police Magistrate'.[63] Farr's career path was also exceptionally brief when compared with other appointees in this period. J.C. McPhee, for example, a Senior Colonel Chaplain on Gallipoli, had returned to Australia in 1917 and was appointed as a Special Magistrate of the War Pensions Branch of Treasury. In January of 1918, he was apparently head-hunted by Lockyer and in April was appointed Secretary to the new Commission. In 1926 he was appointed Deputy Commissioner of Victoria and he remained there until his retirement in 1940, having received his OBE the previous year.[64] R.W. Carswell was one of the staff recruited in March 1918 to work in Vocational Training. He then became Officer in Charge of the Medical and General Section and in 1923 Chief Clerk of the New South Wales Branch. In 1939 he was made Deputy Commissioner of that state. Similarly, F.H. Rowe was a member of the State War Council of Victoria who was recruited in March 1918 to become Officer in Charge of Assistance. In 1920 he became Chief Clerk of the Brisbane Branch and in 1922 Deputy Commissioner of that Branch. In 1933 he transferred to Headquarters as Senior Pensions Officer and in 1935 was appointed a Repatriation Commissioner.[65]

These are not isolated cases. However, the sheer size of the Departmental staff and the destruction of most detailed staff records obscures the careers of all but the most senior bureaucrats. Yet the names of significant figures keep re-appearing over the years: Ovington, Keays, Barrett, Chidgey and many others, evidence that suitable men were indeed found.

One last group of appointees must be mentioned. On 17 January 1918, at a meeting of the Executive of the ASR Fund Board of Trustees, the Chairman congratulated Langdon Bonython on his appointment to the new Repatriation Commission. Bonython, in reply, told his colleagues that he had assumed that Williams and Baillieu had been invited to join as well.[66] Such was not the case. As mentioned previously, only Bonython and Grayndler survived the old Executive. In addition to these two men, the new honorary Commission which commenced work in April, chaired by the Minister, consisted of Robert Gibson, H.P. Moorehead, Lt Col R.H. Owen and John Sanderson.

Scottish Presbyterian Robert (later Sir Robert) Gibson, is described by C.B. Shedvin as a man whose 'economic philosophy placed a high valuation on thrift, saving, giving to those in genuine need, and steady improvement in material conditions' and as a critic of waste and inefficiency in the public service. His career in the Victorian Chamber of Manufacturers, as Victorian representative on the Central Coal Board, as chairman of the Royal Commission on Public Expenditure and other civic appointments culminated in his election as Chairman of the Commonwealth Bank in 1926, a position he held until his death in 1934. Gibson's brother John had formed the Monier Pipe Construction Company with John Monash prior to the War and Gibson himself 'worked harmoniously' with Monash on the Victorian State Electricity Commission.[67] This connection with Monash helps to shed light on a subsequent change to the personnel of the Commission, discussed in Chapter 6.

Harold Moorehead was a journalist with the Argus prior to service in the AIF where he lost an arm and a leg at Gallipoli. After his return to Australia he became active in state run veteran organisations including the Canteen Trust and the McCaughey Trust.[68]

Lt Col Robert Haylock Owen was a career officer. He had served as a lieutenant in the New South Wales Sudan Contingent and subsequently was commissioned in the British Regular Army. In 1914, although aged 52 and retired, he was persuaded to command the 3rd Battalion. Wounded at Gallipoli in June he was invalided home and discharged in May 1916.[69]

John Sanderson, like the Baillieus, represented the inner circle of financial and mercantile elites in Melbourne. He was connected to the Baillieus through membership of the Board of the Mount Morgan Gold Mining Company and through association with Broken Hill mining. A member of the Round Table and the Melbourne Club, he later became a close friend of S.M. Bruce.[70]

Perhaps the most important characteristic of this Commission is the unremarkable nature of its members – and the dropping of Baillieu and Williams from its ranks. It comprised a senior Army officer, an amputee veteran of Gallipoli, a member of the Melbourne ruling class and an austere Scottish businessman and financier in addition to the former Board members. Pryor speculated that the new appointees 'were probably acceptable to Senator Millen because they would raise little opposition to him'.[71] After the altercation between Millen, Williams and Baillieu upon Millen taking control, this seems a plausible explanation. The Commission served only two years until the Act was repealed and a paid Commission of three was appointed. None of these original Commissioners survived the re-organisation.

In summing up this complex, largely hidden activity involved in establishing a new federal Department, a number of points must be made. Overall, the evidence is unequivocal on the seminal role of the senior bureaucrats, with or without the Minister's involvement, in the establishment of the Department. It is also clear that in that setting-up process a particular ideology was fostered in both the staff and the honorary Boards. Analysis of the process and its outcome allows two possible but irreconcilable interpretations.

The first interpretation would see the primary responsibility of the Department as custody of public money, just as Treasury officials took custody of War Pensions. The public would be grateful for money being well spent in a 'generous' scheme while the bureaucracy protected its purse. Within this interpretation there could be dissent – notably from those business elites who saw Ministerial veto and centralised government control as allowing too much power to the state. While this question of state intervention and control was indeed important, in reality the dispute between the Executive of the Board of Trustees and the Minister was rather like an argument over who should drive the train, not its direction.

The second interpretation would see the direction the Department took as one of 'cold-hearted' rationalism designed to forever maintain the veteran in the role of supplicant. Such an interpretation would see the returned soldier as politically impotent at this date, despite a service to the state that often resulted in bodily or mental damage. Both interpretations can be applied to the modifications to the Regulations and to the practices of the Department that took place in the crucial two years that followed the proclamation of the Act in 1918. Both interpretations continue to be voiced in open warfare between veteran organisations and the Department.

However, there was one other group of staff vital to Departmental functioning after the war – doctors. To understand their ambiguous yet powerful position within the Department requires some understanding of the place of medicine and the medical profession within Australia at that time. This is explored in the following chapter.

CHAPTER 5

Doctors and Soldiers: New Chapters in the History of Medicine

Medicine and medical knowledge had an unambiguous importance for the Australian state during the Great War: doctors, in principle, maintained the army as a fighting force through both curative and preventive medicine. In previous wars the embryonic AAMC had been a shadowy, disorganised presence, its principal contribution to warfare being the surgical skills of its members. This clear change in role and stature during a period of less than twenty years demands explanation. In broad terms, the answer lies in the social transformations of the late nineteenth century and early twentieth century, particularly in the 'new' liberalism and the ideology of expertise which saw an increased awareness of public health and preventive medicine. This chapter examines some of the issues involved in terms of the Australian experience during the period under study. It refers particularly to the relationship between medical professionalisation and the crisis of war, and to the doctor/soldier relationship.

The professionalisation of medicine

From the late 1960s until relatively recently, the professionalisation process has been fecund ground for both historical and sociological research.[1] Informed by diverse theoretical perspectives, scholars in the field have nevertheless tended towards consensus in identifying the chief characteristics of professionals. These are: individualism; collegial control; an ideal of social service; and the possession of an esoteric body of knowledge. In the early twentieth century, liberal principles of individualism and social reform by limited state intervention were implicit in the professionalisation process and particularly evident in the professionalisation of medicine.

In *The Rise of Professionalism*, Larson suggests three 'residual' or pre-capitalist components of professionalism: the intrinsic value of work as craft; the ideal of universal service; and, a modern version of *noblesse oblige* – rank imposing duties as well as confirming rights.[2] The absorption of these characteristics into the modem ideology of professions has occurred unevenly and in different historical settings. However, while research into this particular aspect of the professionalisation process is ongoing, it is reasonably clear that in most Western countries the ability of the medical profession to retain its ideal of service has been a direct result of state appropriation of health and welfare functions.

In her study of 'moral contagion' in France, Jan Goldstein has shown how the repeated plague epidemics in the sixteenth and seventeenth centuries, and the public health measures they spawned, 'signified the high-water mark of medical authority and moment of total collaboration between the constituted political authorities and the doctors'.[3] By the early nineteenth century, the term 'political medicine' was in general usage in France. This term described the alliance between the state and the profession both in matters of public health intervention and in courts of law.[4] In Britain, this collaboration between the two oldest respectable professions and the modern state has been examined by Roger Smith in relation to notions of responsibility and insanity and in relation to responses in Britain and France to the insanity defence. On the French response he notes 'the striking willingness of both political society and the legal profession in France to turn to medical conceptualizations of social problems at the end of the [nineteenth] century'. However, while there was a parallel response in Britain, 'medicine commanded less authority both as a worldview and as a decision-making institution in relation to social danger'.[5]

Also of importance in Goldstein's study, however, is the adaptivity of the medical profession to the changing nature of the state itself. A successful alliance was formed in an absolutist regime, maintained through the revolutionary period, and survives to the present. This phenomenon is not limited to France nor is it restricted to the medical profession. Indeed, contemporary studies tend to assume such an integral relationship, whatever the nature of the state, and focus more on specificities in particular historical circumstances.[6]

Yet there are certain modern phenomena which seem to be common to certain countries at different times and to have provided an impetus to the professionalisation process. First, there is the change in perceptions of the population from a collection of individuals to a collective body which could be measured, analysed and managed. Demographics, morbidity and mortality levels, population growth and decline, education and training, and marriage and procreation all became factors for economic management. Second, there is the changing perception of children/childhood and the 'medical acculturation' of the family. Children were no longer simply a product of a marital union, but objects of highly scrutinised management. The locus of attention was in the relationship between parents and child: the family became the provider of the clean, healthy fit bodies, and the cleansed domestic space. The work of the early twentieth-century Australian eugenicists and maternal welfare experts embodied these notions. Finally, there is the politicisation of the health of the body politic; that is, the emergence of programs of hygiene which, by their nature, entailed medical interventions and controls. The ability to dictate the desirable nature of urban spaces, housing, and even personal habits empowered the doctor as a social or political reformer – the progenitor of the modern public health specialist.[7]

These pre-conditions for professional progress necessitated the collaboration of the state for their implementation and it is that collaboration which forms the substance of this Chapter. Although late in coming to Australian society and political culture, compared with their European origins, it will be argued in the following section that these pre-conditions for rapid professionalisation were in place by the outbreak of World War One. War then provided a political, economic, social and health crisis of a scale hitherto unexperienced in the Commonwealth and that crisis, by its nature, served to rapidly accelerate the professionalisation process.

The rise and rise of professional medicine in Australia

The measurement and management of the Australian population commenced with settlement. Musters, censuses, inquiries, registrations of births, deaths and marriages and other statistics-seeking surveys have been increasingly pored over by bureaucrats, politicians and erstwhile social reformers for two centuries. What concerns us here is the shift in emphasis in the data collected in the last decades of the nineteenth century and the first decades of this century. Kerreen Reiger, Desley Deacon and others have established the growing preoccupation with the health and welfare of children and the family in this period, with women, portrayed as producers and nurturers, becoming central to the concerns of reforming social managers.[8]

Simultaneously, 'hygiene', a concept which addressed intimate behaviour, private spaces, individual actions and responsibilities, replaced 'sanitation', an idea linked to environmental reforms, public services and state responsibility. Unlike the French experience of epidemics, effective 'sanitation' at the turn of the century in Australia, when bubonic plague affected nearly all states, was not so much a province of medical expertise as one for Sanitary Inspectors and engineers.[9] 'Hygiene', on the other hand, called upon the principles of scientific medicine, on germ theory as opposed to miasmas, as much as it relied on theories of racial decline.[10]

The Twin Towers published in 1918, a collection of some of the voluminous writings of Dr James Barrett, influential member of the University of Melbourne Council, advocate of 'national efficiency' and of the professions generally, provides a useful summary of the ideas which permeated intellectual and political debate in the period. The role of universities, education, medicine, venereal disease, milk, neglected children, town planning, playgrounds and Empire serve as organising concepts in the work but also as indicators of the evolution of new ways of thinking. In his Presidential Address to the Medical Society of Victoria in 1901, Barrett linked many of these concerns when he commented that

> the propagation of the Anglo-Saxon race has been placed largely under voluntary control, owing to the education of its women. The extent to which this control is resorted to may determine the fate of the Empire; in other words, it is the character of the race which is on its trial.
>
> To what extent then are we, as medical men, concerned in this business? It seems to me that we are concerned to a profound extent. If for no other reason, because we enjoy that confidence of members of the family which no one else can enjoy; because we are consulted on matters which are never heard of by anyone else.[11]

Some military doctors shared Barrett's eugenicist view, particularly in relation to the settlement of the Australian 'frontier': the Northern Territory. In 1920, Colonel Eames, the Principal Medical Officer of 2nd Military District (MD) wrote to the Commandant of 2nd MD that

> At the late Medical Congress held in Brisbane last August, it was shown that there were no Medical reasons why a white race should not successfully populate the Northern Territory. As the necessity for populating the Territory with a virile race is very largely a Defence question, the Medical Services become directly concerned.[12]

Eames' former boss, the Director of Medical Services of the AAMC in Europe, Neville Howse, had a slightly different slant on the problem: sterilised black labour.[13]

Whilst these ideas were being articulated by the educated few in the early 1900s, by the 1920s they were being widely implemented by a variety of new organisations from Baby Health Clinics to the Commonwealth Department of Public Health. Arguably, it was in the same period that medicine in Australia gained full professional status. Key developments prior to the outbreak of war were collegial control from 1912 through a federated professional organization – the British Medical Association (BMA); a National Code of Ethics, promulgated in 1912, which effectively internalised intra-professional disputes thereby reducing the risk of adverse publicity; a national journal, the *Medical Journal of Australia*, which commenced circulation in 1914; and state collaboration.[14] The last development, which is crucial to an understanding of the rise of medicine, is extremely complex.

While the pre-conditions for professionalisation, outlined above, were in place by the outbreak of war, it is clear that the process started to accelerate from about 1908. Various explanations have been put forward to explain this latter phenomenon. Pensabene's pioneering work, *The Rise of the Medical Practitioner in Victoria*, argues that the changing nature of medical knowledge, that is its scientism, described as a series of 'advances', 'breakthroughs' and 'new heights in research', resulted in a favourably altered public perception of the profession.[15] A coincidental lowering of mortality rates, but one unrelated to any 'progress' in medical ideas, is viewed as a second contributing factor.

Arguing that Pensabene's narrative is deterministic, Willis's *Medical Dominance* is implicitly concerned with a sociological explanation of the professionalisation of medicine in Australia.[16] Willis argues for an understanding of the medical dominance of the health division of labour in Australia on the basis of medicine's 'autonomy', 'authority' and 'sovereignty', analytical concepts similar to those widely used in analyses of the professionalisation process elsewhere. He goes on to argue that medicine's position of dominance within the health arena in Australia was achieved by 1908 and consolidated by 1933.[17] Since the medical profession and medicine's authority are critical to the study of the role of doctors in both the AAMC and the Repatriation system, these issues need close examination.

The social history of medicine in Australia has only recently received serious attention from historians.[18] Willis's work reflects this, for although his sociological analysis is wide-ranging, the history is at times misleading and tendentious. This is particularly true in his analysis of state legitimation of medicine. Whig medical history has frequently portrayed the emergence of licensing laws for medical practitioners as evidence of the inexorable progress of medicine during the nineteenth century.[19] Willis's preoccupation with such legislation leads him to explain the rapid rise to power of medicine in the early twentieth century in Australia in terms of the passage of statutes governing the profession. In his pursuit of evidence to support his hypothesis, Willis traces the profession's demands, by way of the Victorian Medical Board, for legislation which would guarantee a number of key regulatory powers: a minimum five years training for registration, an infamous conduct clause, a ban on unqualified practitioners and the right to undertake its own prosecutions.[20] In the 1908 Amending Act to the (Victorian) Medical Act, only the five year training clause was achieved. Other concessions were only minor, yet Willis sees this Act as pivotal.

According to Pensabene, the amending Act was the 'first major legislative success in over fifty years' for the profession. But he is also quick to point out that such legislation 'played a minor role in the rise of the medical practitioner in Victoria'.[21] For Willis, on the other hand, it was 'a major victory for scientific medicine, ensuring a position of dominance within the health arena':

> State patronage of medicine had been relatively perfunctory until 1908 ... [but] the legal framework established in 1908 provided the basis upon which the professionalisation of medicine could proceed and its dominance could be consolidated.[22]

There are a number of serious problems with this analysis. First, a minimum of five years training at a recognised University along with an infamous conduct clause and other significant regulatory powers had been legislated as early as 1900 in New South Wales.[23] Yet the medical profession did not immediately dominate the health sphere as a result. The second problem is Willis's repeated assertion that one piece of legislation created a position of dominance. Willis's vision of one magic moment in the history of the professionalisation process greatly oversimplifies a much longer and more complex historical relationship between the profession and the state.

Examination of legislation passed in both New South Wales and at Commonwealth level from around 1900 to the 1920s reveals a distinct rise in the number of statutes which constituted doctors as determining authorities in a variety of domains. For example, in the 1909 Act to amend the (NSW) Inebriates Act, 1900, a Supervising Board was established consisting of the Inspector General of the Insane, the Comptroller General of Prisons and the Chief Medical Officer of the Government. The functions of the Board included the power to recommend the transfer of 'inebriates' from one state institution to another and to inquire into the administration of any institution or the condition of its inmates. This latter enquiry function had previously been the sole prerogative of the Inspector

General of the Insane. In a somewhat different context, the 1910 (NSW) Workmen's Compensation Act, like the state and federal Invalid Pensions Acts, made doctors responsible for medical certification of potential beneficiaries as eligible or ineligible on the basis of their degree of disability, either mental or physical. The third problem with Willis's analysis is that at no stage does it explain why the state co-operated with doctors to pass the 1908 Victorian Act.

This Act was important but it was not decisive; it was part of a much longer trend. The liaison between medicine and the state in the early twentieth century in Australia was slow to develop and tentative, with each party endeavouring to ascertain the benefits of coupling. It was also characterised by state domination until well beyond the present period of study. Legislation on professional status was only part of this process. Practice was equally important.

For example, doctors were the designated authority in the Invalid Pension Acts. The health of the individual applying for an Invalid Pension was central to the application. There was a statutory requirement to establish permanent incapacity and the decision was reached by the Invalid Pension bureaucracy, that is by Treasury officials assessing the opinion of a Commonwealth Medical Referee (CMR).

Briefly, the regulations governing Invalid Pensions at the time the Act came into effect (1911) were that an individual had to be a resident of Australia with income or property not exceeding limits prescribed by the Old Age Pension Act and without any financial maintenance by relatives. To obtain the Invalid Pension a person had to prove 'permanent incapacity for any work'. The procedure, once established, entailed forwarding a claim to the local Registrar; an investigation by police – including assessment by the police officer of the applicant's health and his or her worthiness; other investigations necessary to determine the financial status of the applicant; certifications of permanent invalidity by two medical practitioners – one a CMR; and, finally, investigation of the claim and a recommendation on award or refusal of the pension by a Magistrate.[24]

The following cases provide indications of the way the system operated and reveal something of contemporary understandings of health.[25]

Case of David H, Glenferrie, Victoria. August 1911.

The CMR certified as follows:

[he] is suffering from chronic arthritis [and] frequent micturition. Has deformed hands, elbows, knees and feet, and walks with crutches. Facial appearance is that of a chronic alcoholic, and he admits to much wine and spirits etc.

The CMR also suggested the condition was within the applicant's control. The Special Magistrate suggested the condition might be self-induced.

The Acting Commissioner of Pensions approved a full Invalid Pension.[26]

Case of Margaret F, Buttlejork, Victoria. April 1912.

The applicant is described in the report as

a single woman 58 years of age [who] ekes out a precarious existence by hunting rabbits and disposing of them to the rabbit factory. From police report it would appear that claimant is mainly dependent on rabbits for her food.
The Police Report also noted the applicant's claim to severe rheumatism.

The CMR certified that

[she] is suffering from no particular disease or injury... The alleged invalidity is such as not to incapacitate her for work... She is in good enough health ... to catch a few rabbits.

The Commissioner approved a full Invalid Pension.[27]

Case of Michael P, Annie T, Mary K, John S, Melbourne. May 1912.

All suffered from Tuberculosis: two refused treatment; one was an inmate of an institution; one was prepared to be institutionalised. The report to the Commissioner requested clarification as to whether the Pension should be withheld from applicants suffering from an infectious disease if they were not prepared to undergo treatment.

The Commissioner approved unconditional full Invalid Pensions for all applicants.[28]

The case studies above represent Rulings by the Commissioner and Assistant Commissioner of Pensions during the years from 1911 to 1913. These early Rulings established precedents which were circulated to all States for the guidance of Pension adjudicators and administrators; that is, they became Pension policies. If one had to define health according to these and other rulings of the period then it would be broad indeed, taking account of factors such as poverty and destitution while respecting individual rights and freedoms: recalcitrance in the face of perceived public health risk was tolerated as much as was drunkenness. Interestingly, the opinions of the CMR and other doctors on somatic matters appear to have been of secondary importance.[29]

By the end of June 1913, there were just under 14 000 recipients (compared with around 83 000 recipients of the Old Age Pension).[30] In the ensuing years this number rose steadily. At the same time medical practitioners rapidly gained ground in terms of their professional status. In 1911 the instrumentality of doctors to the assessment and decision-making process in the Pensions bureaucracy as evidenced in the Invalid Pensions Rulings was clearly marginal.[31] By the end of World War One this had changed significantly. The reasons for that change are examined below. However, this was not the only social change occurring.

The following cases, referred to the Pensions Commissioner for determination, occur *after* 1913.

Case of Coral I, Geelong, Victoria. June 1917.

The claimant is described as 22 years old, suffering from pronounced syphilis, mental deficiency due to a kick in the head from a horse at age 7 and bedridden. The CMR considered she should be hospitalised.

The Assistant Commissioner rejected the claim on the grounds that she was considered 'not deserving' and recommended state charitable relief and action under the Venereal Diseases Act.[32]

Case of Richard C, Rookwood, New South Wales. June 1917.

The claimant is described as having been hospitalised for eight years for pulmonary tuberculosis.

The Assistant Commissioner refused the claim on the grounds that it was in the applicant's best interest to remain in an institution (the pension interpreted here as inducement to leave hospital).[33]

Case of Frederick H, Murrambeena, Victoria. October 1917.

The claimant, born in Germany but a resident of Australia since 1869 and naturalised August 1914, was granted an Invalid Pension in July 1917 on the grounds of permanent incapacity.

The Commonwealth Treasurer considered the pension should not have been granted because the claimant obtained his naturalisation after war had broken out. The Crown Solicitor ruled that the Minister or the Commissioner or a Deputy Commissioner had power to cancel the pension.

The pension was cancelled in October 1917.[34]

Clearly by 1917 there was a change in the direction of policy. Xenophobia in this period has been well documented and appears to account for the treatment meted out to Frederick H. Indeed there are numerous rulings similar to this throughout the war years. However, there are other more complex reasons for this change.

Procedures and practices, just like policies, are shaped by ways of thinking. They are imbued with attitudes and beliefs that emanate from the nature of social organisation at a particular time. In 1913, the Commissioner of Pensions was also the Secretary of Treasury and the incumbent at that date was George Allen. Then in his early sixties, Allen was the 'tutor' of all the early Treasurers. With his brother, Sir Harry Allen, the eminent pathologist, medical administrator, Dean of the Faculty of Medicine at Melbourne University from 1897 to 1924 and President of both the Victorian Medical Associations (1892) and the Victorian Branch of the BMA (1907), he was also very active in charities. Allen formally retired in March 1916.[35] However, from early in 1914, he was only rarely involved in decisions on Invalid Pensions. Instead, the Assistant Commissioner – who was simultaneously Assistant Secretary of Treasury – emerges as the ultimate adjudicator and policy-maker.

James Collins had been Allen's assistant for many years and prior to Federation he had organised the Victorian Old Age Pension Office. Unlike Allen, whose middle class background perhaps accounted for his philanthropy, Collins was the son of a miner who joined the Public Service at age seventeen and worked his way indefatigably to the top: his only known leisure activity being voluminous reading on finance.[36] The decisions on the last three cases reveal something of Collins's approach to invalidity.

Yet the change in policy direction is not solely attributable to Collins's position. He was not alone in his views and the fact that he was surrounded by a number of like-minded men was not due to chance.

Collins was appointed Secretary of Treasury on Allen's retirement in March 1916. He was then rapidly joined by his long-time friend C.J. Cerutty as Assistant Secretary.[37] Cerutty went on to become Auditor General from 1926 to 1935 during which time his harshly judgemental views on the undeserving sick and poor and Australia's so-called 'pension burden' were unambiguous.[38] However, while acting as Assistant Secretary, Cerutty frequently acted for Collins, thus ensuring a continuity of approach.[39]

This was not the only example of cronyism within Pensions. From late 1917, C.J. Cornell held the position of Assistant Commissioner of Pensions. Cornell had previously been Deputy Commissioner of Pensions and Maternity Allowances in Brisbane – a position he held thanks to the intervention of Collins who persuaded the Public Service Commissioner of Cornell's appropriateness for the job on the basis of his alleged ability to detect fraud.[40]

Bureaucratic networks, then, knitted together by a common ideology, produced a formidable uniformity in policy-making. Yet these individuals did not have absolute discretion. The ideological persuasion of the incumbent Treasurer, who could and did overrule the Commissioner, was another critical factor as evidenced in the case of Frederick H.

However, the importance of medicine and medical knowledge in this policy-making process grew exponentially during World War One. Once War Pensions were added to the portfolio of the Pensions Commissioner and Treasury administration, and the total cost of pensions ballooned beyond Treasury's wildest estimates, new means of rejecting applicants had to be found. An ex-soldier could hardly be labelled morally undeserving by the government that had sent him to fight even if he drank or had syphilis. But if doctors could argue that his medical condition was self-induced then his application could be rejected on medical grounds. The value of such professional authority to the state was immense and, it will be argued, immeasurably assisted the professionalisation process.

Clearly, medicine's value to Treasury was instrumental. By 30 June 1920, there were more than 225 000 War Pensions being paid at a cost of over £6 million. Of this number, over 90 000 were incapacitated members of the armed forces.[41] At the same date there were over 35 000 Invalid Pensions being paid. So from 14 000 Invalid Pensions requiring medical examinations in 1913, there were now well over 125 000 Australians who were forced to attend medical practitioners on a regular basis in order to qualify for a pension benefit. In 1924, over 50 000 widows, orphans and certain other dependants of deceased soldiers were added to the list of pension beneficiaries eligible for medical benefits.[42] This was by far the most important contribution made to the professionalisation process in the period and the most important expression of state cooperation and legitimation.

But who were these doctors? Against the pre-war background etched above the Australian Army Medical Corps (AAMC) was formed. The citizen-soldier-doctors of the medical corps had seen some perfunctory action in the South African campaigns but one would be pressed to see the corps as composed of experienced military doctors. Yet military values and militarism have particular significance within this work. In a scathing review of Chris Coulthard-Clarke's *Soldiers in Politics*, Brian Dickey states that 'there is no such thing as "the military" in Australian history'. Rather, he says, 'the sort of people who joined and succeeded in "the military" were already deeply conservative in a variety of ways. Their military behaviour was more outcome than cause'.[43] Is this judgement also true of the members of the AAMC or of the many former AAMC doctors who assessed veterans as part of the pensioning process?

The AAMC

What a different history the mercilessly true one would be – is there ever such written?[44]

The history of the AAMC in World War One, Butler's life work, has been revisited quite recently by Tyquin and is not attempted here.[45] However, there are a number of key issues within that history that have particular significance for the purposes of this work. First, it is clear from Tyquin's work, from the biographical details of former AAMC doctors who later worked for the Repatriation Department, and from other sources used here, that within the profession there was a group of doctors who were greatly enamoured of the soldier's uniform. Indeed some were soldiers first and foremost: Dr Charles Courtney, Principal Departmental Medical Officer of the Repatriation Department from 1922 to 1935, enlisted in 1914 and was sent abroad not as a member of the Medical Corps but as the Officer Commanding 'C' Squadron of the 4th Light Horse, that is, as a combatant not a doctor.[46] Paid permanent positions for doctors in the AAMC were few prior to the war so there was no incentive for doctors attracted to the military life to give up lucrative practices or positions. However, they could and did join the militia units, being paid between £1 and £2/2 per day for examination of recruits and enlisted men, instructing stretcher bearers, and attending educational camps.[47] After 1909 they could also join the AAMC Reserve. According to Tyquin, in 1910 there were approximately 700 (mostly) militia doctors attached to the AAMC. In 1914, according to the Commonwealth statistician, there were approximately 2600 to 2800 doctors *in practice* in Australia.[48] Assuming no *significant* growth in numbers between 1910 and 1914, that means that in 1910 approximately 25% of doctors in practice in Australia were participating in military activities in a period when no conflict was anticipated.

The second key issue to emerge is that most if not all of the *senior* doctors of the AAMC during the war were drawn from these ranks. According to Tyquin, in September 1914 there were only 8 doctors in the AAMC who had no military experience. Yet a significant percentage of the junior doctors who served in the AIF, the Regimental Medical Officers (RMOs), had no military training or background aside from rapid training at and after enlistment. These last two facts explain, in part, the palpable tensions that existed between the two groups, especially during the latter years of the war. As Tyquin and others have noted, in the army loyalty to the needs of the state took precedence over those of the individual soldier.[49] As valid now as it was in World War One, frontline RMOs had to manage an ethical quandary: obey orders from far-removed medical Commanding Officers or treat patients as they had at home. That difference in treatment is abundantly clear in the boarding process explored in Chapter 7.

Finally, senior AAMC doctors were primarily administrators rather than doctors. Their age, personality, professional background and military experience helped shape their values and attitudes. It becomes clear in delving into the mass of archival material available that age had considerable significance. The older doctors, those in the most senior administrative positions and the 'Consultants', were largely Victorian gentlemen, born and educated in Britain and serving Queen (or King) and country, by default, from the antipodes. Most were steeped in Empire, in soldiering as vocation, in Victorian ethics and values and their administrative styles reflected this. They were, in one historian's astute observation, a 'social anachronism': 'no matter how bad or even feudal conditions of labour might be in the mines, for example, contravening the mineowners' instructions could not actually lead to flogging, spread-eagling, or being tied to the tail of a travelling wagon – methods of discipline employed during the Boer War …'.[50]

Many of the younger administrators, however, those sometimes only a few years out of Australian medical schools, were 'modern' army men. They understood administration as a career in itself. They were imbued with modernist values – efficiency, economy and consistency. They were archetypal bureaucrats and this fitted well with army imperatives and with the modernising or engineering approach of those like John Monash. In this respect they had much in common with other medical specialities in the late 19th and early 20th centuries. Cooter has commented that such specialists 'are to be seen as ideologues of corporatism, rationalization, and statism: at a time when the state was reaching out to embrace professionals in its effort to efficiently manage its welfare, these were professionals embracing the state'.[51]

There are two further distinctions that can be made amongst the AAMC fraternity, particularly amongst its elite. In very broad terms, the older doctors, with some notable exceptions, practised the 'art' of medicine, while the 'science' was ignored and neglected. Nowhere was this more apparent than in Britain and France under the Directorship of the DMS Neville Howse. However, the final distinction, and one of immense importance to soldiers, is one of world view. Most doctors came from middle class backgrounds and their world views were shaped by that. The primary distinction within the group was between reformist liberals, those who believed the state had a role to play in improving society, in assisting its more vulnerable populations, and the classical liberals who embodied those characteristics described earlier: economy, productivity, and the selection of 'suitable men' to implement these imperatives.

All of these factors had a bearing on the relationship between doctors and soldiers throughout the war. They also created hostilities and divisions within the AAMC. This tension is most readily appreciated by looking briefly at a handful of men who, whilst hardly representative, were either keen observers or aggressive participants in this drama.

Sir Neville Howse VC, DMS overseas of the AAMC, has had his share of biographers and hagiographers, perhaps his most ardent fan being Butler himself.[52] His illustrious career within and without the AAMC need not detain us here. Of more interest is the voice of his critics, a voice more or less suppressed by his biographers. Perhaps his most vocal critic, both during and after the war, was a man whose distinguished career in medicine almost equalled Howse's career in politics. While Howse, the son of a doctor, was educated at London Hospital, John William Springthorpe, 'Springy', although born in England was educated at Melbourne University. Indeed he formed a long friendship with John Monash as a result of their work together in setting up the Melbourne University Union.[53] Springthorpe was highly qualified: he graduated MA and MB BS in 1879 then an MD in 1884 and was the first Australian graduate to become a member of the Royal College of Physicians.[54] He was also, like Monash, something of a polymath, having a keen interest in the arts, literature and myriad professional interests. His writings, which were prolific, reveal a man who was by nature an advocate, deeply compassionate, egalitarian, committed to the science of medicine, and an insightful observer. Unlike Monash, Howse and many of his AAMC contemporaries, Springthorpe had no military training or background. He was first and foremost a doctor. And it is probably this last fact, as much as his personality, that resulted in his outrage at the treatment of soldiers, and contempt for many of the other senior doctors of the AAMC.

Springthorpe enlisted in October 1914, aged 59, with the rank of Lt Col and was demobilised in May 1919. He served in Egypt and England (No. 2 AGH and No. 3

AAH), with a brief visit to France (he repeatedly requested time in France but was denied the opportunity).[55] He was generally posted as the Senior Physician. Springthorpe kept a diary from 1914 to 1918 and a typescript of the diary, with his 1926 handwritten comments, along with other correspondence is held in the Australian War Memorial. His writings contain a number of passionate themes. In no particular order these were: the poor medicine practised by the AAMC and its lack of interest in science and/or research; the appalling treatment of soldiers on all fronts and in England (and, later, of former soldiers in Australia); the lack of 'modern' leadership in the AAMC; the significant distinctions in treatment and handling made between officers and other ranks; and, his bête noir, the medical boarding process (on which see Chapter 7).

He began his critique of conditions and campaigns for change in Egypt and it continued throughout his career in the AAMC. To do him justice, and not dilute either the sense or passion of his own words, excerpts of his writings on some of these themes at different dates are reproduced here.

On the value of medical statistics of the war and the practices of AAMC doctors:

> 19 September 1917
> Tebbutt confirms my view of front dealings with Shell Shocks 'so many, no time to diagnose, even if able, MOs not permitted to send back, except as N.Y.D.N. [not yet diagnosed nervous] to special hospitals where, after memo from the front, they are diagnosed "Shell Shock – Sick", "Shell Shock, Wounded", or otherwise by experts' (the difference being apparently because the Wounded and not the Sick were eligible for a gold stripe – strange discrimination!) ... for some time the 'Shell Shock, Sick' were considered and even dealt with as – malingerers![56]

> 20 October 1917
> Boarded 13 cases – one from Cambridge with fracture of skull ... sent in as 'GSW [gun shot would] of Shoulder' – such is an Army Record – even from a University. (And on the Record is based their future pension. Often not worth wrapping up a bar of soap!)

> 25 January 1918
> Histories of fresh cases – poorer notes with them than ever – (is treatment also?) – more than scandalous – but – on it goes, much the same as ever...

> 20 July 1923
> The Statistics. I can hardly see how they can do anything but seriously mislead. Diagnoses were almost as a rule made by a Junior Admitting Officer partly on scanty notes from RMOs who had neither time nor experience to disentangle symptoms from disease or to attribute true causation or to state the actual even dominating facts. I could give you countless instances of such imperfect and untrue conditions as jumbling up of Influenza with ... Pneumonia, cases treated as surgical sepsis where they were really paratyphoid, jumbling of Colitis ... with Dysentery, typhoid with Dysentery ... I could prolong the list ... [57]

On the administration of the AAMC and its senior doctors:

15 January 1917

The more I see of the regulational treatment of the men the less it seems just, necessary or advisable – it is shocking to men who have volunteered, and given up so much, if not all. And the cruel, unnecessary difference made between officers and men, justifiable only if they were a different and superior class of beings, and as if the men did not deserve and could not be trusted. The result is they are denied justice, treated inconsiderately, harshly and unfairly and apt to return badness for injustice and go to the devil.

30 June 1917

I fancy after the war, there will be an Enquiry into the treatment of our men here, and deservedly so … the Dumping of men down – the methods of Boarding, the unjust Decisions, the useless Records, the absence of Supervision, the Delay in Transporting, the detention at Weymouth for so long – the attitude of H.Q. towards the patient as distinct from the fighter – the sending of unfit men back from CCS [Casualty Clearing Stations], back from Base, from England, its cost, financial and personal … the unfairness, unnecessity and inhumanity of it all.

Springthorpe left Sydney on 28 November 1914 on board the *Kyarra* transport. With him on the ship was Captain James Reiach, then aged 45, a medical practitioner from Windsor, New South Wales. Reiach served with Springthorpe in Egypt then proceeded to France where he witnessed the Somme winter. Reiach suffered with acute rheumatism and bronchitis during the war. By early he 1917 he was described as 'pale and thin', as having swollen, tender wrists and finger joints, and having 'marked general debility due to carrying on his work while unfit to do so'.[58] After a month in a London hospital, on 10 January 1917 he was posted to the No 3 AAH where he met up once again with Springthorpe.

Springthorpe's diary continues:

10 January 1917

Major Reiach from the front – quite knocked out – for the men every time (as in Egypt where he sent back cases R[yan] had sent on – one of the best – no decoration …[59]

20 July 1917

Reiach's view of things 'since Egypt bad management – always second place – Canada fought for and gained hers – we still secondary at the front… Howse power only over personell (sic) – selfish – unforgiving – aim parliament and Minister of Defence …'

13 August 1917

Reiach says 'Howse cunning and treacherous, all for money and advancement, no bowels, not a fresh brain – reads nothing outside newspapers'.

22 November 1917

In to see DMS [Howse] – long talk – his aim to go back and take charge of Pensions … Pensions to be the main after war work.

Clearly these views are at odds with the celebrations of the AAMC and of Howse published in recent years. And perhaps they were a minority view. It is beyond the scope of this work to examine all the war diaries and other first hand accounts in order to find concordant (or conflicting) views. Yet there is a veracity to Springthorpe's views. As will be seen in Chapters 7 to 9, his complaints about the quality of service records and about misdiagnoses would have far reaching consequences for former soldiers. As for Howse, he did indeed enter Parliament (in 1922) and went on to hold Ministries in Defence, Health, Home and Territories, and Repatriation. Reiach never received a decoration. Indeed, the work of the Regimental Medical Officer on the Western Front has yet to be told in human terms.

What can be known with greater certainly, however, is that promotion through the AAMC under Howse was primarily based on 'a nudge and a wink'[60], and favoured the administrators – as did the honours and awards. Being posted to a less than salubrious administrative position in a non-combat field, for example, could reap its own rewards.

The First Australian Dermatological Hospital, Bulford

Neville Howse made clear his abstemious values regarding alcohol and venereal disease repeatedly in both official and unofficial correspondence.[61] Although Butler suggests he was active in setting up a prophylactic 'scheme' to attack the high incidence of venereal disease in Egypt, it seems the initiative for this came rather from Dr (later Major) W.E. Grigor. Grigor together with Major A. Morris, a venereologist, and Major G. Raffan, a dermatologist, formed the first Australian Venereal Disease 'unit'. Grigor and Morris left Australia about October 1915 and toured similar units in France and England. The full establishment of the VD unit embarked for Cairo on 22 December 1915, one month after Howse had been appointed temporary Surgeon General and Director of Medical Services for the AIF. Grigor and Morris then returned to Cairo where Dr C.J. Wiley was pathologist in addition to a number of other medical officers, only one of whom apparently had any knowledge of this particular clinical speciality. According to Wiley, who wrote a lengthy 'Private & Confidential' account of VD in the AIF for Butler, this unit was initially to be called the Australian VD Hospital, but, as Wiley noted, 'this designation had certain obvious disadvantages'. It then became known as the 1st Australian Dermatological Hospital (1st ADH).[62]

Howse attached Raffan, the dermatologist, to his own staff as special adviser and supervisor. Wiley, the pathologist, told Butler that the 'standard of cure' set for gonorrhoea was difficult. In fact it was so high that more cases were admitted to hospital than were discharged. This meant that when the AIF was ordered to France in early 1916, the 'accumulation of soldiers suffering from venereal disease offered a difficult problem to medical headquarters'. The order given by headquarters (for which read Howse) was that all soldiers were to be discharged to their units, provided they met two standards: 'no

91

disabling complications' and no microscopic evidence of gonococci. Retrospectively, and understandably protecting his science, Wiley wrote that:

> The discharge from hospital of these patients might have been left to the clinical acumen of the physician, for there is no reasons why laboratory tests should have to bear the responsibility that medical headquarters should have taken. An examination of a slide is of no real value under these circumstances, – but perhaps it satisfied some of the patients, and if headquarters felt any misgivings about the infectivity of these men, they doubtless felt they had all the support of laboratory science behind them.[63]

Howse left Egypt for London in mid April 1916 and by May had established his headquarters in Horseferry Road. The 1st ADH arrived in August and took over the British VD hospital at Bulford on the Salisbury Plain. Wiley reported that the hospital was 'very conveniently disposed' and that soon large numbers of patients arrived – 'it was always the lot of the A.D.H. to treat large numbers of patients'. Yet there was something not quite right at the ADH. Butler is quite blunt about the problems but extraordinarily cagey about naming names. His description of the history of this establishment is important and worth quoting in full.

> *The Australian Dermatological Hospital.* The history of the 'ADH' reflects the banal tragedy and social cruelty that surrounds venereal disease. Only to the initiated few does 'Bulford' conjure a picture of scientific enthusiasm, earnest endeavour and clinical work of conspicuously high standard.
>
> And it must be confessed that the forlorn and unhopeful outlook, imposed on these hospitals by social custom in civil life and continued in the war, was not relieved in this AIF unit by any obvious sympathetic consideration from AIF Headquarters. Neither the difficulties of clinical treatment, nor the already sufficient disabilities imposed upon the patients by the nature of their disease appear to have been realized there. Admirably staffed in Australia, the unit, when in Europe became to a considerable extent the unhappy dumping ground for the disciplinary posting of medical officers and other ranks regardless of their special qualifications. The CO was chosen by seniority in the service and took no part in the technical work. Like the bulk of the profession, Gen. Howse held (rightly or wrongly) that the specialists in venereal disease brought to the treatment, in particular of gonorrhoea, refinements of technique that had little reflection in clinical advantage over simpler methods. It must be said that these refinements were perhaps unduly exploited.[64]

Howse never inspected the ADH since, according to Butler, 'he had the strongest prejudice against VD and drink'.[65] Yet we know that he took total personal control over the movements of all medical staff in the AAMC, being ably assisted by the highly decorated Colonel Douglas McWhae.[66] Who, then, did he place at the ADH? This question deserves a minor study in itself. For the purposes of this work it is worth noting briefly the postings of two doctors in particular. The first, Lt Col Piero Fiaschi, arrived at the ADH in April 1917.[67] Fiaschi was fondly remembered by Wiley as the first medical officer to take an interest in prophylaxis and early treatment of VD, having started this in the 1st Light Horse Brigade from its inception until the evacuation from Gallipoli. In later years he was a genito-urinary specialist and authority on venereal disease. It therefore sounds quite natural that Fiaschi should be posted to the ADH – until we examine Howse's correspondence. Tucked away amongst many other letters to various individuals arranging promotions or exploring ways to rid himself of officers he didn't want or like, was this note:

> Howse reports Lt Col Fiaschi is a very good officer but he possesses many objectionable traits, … He would be pleased if Fiaschi asked permission to leave the A.A.M.C. with the object of joining the Italian Service.

Piero Fiaschi was the son of Col Thomas Fiaschi. Both were highly qualified doctors (Piero also had qualifications in dentistry) and both were keen on military life.[68] However, Thomas Fiaschi had been a bitter enemy of Howse during the South African wars. Indeed he had been the PMO of the 2nd Military District when Howse attempted to enlist and was unable to obtain what he perceived as an appropriate commission.[69] Ironically it was not Piero who joined the Italian Service, but his father, Thomas, who resigned his commission as Colonel in the AAMC and went to Italy to work as a surgeon in a military hospital. Piero spent all of his war service (20 August 1914 to September 1918) at the front – aside from his time at the 1st ADH. In 1919, when awards for high-ranking officers were showered on the AIF, he was mentioned in despatches and appointed OBE.

If Butler is correct in saying that the 1st ADH was the dumping ground for recalcitrant medical officers then Fiaschi's posting in 1917 could certainly be read that way. If he is also correct about COs being appointed on the basis of seniority – and little else – then one particular CO warrants attention. In February 1917, Lt Col Kenneth Smith was appointed the CO of the 1st ADH.[70] Smith was born in Sydney in 1885. He was educated at the Brisbane Grammar School and took his medical degree in 1908 from Sydney University. He joined the AAMC in January 1911 as Captain and was appointed Adjutant to the AMC 2nd Military District early in 1912. He was mobilised on the outbreak of war in this latter capacity and employed in full time service until May 1915 when he was appointed to No. 3 AGH. Quickly promoted to Major, he was appointed Registrar of No. 3 AGH in September and remained in this position with a promotion to temporary Lt Col until he was transferred to No. 2 AGH in October 1916 as second in command. In November his rank was confirmed. At the end of February 1917 he moved to the 1st ADH with the rank of temporary Colonel. He remained as CO of the ADH for nearly a year only departing for France, and for 'the Field' for the first time, in February 1918 as CO of the 15th Field Ambulance. By April he was back in England and in July appointed ADMS 4th Australian Division. He returned to England in October and remained there, being attached to the Demobilisation Department under Monash in February 1919.[71]

Smith's was the archetypal administrative career of a young military-minded doctor. His only experience as a frontline medical officer was two months as CO of the 15th Field Ambulance in 1918. After his twelve months at the 1st ADH, and *before* he went to France, he was awarded the CMG. The recommendation was made by Douglas McWhae. We shall meet Smith again as Senior Medical Officer in New South Wales and Principal Departmental Medical Officer within Repatriation in later chapters.

Of more immediate interest are various contemporary assessments of treatment of soldiers at the ADH during his period as Commanding Officer. Since most of the information we have comes from Wiley and his colleague Gibson, both of whom served there along with Raffan (when he wasn't with Howse at Headquarters) and Morris, it is rather explicit and technical in its description of treatment. In brief they describe a period prior to 1918 when, as Gibson puts it, he 'often wondered how the hospital managed to get through without rioting on the part of the patients'. Aside from rapid turnover in medical staff, medical staff with no knowledge of treatment of venereal disease, absence of any research, and discouragement of publications, the treatment at times did 'more harm than good'. Metal instruments were used to dilate the urethra of patients 'to excess', and infections as a result of less than optimal surgical practices were 'prevalent'. As well, Butler notes that '(in 1917?) the DMS [Howse] issued an instruction that all cases of VD were without exception to be diagnosed gonorrhoea. He had to rescind this soon after on the representation of the Specialists'.[72]

In his published work Butler's final words on clinical work at the 1st ADH are those of 'an officer': 'from the military point of view it was "OK", from the clinical "*pas bon*"'.[73] However the final word should come from Smith himself. In a military profile of senior ranking officers collected by Defence at the end of the war, officers were asked to describe the 'Period during service in A.I.F. considered most important or interesting'. Smith wrote of 'three particularly interesting periods of service': on Lemnos, as Registrar with No. 3 AGH; as ADMS 4th Division 'during the advance to Hindenburg Line'; but the last is perhaps the most revealing: 'Period as O.C. 1st A.D. Hospital as regards the disciplinary handling of patients'.[74]

Doctors, then, were far from a homogeneous group, despite their middle class backgrounds and relative affluence. By far the most profound difference was in world view. Yet despite Dickey's assertion to the contrary, military values also differentiated doctors, both those who served in the AIF and those who went on to work for Repatriation after the war. Part of the problem with Dickey's critique is that it defines 'the military' rather narrowly as a 'tiny band of full-time soldiers'. This work seeks to tease out *militarism*, and military values. There is no question that militarism was alive and well amongst most of the senior members of the AAMC. Their 'command' careers were characterised by demands for discipline and obedience, as much as regularity and order. These characteristics have been described by Hume, Adam Smith, Comte, Spencer, Weber and others as intrinsically concerned with military institutions, structures and values.[75]

Military discipline as model for industrial discipline was explored at length by Weber and more recently by Foucault. What militarism does for the conservative liberals of the AAMC, and others, is add discipline (and its corollary, punishment,) and obedience to the emphasis on economy and productivity. War simply re-invigorated these long-standing hallmarks of classical liberalism.

The homefront

During the course of the war came rapid, often improvised changes in the Australian health system which reflected the strategic importance of soldiers to the nation. As Pearce, then Minister for Defence, informed Millen in early 1918, the function of the Australian Army Medical Service was to return soldiers to Active Service with maximum speed.[76] In order to do that, staff and facilities were needed.

In 1914, the Director General of Medical Services (DGMS), Dr R.H.J. Fetherston, was required to find personnel for three fields of service: the AIF, the Sea Transport Service and the Home Service. According to Butler, the experience of South Australia is typical of the profession's response to war. In that state over 90% of doctors joined the AAMC Reserve. As if that was not enough, in April 1917, after the failure of the Conscription Referendum, the Federal Committee of the BMA asked the Commonwealth government to introduce a Bill for the compulsory enlistment of medical practitioners for service in the AIF. The proposal failed to gain approval of members by ten votes but the patriotic spirit, and perhaps also the attraction of practising medicine at war, was overwhelmingly clear. Weindling has described the 'enthusiasm' of medical mobilisation at this time in Germany where 24 000 out of 33 000 male doctors served.[77] While the precise number of doctors who actually embarked from Australia for service overseas is unknown, by the end of 1917 around 1000 were employed by the Department of Defence in Australia.[78]

Some indication of the increased demand for medical professionals during the course of the war can also be seen in the number of hospitals created. Throughout Australia 20 General or Auxiliary Hospitals were opened with a capacity of around 3 500 beds. In addition to this were 14 'Special Hospitals' for treatment of 'mental', 'TB' or 'VD' patients with a capacity of around 750 beds. This does not include Red Cross institutions or camp hospitals. Records for staff of these institutions are incomplete, but where available they indicate employment of 83 full-time and 64 part-time doctors, 123 Sisters and around 300 Nurses.[79] Clearly war provided many employment opportunities which only strengthened the professionalisation process.

Another indication of the increased importance of medicine to civil authorities in wartime emerges from the arrangements for the supervision of these institutions. In October 1915, by which date most of the new Australian General Hospitals had been opened, the Federal Parliamentary War Committee (FPWC) set up Advisory Committees in each state to inspect and report on the management and operation of all military hospitals and convalescent homes in Australia. The Committees were also empowered to inquire into complaints over treatment of patients. Each state had a Committee of seven members, and the FPWC advised that two such members should be 'ladies'. The recommended membership was two members of the FPWC, the Lord Mayor of the city, two nominees of the Red Cross ('ladies'), one member of the Chamber of Commerce and a nominee of the Trades and Labour Council.[80] By 1921, when these Committees were disbanded, the functions were performed by a Medical Advisory Committee with supervision by Repatriation Deputy Commissioners.[81] In other words, the war years saw the demise of lay authority, including that of the 'lady', over institutions caring for the sick and wounded. By 1921 such institutions were seen as *medical* institutions and were supervised by doctors and departmental bureaucrats. Similarly, in the repatriation process, the role of doctors enlarged as the war progressed

Following the 1918 Repatriation Act, a medical bureaucracy had to be created to provide treatment and services for soldiers after their discharge from the AIF. In brief this consisted of a Principal Department Medical Officer (PDMO) in Melbourne, Departmental Medical Officers (DMOs) in each state and Local Medical Officers (LMOs) in each local committee area. These doctors were responsible for examination of former members of the AIF for Vocational Training, employment and other purposes and for treatment in hospitals, convalescent homes and elsewhere. By 1920 there were 622 LMOs in country areas.[82]

Doctors also performed less visible functions within the new Department. For example, in June 1919, the troopship *Benalla* arrived in Sydney from London with a number of soldiers, their British wives and munition workers. The Customs and Excise Boarding Inspector was informed that a soldier and his wife had been suspected of having active venereal disease but that after both were examined by the Customs Health Officer and by the Military Doctor, it was determined that only the wife was 'infected'. The soldier was subsequently discharged. The Boarding Inspector wrote to the Collector of Customs seeking clarification as to who should be held responsible for allowing the woman 'entry into the Commonwealth', the Master of the ship or the 'military authorities'. The question was referred to Atlee Hunt, then Secretary of Home and Territories Department, who wrote to Gilbert in an attempt to settle who was responsible for treatment in this and similar cases as he believed it was impossible to send the woman back to England or to make the ship's Master responsible. The file and Atlee Hunt's letter were forwarded to the PDMO for comment.[83]

At this date the PDMO was Dr (Captain) James Francis Agnew. Agnew, a Scot and Presbyterian elder, had been government health officer in Collingwood, Victoria, and a member of the AAMC Reserve when war broke out, at which time he was 52 years of age. As a later obituary noted, 'a term of duty as a Hussar in a crack regiment of the line [gave] him an introduction to a side of life which deeply interested him, and added to his later influence with men'.[84]

Agnew served briefly in No. 2 AGH in Egypt but was discharged from the Army in March 1916 and by 1918 was DMO to the Victorian office of the Repatriation Department.[85] Agnew's response to Gilbert was characteristic of his brief tenure as PDMO (he died in 1922). He insisted the Department had no responsibility for treatment of former soldiers' wives and, further, believed that a new system should be instituted in England to prevent ex-soldiers' dependants from coming to Australia if they suffered from any infectious or contagious disease.[86] As for the case in question, he believed the woman should be 'instructed to seek treatment' at a venereal disease clinic or at a public hospital. Gilbert approved these recommendations which were then forwarded, under his signature, to the Departments of Home and Territories and Quarantine as a means of dealing with 'these women'.

Agnew also played an important role in determining early Departmental policy on medical treatment of soldiers after their discharge. A lengthy report submitted to Gilbert on this subject in September 1918, a report which reflected Millen's wishes and subsequently formed the basis of the early Repatriation structure, reveals the principles guiding his suggested organisation. Of primary concern was cost. While he advised Gilbert that the 'interests of the discharged man' were of paramount importance in setting up any new medical machinery, nevertheless 'the total provision must have relation to a reasonable expenditure'.[87] 'Expenses' associated with the system needed to be carefully controlled. For example, Agnew was extremely critical of the early discharge of soldiers from military hospitals before the completion of 'active treatment'. This was not simply a complaint on medical grounds, rather it was a complaint about a process which, in Agnew's view, benefited no-one. His description of the problem bears quoting at length:

> Under the existing system many men are discharged … before their active treatment has been completed … The practice is to require these men to return to military hospitals periodically for further treatment. In the interim they become a charge upon the Repatriation Department. Because of their immediate physical condition, or because of the interruptions which periodical returns to hospital involve, they cannot be placed in any definite employment, nor can they be submitted for vocational training. While away from the hospital they are free of restraint and develop a habit of idleness, the subsequent cure of which is difficult to the man himself, and incidentally expensive to the Repatriation Department …
>
> The drift, and perhaps wastage, which is here indicated would be arrested if the man were kept under military discipline until the completion of his active treatment … Similar considerations apply to men suffering from shell-shock, neurasthenia, chronic alcoholism and allied diseases or tuberculosis.[88]

'Wastage', a 'habit of idleness', 'military medical discipline', 'control', all of these concepts resonate throughout the report. For Agnew, the solution was simple: employ more doctors, especially ex-AAMC doctors. Ex-army doctors, he argued, could spot malingerers, could 'handle' soldiers, and if their advice was refused, the Department could be absolved of responsibility, not just for medical treatment but also for sustenance.

Agnew's arguments did not go unheeded. The appointment of Departmental medical officers under his careful supervision is analysed in later chapters. However, the policies and procedures he helped to establish had long-lasting structural effects, not least of which was the extended use of doctors to control Departmental costs. Departmental doctors had a wide range of tasks to perform, many of which related to eligibility for benefits such as medical examinations for War Pensions, for land settlement for vocational training and the examination of widows of soldiers for sustenance and other benefits.[89] In most of these matters Agnew was all too ready to collaborate with the Department and its pecuniary motives. For example, in February 1919, the Brisbane DC wrote to Gilbert wanting direction on a case where an ex-soldier suffering from tuberculosis was discharged from a military hospital but the DMO believed him to be a 'disquieting element' and thus inadmissible to a Departmental sanatorium. The DC had referred the case to the State Board which pointed out that New South Wales law provided for the institutionalisation of persons perceived to be 'a menace to the Community' provided there was agreement between two doctors and a Police magistrate. It now sought the advice of the Repatriation Commission. The matter was referred to Agnew who completely reconstituted the question. While the DC and the State Board perceived the issue in terms of the ex-soldier's health and a crude public health mentality which sanctioned incarceration on the ground of possible contagion, Agnew saw the problem purely in terms of discipline and of Departmental and individual responsibility. He advised Gilbert that

> It is not recommended that this Department should involve itself in the committal of men to State Institutions. If a man persistently refuses to avail himself of the provisions made for the treatment of his war disability or, being an inmate of a hospital, refuses to conform with the regulations, thus retarding his own, or the recovery of others, this Department may, in these circumstances, refuse further assistance or responsibility.[90]

While these values were being embedded in the new medical structure of the Department, the profession was reaping other Departmental benefits. Assistance with university fees, with purchasing medical instruments, with purchasing cars and with setting up practices was available through the Department to ex-AAMC doctors, to ex-AIF medical students and to ex-soldiers wishing to study medicine. Assistance to this latter group had a significant effect on the number of medical graduates practising in Australia from the late 1920s.[91] In passing, it is worth noting the nature of the 'suitable instruments' compiled by Agnew and his colleagues for issue under the 'Tools of Trade' regulations to 'young medical officers taking up Practice'. Approximately 25% of these instruments were concerned with women's reproductive organs, thereby indicating the extent of intervention in childbirth and possibly the extensive practice of uterine curettage in this period.[92] Again, these practices require further study.

Overall, it can be seen that new structures of medical power proliferated during the war years in response to state requirements first of all for a fit Army and then as part of a bureaucratic organisation for handling ex-soldiers. The medical profession also benefited from the Vocational Training provisions. The range of structures included organisational ones such as hospitals and convalescent homes and procedural ones such as assessments for Repatriation benefits. These were accompanied by the invisible permeation of processes and procedures with a particular ideology which vested authority in the profession by virtue of the medical definition of a vast range of problems affecting returned soldiers and drew on military discipline as a source of power. In Agnew's words, it was often 'considered advisable on medical grounds for military control to continue'.[93] In many of these areas, particularly the enthusiasm of the profession for army service and the extent of military values within medicine, there is a striking parallel to be found in Weindling's account of German medicine and public health in the same period.[94]

As a result of the new power war conferred on the profession, doctors were well placed when it came to debates over conditions of service both within and outside the Department. Yet while there was a gloss of victory on the profession in these negotiations, such superficial assessments fail to take account of state power over the profession.

A marriage of convenience: state-subsidised medicine

In December 1917, one of Lockyer's inner circle of bureaucrats, R. Ovington, wrote prophetically that

> [if] financial aid is given to the sick and bereaved members of the A.I.F. who are not members of a Friendly Society, by the Department of Repatriation, or by Local Committees of Repatriation, it is not likely that other soldiers with equal claims to its receipt, will continue to pay for these benefits. The result will be that they will withdraw from the societies and look to Departmental or Local funds for assistance. Therefore, the Department will have to extend this form of assistance to all, or withhold it altogether.[95]

The fortunes of the Friendly Societies, always a 'target of hatred' for the medical profession, accurately reflect the increasing power of certain sectors of the profession in this period.[96] The Societies were essentially non-profit co-operatives which carefully controlled medical fees as part of their responsibility for contributors' funds. Membership in Victoria had grown steadily from 1870 until 1914 when it stood at around 160 000, of which around 147 000 were male members. This membership level was not surpassed until 1926-7 and indeed declined by some 10% in the intervening years.[97] According to Pensabene, 25-30% of the decline was due to war service mortality. However, he attributes 'most of the decline in membership' to the outcome of a long-running dispute between the lodges and the British Medical Association.

In late 1913, the Victorian Branch of the BMA had demanded an increase in capitation fees, an income limit for members and, importantly, an increase in the number of services not forming part of the lodge service. War intervened and the matter was only partly resolved when a Royal Commission was appointed in 1918. The BMA claimed the outcome of that Commission as a major victory. Fees were increased and an income limit was introduced, although in neither case were the BMA's full claims granted. Fee increases ranged from 15-30% and, according to Pensabene, lodge members were forced to pay additional fees for anaesthetics and midwifery. In New South Wales the new agreement excluded surgical operations and treatment of fractures as well.[98] Willis sees the Victorian experience as another 'moment' in the professionalisation process, claiming that the Societies were forced to 'give in' to doctors and that 'in economic terms it represented gaining control over the demand for medical services in the medical market place'.[99] In a more historically informed analysis, Gillespie has argued that, contrary to Willis's view, medical opposition did not seriously affect the lodges in the short term. Instead Gillespie highlights the doctors' control of certain services as the means whereby 'a slow erosion' of lodge services took place. By excluding so many vital services increasing numbers of working class contributors were forced to use the free public hospital system while those on higher incomes were forced to pay the full private fee. Yet despite this movement out of the lodges, 40% of doctors still earned their capitation fees in 1925 and this situation had not seriously changed twenty years later.[100]

Instead of viewing this situation as 'medical dominance', the dispute can be reinterpreted as the articulation of intra-professional power struggles, the principal outcome of which was to give massive support to the medical specialisations of obstetrics, surgery, orthopaedics and anaesthetics because, despite their fundamental importance to the practice of medicine, these services were henceforth largely available on a fee-for-service basis only. At the same time, two-fifths of the profession still relied on the capitation fees as an important source of income. What Pensabene, Willis and Gillespie fail to address is the sheer number of returned soldiers and, after 1924, widows and other dependants of deceased soldiers, who were eligible for medical treatment at no cost through the Repatriation system.[101] While the nature of that 'care' is critically examined in subsequent chapters, and the notion that this was a 'welfare' system has already been seriously questioned, it remains that this state-enforced patronage of doctors was of immeasurable assistance to the professionalisation process. Between them, by the early 1920s, the Department, the Friendly Societies and Treasury provided doctors with well over 600 000 clients of whom nearly one-third were state subsidised.[102] As far as war pensions are concerned, this historical process provides an explanation for the buoyancy and confidence of both individual doctors and the BMA in their dealings with the Depatment from 1918.

CHAPTER 6

Demobilisation, Repatriation and Australian Productivity

The repatriation scheme which came into effect in April 1918 consisted of a range of benefits or forms of assistance that had evolved in the voluntary organisations and the State War Councils since 1915. These benefits were now centralised, rationalised and tightly controlled in the departmental organisation, but the emphasis remained a short term one of providing rapid ameliorative aid and effective procedures for re-integration. The scheme was put together at a time when there was no end to the war in sight. Indeed twenty-five per cent of Australian casualties occurred in 1918 and as late as June of that year Hughes was anticipating two further years of warfare.[1] Australia's commitment to the war effort meant that there would be an ongoing demand for recruits from the Imperial War Office yet the numbers volunteering in Australia continued to dwindle. As Hughes wrote to Pearce en route to London in May, 'A Referendum is hopeless, a coup d'état impossible: We must just make the best of a very bad job'.[2] The longer the war went on, the longer the AIF overseas – already suffering from attrition – would be called upon to endure and the greater the attrition. Each year of service could be seen as widening the chasm between civilian and soldier; army discipline and army pay could not be reproduced readily in civilian society. There was a consciousness of this expressed both in Australian political life and overseas amongst the senior members of the AIF.

Neither issue was perceived to be of immediate importance by Hughes, or most of his colleagues, when he sailed for London in April 1918. At that date soldiers remained a precious commodity needed to win trade deals from Britain. The war loans that were part and parcel of Australia's war effort of raising and maintaining an army overseas needed to be balanced by favourable trade agreements. However, there was a growing concern in Australian political circles at the human cost of the damage. Never at a loss for words, Hughes pleaded with the Imperial War Cabinet to use air power and conserve manpower since it would bring victory 'at an infinitely lower price in blood than anything else'.[3]

Like Hughes, Millen feared the economic effects of high casualty rates both in terms of the immediate cost to the Repatriation Department and the longer term labour consequences. Unlike Hughes, he foresaw the possible economic effect the cessation of hostilities might have. On moving the second reading of the Australian Soldiers' Repatriation (ASR) Bill in the Senate in July 1917, he commented on the effect on the

Australian economy of having 250 000 'idle' men: in one week, he argued, the loss in wage-earning capacity was between £600 000 and £700 000.[4] Yet Millen was practically alone amongst the key political figures in power at this date in seeing demobilisation in these terms.

That was all to change and with unexpected rapidity. Between July 1918 and the Armistice, from being seen as 'cannon fodder' or as commodities to bring to the Imperial bargaining table, the AIF abroad came to be seen as cogs in the wheels of Australian industrial and agricultural production. For those responsible for their management and control, the Repatriation Department and the 'Generals' union' of the AIF, the question of rapid demobilisation was intimately linked to the question of Australia's war debt, and the matter of educating and re-training the disabled was linked to the imperative of increasing Australian productivity and productive efficiency.[5] Both were seen as necessary to the maintenance of civil order. This was a profound shift in the focus of government at a time when war had fostered a conservative hegemony and a constitutionally sanctioned state control of political, economic and social life. How this shift in emphasis occurred and its effects on the returning AIF forms the substance of this Chapter.

The occupation and preoccupation of 'idle' men

From April to the Armistice the question of who would control the demobilisation and repatriation of the AIF and the nature of the process involved became increasingly important to those with vested interests in the issue: the commanders of the AIF, the Prime Minister and Cabinet. General Birdwood, who in this period was promoted to command of the British Fifth Army, repeatedly cabled Defence in Melbourne in April and July on the need for a plan and for some staffing arrangement. On 6 August, Defence finally replied that Cabinet considered no action was necessary and that the government was awaiting a communication from Hughes, then in London.[6]

Hughes, on the other hand, saw the issue as one intimately connected to the changes being made to the command of the British and Australian armies. In his view, Birdwood's appointment to the Fifth Army, while formally remaining General Officer Commanding (GOC) the AIF, meant that he was serving two masters, the British War Office and the Australian Defence Department, an untenable position according to Hughes and one which he and Cook believed would prejudice the AIF. On 1 August Hughes cabled Watt, then Acting Prime Minister, that he and Cook believed the interests and welfare of Australian soldiers were not properly safeguarded under the existing administrative arrangements. Further, he suggested that Australian casualties were higher than Canada's because Australia got 'more than her share of fighting' and this because, unlike Canada, there was no Australian General in charge of Administration and officially separate from the office of corps commander.[7] Hughes went on to suggest that John Monash, then commander of the Australian Army Corps, should be offered the position of GOC AIF. However, rapid changes in the military situation on the Western Front after the launch of the Allied offensive in August brought the matter to a head.

In early September a conference of senior AIF personnel was called in order to make recommendations on repatriation and demobilisation to the respective Ministers and to the GOC AIF. The discussion paper circulated prior to the conference commenced by arguing that women who had replaced soldiers in Australian industry must not be displaced from their jobs by the repatriation of the AIF. This was not argued on the basis of some proto-feminist view of equity in the workplace, but rather on the basis of a passionate belief in the need to increase Australian productivity. Soldiers, it argued, should be found 'other productive work of heavier nature' since there was an imperative to increase post-war production 'immensely' to cover the total Australian debt of £156 million.[8] The second major preoccupation of the paper was with the order of troop demobilisation. In line with its obsession with productivity, the paper contained a suggested hierarchy of trades as the basis of ordering demobilisation. While this hierarchy, one similar to that employed by the Imperial authorities, did not become the basis of demobilisation it did remain as a loosely based system of categorising the employment potential or skill of returning soldiers within the Repatriation Department.[9] However, the biggest problem identified in the paper, and one 'bristling with difficulties', was that of 'filling in time', of how to preoccupy nearly 200 000 soldiers abroad.

The AIF Education Scheme, headed by G.M. Long, Bishop of Bathurst and father of Gavin Long, official historian of World War Two, had been in existence for some time as a result of much earlier concerns amongst the Generals of the AIF about the effects of demobilisation.[10] In Hughes's opinion, however, Long's scheme was ineffectual and inadequate.[11] On 23 October he demanded a meeting with AIF Administrative staff in London over the whole issue of repatriation and demobilisation. Brigadier-General T.H. Dodds, then Commandant of Administrative Headquarters, reported the outcome of the meeting to his superior, Birdwood, the following day, expressing his frustration:

> I was rather disappointed with regard to the attitude he took up in connection with the Education Scheme and regarding the whole scheme generally he thought it was pretty useless and likely to have no greater effect either in the benefit of the men or to Australia than would 'a camel piddling against a pyramid have in boring a hole in the pyramid'. What can you do with a man like this?[12]

Yet the question of education as a means of passing time was really only part of a much broader problem, that of returning the troops to Australia. In particular, it was a question of the rate and order of return. October and November saw a flurry of sometimes heated exchanges between Hughes in London, and Watt and Pearce in Melbourne. Of primary concern was shipping. For Watt and Pearce, the ship-building activities of the Allies together with a forecast demand for Australian raw materials and primary produce after the war, translated into rapid repatriation of the AIF over a period of around nine months. Pearce informed Cabinet that the original demobilisation time, estimated at two to three years by the Army Council, had been revised and that Birdwood now believed six to nine months was realistic.[13] At his meeting with Hughes, Dodds also noted that the Ministry of Shipping had undertaken to return AIF troops within nine months. Hughes, on the other hand, insisted on slowing this process and initially demanded it be stretched over 18 months. This intentional delay – denied by Monash in his official history of demobilisation although intimated in personal correspondence – was represented officially as due to a concern for the comfort and welfare of troops on the returning transports.[14] Yet it is clear from the available evidence that the only serious concern of all the political figures involved was to balance a politically acceptable rate of return while concurrently maximising the number of ships coming to Australia, ships they believed would return to Europe full of Australian produce.[15]

The second most important concern was the control, discipline and employment of the troops in England after their return from France.[16] 'Disgruntled and discontented' men needed 'sympathetic consideration' or, as Watt cabled Hughes, the political consequences in Australia would be 'ugly'.[17] For Hughes, however, the administrative arrangements for demobilisation were of secondary interest. Of primary importance was the conversion of soldiers to 'wealth-producing citizens'. In line with the earlier AIF Generals' discussion paper, Hughes believed adamantly in the necessity to re-train soldiers to 'habits of industry'. His grandiose ideas – freely admitted as deriving from Canadian practice – for organising vocational training in national workshops to assist emerging industries in Australia were ultimately compromised by the implacability of British unions to foreign and un-unionised labour.[18] A simpler scheme of 'non-military employment' along lines originally envisaged by Long and incorporating some element of industrial training was instituted but by April 1919 the number of soldiers undergoing such training was viewed as 'disappointing'.[19] For Monash, then in charge of the scheme, the primary function was clear – one of 'keeping the mens' minds occupied' and increasing 'their economic value'.[20]

While the Defence Department, the Generals and Hughes continued their discussions on the principles that should govern repatriation, the Repatriation Department was busy bombarding soldiers with propaganda about the benefits that awaited them on their return to Australia. This was one of the most important instances of war time propaganda emanating from the federal government. Unlike the propaganda produced for the referenda, that issued to the AIF in 1918 and early 1919 had multiple concerns. Employment, 'sustenance', land settlement, education, medical benefits, loans, gifts and care of the disabled were just some of the subjects covered. In August 1918, a one page circular entitled 'What the Government is doing' was issued from the London office of the AIF Administrative Headquarters. At the same time 200 000 copies of a pamphlet entitled 'What Australia is doing for her Returned Soldiers' was ordered from the Government Printer and subsequently circulated to all troops. Also in August, the *Kia Ora and Coo-ee Magazine* and *Kia Ora and Coo-ee Newsletter* (respectively monthly and weekly publications) containing information on Repatriation benefits, were circulated in Egypt. In September, directions went to AIF Headquarters and to the AIF 'Printing Section' to include a notice on the Repatriation scheme in all journals published by the UK Depots or in the official journal *Aussie*. In November, 25 000 copies of a pamphlet covering the whole scheme went to Egypt. After Monash was put in charge of demobilisation in late November, propaganda issued from both sources.[21]

As well as this propaganda war in print, the Repatriation Department despatched one of its Honorary Commissioners and a key bureaucrat to London to look after its interests. In March 1919, Lt Col Owen, formerly Commanding Officer of the 3rd Battalion, was offered £2.2.0 per day plus travelling expenses for 'propaganda work among the troops' over an anticipated five to six months. In May Owen's place on the Commission was offered by Millen to Major J.H.P. Eller. However, the offer was withdrawn by Gilbert when it was discovered Eller was also an applicant for a staff position within the Department. Instead an invitation went to Lt Col James Semmens.[22] Given Semmens's importance to the repatriation process during the first fifteen years it is worth digressing briefly to examine his background.

Born in Rushworth, Victoria, Semmens was a career Public Servant who started out as a clerk in the Victorian Income Tax Office and, after a stint at Melbourne University, progressed to become Chief Inspector of Fisheries and Game for Victoria by 1920. Around 1890, Semmens joined the Militia and in 1908 transferred from the 1st Battalion, 5th Australian Infantry Regiment, to the infant Australian Intelligence Corps (AIC) which came into existence that year under the supervision of J.W. (later Hon Sir James) McCay, and under the immediate command of John Monash. All three men appear to have been at Melbourne University in the same period, with McCay and Monash both doing law in the early 1890s. In 1913, Semmens was chosen by McCay to succeed Monash as head of the AIC in Victoria and promoted to Lieutenant Colonel. On the outbreak of war, Major General Bridges chose McCay to command the 2nd (Victorian) Brigade and McCay chose Semmens to command the 6th Battalion – the Melbourne Battalion. Semmens, in turn, recruited H. Gordon Bennett, another long-time militia man and one destined for a troubled career in the 2nd AIF, as his second in command. According to the historian of the AIC, Semmens's Battalion also had the greatest AIC representation of all AIF units. Semmens accompanied his Battalion to Egypt but was shortly thereafter returned to Australia as permanently unfit for service abroad. From the date of his return to Australia he was in charge of various AIF training camps as well as being sometime Vice President of the Returned Soldiers Association of Victoria when he was outspoken on the undisciplined nature of returned soldiers. He also acted as a member of the Qualifications Committee for Soldier Land Settlement in Victoria and was active in this position at the time he was recruited to the Repatriation Commission.[23]

Semmens's AIC association may partly explain his offer of a seat on the Commission. As noted previously, one of the most important members of the small bureaucratic inner circle in early 1918 was Major M.B. Ryan. Ryan is a shadowy figure but it is at least certain that he was a member of the AIC in Melbourne from 1912 until he was recruited by Semmens as a Lieutenant in the 6th Battalion. Of more importance here is his appearance in March 1919 in London as the Departmental representative – two months ahead of Owen – acting as liaison officer with Monash, his previous Commanding Officer in the AIC. Indeed, at this date, AIC representation in Australian repatriation and demobilisation matters in London was remarkable. McCay was GOC AIF Depots in the United Kingdom, Monash was Director General of demobilisation and Ryan the only official representative of the Repatriation Department.[24] Ryan became a member of the Commission in 1926.[25]

The reaction of soldiers to this propaganda war was mixed. In part reactions were determined by the propaganda itself. For example, in Egypt, the *Kia Ora Coo-ee News* was quick to remind soldiers that 'when the crisis of war is past, and the crisis of settlement arrives, the hero who did all the fighting is apt to be forgotten'. It went on to single out the voluntary forces of ANZAC as more deserving than their British counterparts:

> Those citizens who have voluntary [*sic*] enlisted for the defence of the Empire, have greater need, and more right, to an extensive repatriation scheme, than a Democracy that has adopted conscription.

It also created a new enemy:

> one half of the population [in Australia] has offered all, whereas the other half has remained behind, to its own profit; ... It is only just that he should be helped, and that the other man should pay.[26]

This was in August. In January 1919 all Brigade Commanding Officers in Egypt were circulated with a confidential report on morale 'as gathered from correspondence of troops in the Egyptian Expeditionary Force' (EEF).[27] While the report noted that 'Colonial troops' *seemed* to be more content – attributed by the compiler to their 'much larger' pay – the complaints by British troops were still deemed important to senior AIF ranks. The chief complaint concerned the timing and order of demobilisation and the lack of clear information. This was certainly true of the AIF abroad as much as the BEF or EEF.[28] But the most worrying problem for the soldiers was economic. Would 'home slackers' have taken their old jobs? Would there be a job for them at all? Would the government keep its promises of special treatment?

A justifiable suspicion also characterised the soldiers' response to the training and educational schemes. As Pearce informed Millen, they viewed the schemes as 'an attempt to justify their retention in England for a longer period that [*sic*] would otherwise be necessary'.[29] And there were other complaints. At the end of January a letter signed by sixty-six members of the AIF was published in the *British-Australasian* complaining of a shortage of mattresses, blankets and food – particularly meat, which they claimed 'walked on stilts' through the stews. McCay, as Officer Commanding the Depots, was immediately sent to investigate and found that the meat ration was indeed too low, but that the biggest problem was with the fuel supply for the stoves. The coal supplied did not heat the stove sufficiently to cook food and as a result palliasses of men on leave were emptied of straw and filled with illegally obtained better quality coal.[30]

Yet perhaps the most important response of soldiers to these repatriation activities was their refusal to fill out or sign the repatriation registration form. The 'General Registration' form which had been issued by the Repatriation Department in at least April 1918 was designed to be filled in on the transports returning to Australia.[31] By mid May reports were going to Gilbert of soldiers refusing to fill them in. The Deputy Comptroller in Perth, for example, reported that only 27 completed forms had been received from the hospital ship *Kanowna* which had 397 soldiers on board. To Lockyer such refusals were 'incomprehensible'.[32] The reports of officers on the transports indicated that this refusal was linked to the other great concern of all soldiers at this juncture: war pensions.

The form sought information on the soldier's pre-war employment, including pay, whether or not there was a promise of re-instatement, and if not what occupation the soldier desired to follow after discharge. It also asked whether the soldier wanted assistance from the Department in finding employment and, in the case of physical disability, what kind of 'light' employment the soldier would prefer. At the bottom of the form there was a section entitled 'Physical Condition'. Here the nature and extent of incapacity (expressed as a percentage) and its duration were to be verified from the individual's Medical History sheet and recorded. It will be remembered that the percentage of incapacity formed the basis of a war pension. The Registration form therefore asked for significant information that bore on the two issues of greatest concern to returning soldiers: employment and pensions. Indeed, to all intents and purposes, it linked the two. The Department was representing itself as intent on finding work for soldiers, whether able or disabled. But additionally it was asking for information on the extent of that disability. The reason men gave for not signing the form was that the information would affect their pension.

War pensions were seen increasingly as a right, the least a grateful nation could do in return for loyal service under horrific conditions. Anything which might interfere with that 'right' was treated with suspicion. In this case a Department bent on getting men back to work, when incapacity to work formed the definitional basis of a war pension, presented soldiers with a terrible dilemma. It is clear from the files that most wanted to work but that a significant majority suffered from some kind of pensionable disability. By filling out the Repatriation form soldiers were effectively forced to make a choice between payment for a disability and employment. Their refusal to do so suggests a clear understanding of what was going on, but in the end the choice was going to be made for them.

The history of employment as a Departmental responsibility in this brief period reveals a great deal about the nature of the state in Australia at the end of the war.[33] Raising productivity was of paramount importance to the Nationalist coalition from late 1918, once the end of the war was in sight and the nature of post-war international trading relations were contemplated. Bearing in mind that nearly 50% of Australian males of military age enlisted and more than half of those suffered some form of injury or illness, it is easy to understand just how critical the Department's activities were to economic planning. Every effort was directed towards transforming soldiers into productive economic units. C.B. Macpherson's analysis of the seventeenth-century origins of liberal political economy resonates more strongly through both Ministerial and Departmental correspondence than does any democratic concept of citizenship: 'the working class were regarded not as citizens but as a body of actual and potential labour available for the purposes of the nation'.[34] In this regard, the portrayal of Repatriation by some welfare historians and sociologists as a 'generous' welfare system and one that constituted a new citizenship is misguided.[35] What we are witnessing is the careful manipulation of demobilisation and repatriation through a massive propaganda campaign which tapped into nationalist sentiment while portraying the state as grateful benefactor. The propaganda served to allay, in part, soldiers' legitimate fears over the nature of the society to which they were returning. But it also promised employment. The gap between this promise and reality widened as the economic and logistical problems associated with finding jobs assumed critical proportions. As a result, ways and means were found to limit assistance while maintaining public credibility. In so doing, the scope of 'civil re-establishment' and of 'repatriation' narrowed.

The federal government largely failed in its efforts to expand capital works through loans to the states to create jobs for ex-soldiers. It was reluctant to invest in new industries, a reluctance that is understandable given the futility of trying to raise loans and the immature nature of manufacturing in Australia. Furthermore, although public service preference was officially instituted, complaints of returned soldiers being overlooked or not employed were widespread and the advocacy of the RSSILA was singularly unsuccessful.[36] The Commonwealth public service resented giving preference to soldiers and, adding to the problem, from the end of 1917 the Prime Minister's Department directed all Commonwealth departments not only to vet soldiers' military records but to undertake 'personal confidential enquiries' of their previous employer regarding the 'character' of the individual.[37] Moral or political judgements on the soldier's pre-war behaviour could thus be used to exclude him from 'sensitive' positions; Millen's plans for employing ex-soldiers in the Commonwealth Public Service were also undermined by a Prime Ministerial sensitivity to certain kinds of former soldiers in his immediate surrounds.[38]

Attempts to circumvent the system by appealing to 'sympathetic' Members of Parliament were unsuccessful, including those to Hughes who appears to have done nothing materially for those soldiers who applied to the 'little digger' for assistance.[39] Complaints via other Members of Parliament on behalf of soldiers were met with a well-reasoned and economically seductive Departmental response, as when W.H. Kelly, National Member for Wentworth, asked why soldiers had to report daily for sustenance payments. Gilbert informed him that this procedure stopped the men defrauding the Department.[40]

The transformation of soldiers into productive labour was thus beset with problems. However, the other major concern in the propaganda campaigns, as much as in the demobilisation and repatriation schemes, had been the maintenance of civil order. Here the propaganda used during the war had some unexpected consequences. As well as appeals to nationalism, recruiting had utilised the artificially created social division between 'loyalists' and 'disloyalists'. A useful recruiting device became, in the post-armistice period, a cause of dissent and even violence amongst returned soldiers. 'Slackers' got jobs while 'dinkum diggers' were unemployed.[41] This civil disorder and antagonism was largely unanticipated, as was the politicisation of returned soldiers seeking a better deal on employment.

Marilyn Lake has described the proliferation of returned soldier political organisations during the latter years of the war, noting in particular the early history of the Soldiers National Political Party (SNPP) and its leader, M.P. Pimentel.[42] Lake uses the SNPP to suggest 'federal government connivance' in the establishment of returned soldier political parties in opposition to the RSSILA. This may indeed have been true of Hughes prior to his departure overseas, but it is clear that neither Watt as Acting Prime Minister nor Millen knew anything about either Pimentel or the SNPP until George Steward, then head of civil intelligence (the Counter Espionage Bureau), wrote to Watt in July 1918 warning him that returned soldier organisations, notably the SNPP, would be nominating candidates at the next election. Pimentel's party stood for preference for soldiers, the destruction of Bolshevism and opposition to the use of strikes. It was hardly a threat to the status quo. Indeed Cain notes that it was 'the first right-wing grouping to come under the notice of the Bureau'.[43] The only real threat it posed was an electoral one. As will be seen, the election of December 1919 and Hughes's stake in it played a significant part in shaping the new Repatriation Commission and in further limiting benefits to returned soldiers.

The "Economy" government'[44] and 'the soldier question'[45]

Hughes returned to Australia at the end of August 1919 and almost immediately called an election.[46] The returned AIF represented around thirty to forty per cent of male wage-earners and about twenty per cent of those eligible to vote. Although some soldiers joined left-wing returned soldier organisations with political aims, at the end of 1919 the organisation with the greatest numbers was the RSSILA.[47] Given its membership of around 150 000 out of a total of 250 000 soldiers returned to Australia at that time, it was a small step for Hughes to treat the League as the most representative body, albeit reluctantly.[48] As he reminded the Chairman of the Repatriation Commission, Robert Gibson, 'for all practical purposes the Returned Soldiers' Association has sufficient of the soldiers in it to make it representative'.[49]

109

The Nationalist government had won power on a 'Win the War' platform in a time of crisis. It was an increasingly uneasy coalition and in order for Hughes to maintain his control over the leadership he needed a strong show of personal support from the electorate. The returned soldier vote was therefore of immense importance. During September, October and November, Hughes held conferences with the Executive of the League to find out what they wanted. Their list began with a paid Repatriation Commission of three which included one returned soldier nominated by the League and which was 'removed as far as possible from Ministerial control'. They also wanted co-ordination of the relevant functions of Defence, Treasury and Repatriation under one Department, a suggestion which Hughes applauded and which drew no opposition from Cabinet. Next was an increase in War Pensions according to a scheme prepared by the League, one which proposed 'no material increase' in government expenditure. Preferential employment was discussed again as was the funding and support of the 'Anzac Tweed' and other co-operative industries. Finally, the question of War Gratuities was raised. Of these issues, the value of War Pensions, the issuing of War Gratuities and the nature of the Commission were most important to electoral success, to Treasury and to returned soldiers.[50]

Debates between Hughes and the Repatriation Commission and the League over these matters reveal the disingenuousness of the claim by both the League's Executive and the federal government to be the champions of returned soldiers. It becomes increasingly clear that both groups were primarily interested in votes, in maintaining their numbers and thereby retaining power. For Gilbert Dyett, then leader of the League and a paragon of conservatism, the public announcement of government concessions often appeared more important than the concessions themselves.[51] As the Tasmanian representative put it to Hughes in a diplomatic attempt to defuse his confrontation with Dyett,

> May I suggest that the reason the President is emphasising that particular point will be clearer if I put it this way, amongst returned soldiers there is a certain amount of differences of opinion … It strengthens our unity and the hands of the Executive of the soldiers, if the returned soldiers can … receive some intimation so that we can make an announcement to the various State Branches that some of our work has reached a successful conclusion.[52]

Hughes's response placed equal emphasis on the political utility of making the first announcement:

> I myself have said to the soldiers of this country that I will see they get justice … I have to let the soldiers see that I have his interests at heart.[53]

How these interests were managed by the soldiers' friends requires detailed analysis.

War pensions

In the lead-up to the November election, Hughes made a number of rash promises to the Australian voting public. One of these was the appointment of a Royal Commission 'to inquire into the cost of living in relation to the minimum or basic wage'.[54] At this date real wages were less than the equivalent of the 1907 Harvester judgement in relation to the cost of living.[55] According to Macarthy, in 1919 the Harvester equivalent in Victoria was £3/17/3 per week while the average weekly wage of the lowest paid adult male in Victoria was £3/1/1 or 79% of the Harvester equivalent.[56] In 1920 this fell to 75%. But the Royal Commission's findings reveal the gross inadequacy of even the Harvester equivalent. According to their *Report*, the cost of living in 1920 for a couple with three children was about £5/16/6, that is, a 70% increase since 1914 and approximately 50% more than the Harvester equivalent.[57] But despite this enormous inflation, the lowest paid male worker in 1920 was being paid an amount only marginally higher than the cost of living in 1914. These rates and the Commission's findings have considerable significance when we look at the rates for War Pensions. (Figure 15)

Dyett's pension scheme proposed that, as in England, when the cost of living went down, so should the value of pensions. This suggestion was not acted on. It also allowed for a 20% increase in the pension but the increase was counter-balanced by a reduction

Figure 15. The cost of living and the basic wage, 1919-1920

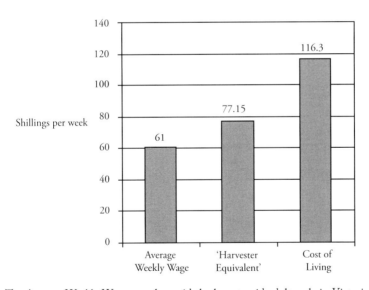

Note: The Average Weekly Wage was that paid the lowest paid adult male in Victoria in 1919. The 'Harvester Equivalent' is the 'monetary amount which at different times and in different parts of Australia was needed to buy the same "bundle" of goods and services which 7s a day (42s a week) could buy in Melbourne in 1907'. The Cost of Living is that arrived at for Victoria by the Royal Commission on the Basic Wage 1920.

Source: P.G. Macarthy, 'Wages for unskilled work, and margins for skill, Australia, 1901-21', AEHR, Vol.12, No.2, September 1972, pp.142-160; CPP, 1920, Vol.4, *Report of the Royal Commission on the Basic Wage*, 23 November 1920.

Figure 16. Comparative rates for war pensions by country 1920:
totally (temporarily) incapacitated Privates

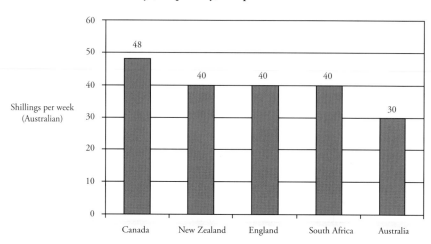

Source: AA(ACT): A2487, 21/372, Amendments to the Australian Soldiers' Repatriation Act
1917-1918

in the Sustenance allowance. The highly visible and politically volatile issue of War
Pensions was thereby made an electoral plus for both groups without any anticipated
strain on Treasury.[58] Hughes supported the proposal and, using figures quoted in an
unofficial Treasury appraisal, announced the 'new scheme' in a campaign speech in
Brisbane.[59] His announcement promised an increase in expenditure on War Pensions
of £650 000 and a new rate for blinded soldiers, a group who, like those who had lost
limbs, figured prominently in the rhetoric of repatriation. However, Treasury had made
an error. A Repatriation payment to widows supplementing their pensions had been
overlooked in the assessment of Departmental expenditure and the real cost of the
increase was subsequently estimated to be around £1 000 000. The Chief Accountant
of the Department estimated an increase of £1 500 000 above the then current annual
liability of £5 508 568.[60] After the election, these promises needed to be redeemed.

The December election gave the Nationalists a landslide victory in the Senate but
they lost ground in the House of Representatives. Indeed it was not until a by-election
in November 1920 that the government had a safe majority over Labor and the Country
Party.[61] During February and March of that year, Millen, the Commission and the
bureaucrats wrangled with Treasury and Cabinet over War Pensions. The battle was
over cost versus political backlash. For Millen, the key considerations were the value
of the Australian War Pension compared with other countries (Figures 16 and 17), the
demands of the RSSILA and avoidance of any real decrease in benefits. Treasury simply
reiterated that the total increase in expenditure had to be kept within the original 1919
assessment of £650 000.

Figure 17. Comparative rates for war pensions by country 1920:
totally (temporarily) incapacitated Privates with dependants

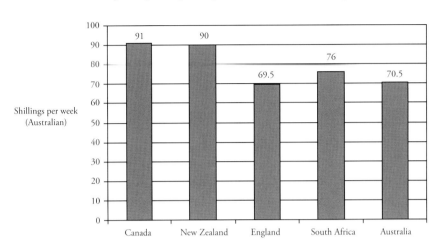

Source: AA(ACT): A2487, 21/372, Amendments to the Australian Soldiers' Repatriation Act
1917-1918

This intransigence provoked some imaginative proposals from the Department. Perhaps the most interesting was a sudden interest in democracy. War Pensions were still paid on a scale which was related to rank and army pay. In a Cabinet submission of 20 February, based upon suggestions of the Commission and key bureaucrats, Millen argued that

> discrimination in rate of pension as between privates and higher rank is not demo-cratic and should be abolished as far as possible in providing for benefits to members of a Volunteer Citizen Army.[62]

Such ideas do not appear to have penetrated the Defence Department when it raised and paid the 'Volunteer Citizen Army'. Their sudden appearance, in the midst of a dispute over the cost of War Pensions, is clearly a matter of pragmatism and not a visionary commitment to egalitarian ideals. In the ultimate Schedule, minor changes were effected by levelling out payments to all ranks below Captain while retaining the existing rates above that rank for the totally incapacitated soldier and his wife. (See Appendix 1). All pensions paid to widows and widowed mothers remained on the old rank-related basis. This system persisted until the provisions of the Financial Emergency Act took effect in 1931 when a common rate of pension for wives and children was introduced along with hefty cuts to all pensions. These new non-differential rates for dependent women and children were maintained after 1934 when other categories were restored to approximate pre-1930 rates. There were no other serious changes to the rank differentials until 1973.[63]

Gender also played a part in constraining costs. Widowed mothers of soldiers, it seems, were not perceived as a significant electoral bloc. In 1919, Pensions paid to widowed mothers of Privates were £1 per week while a totally incapacitated Private received £1/10/0. In the proposed schedule of new rates it was noted that 'under existing rates Widowed Mothers are amply provided for, and it is not desirable to provide any increase'. Allowances paid to children of widows were also maintained at original levels.[64] Pensions paid to widows of Privates were £1 per week but were calculated on the basis of '⅔rds of the lowest rate for incapacitated soldiers'. With an increase in the base rate of Pension paid to incapacitated soldiers, widows received an automatic increase. Given that the base rate was still significantly below the basic wage, paying a widow two-thirds of this inadequate 'wage' was tantamount to condemning her to destitution. The net increase in reality was a mere 3/6 per week, enough to buy 6 lbs (approximately 3 kg) of sugar or about one week's fuel supply for heating and cooking.[65]

Clearly the nature of these reforms to the pensioning system was piecemeal. Widows and widowed mothers received a rate of pension tied to rank which reflected a class differential, a gendered division of labour and a social framework which devalued women's work, both paid and unpaid. Worse, the changes brought no increase at all in pension income for widowed mothers or dependent children and only a token increase for widows despite the 70% increase in the cost of living since 1914. Yet perhaps the most imaginative sleight of hand in this figure conjuring business was the 'new' Pension rate for totally incapacitated soldiers.

As noted above, the War Pensions they received were £1/10/0 per week. However, in addition to the Pension, these soldiers received a supplementary allowance from the Repatriation Department in order to bring their income up to £2/2/0 per week, somewhat closer to overseas pension rates for the same category. In creating 'new' pension scales it was impossible to reduce this amount. The League's proposed scheme had taken account of this and suggested a new pension rate that combined both payments. This was precisely the scheme put forward by Millen. In other words, while the total monetary benefit paid to a totally incapacitated soldier remained the same, in the new Schedule the 'War Pension' was actually increased from £1/10/0 to £2/2/0 per week. Millen's explanation of the new Schedule bears quoting at length for what it reveals of the political and economic expediency underpinning the changes.

> The apparent anomaly that while there is an increase of a million and a quarter in the total expenditure there is, at the same time, no increase in the combined payments to any class (other than the small class represented by the blinded and the totally and *permanently* incapacitated) is explained by the fact that an increase in the basic rate for total (temporary) incapacity involves consequential percentage increases to the partially incapacitated. The partially incapacitated, much the most numerous class, do not, at present, receive supplementary living allowances under the Repatriation supplementary scale, whereas under a raised pension scale they would benefit proportionately.

Figure 18. War pensions in relation to cost of living 1920

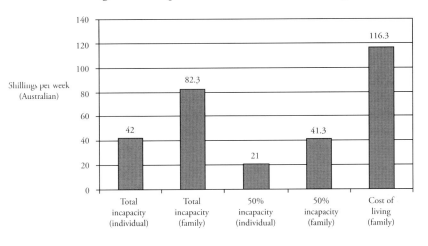

Note: 'Family' payments represent the pensions paid to a veteran with a dependant wife and three children. The 'family' cost of living is that cited by the Royal Commission on the Basic Wage for the same family unit in Victoria in 1920.

Source: CPP, 1920, Vol.4, *Report of the Royal Commission on the Basic Wage*, 23 November 1920; CPD, Vol.91, p.657, 24 March 1920.

In other words, the largest group of beneficiaries, the partially incapacitated soldier, who had previously been receiving only a fraction of the total incapacity pension of £1/10/0 and had not been eligible for a supplementary allowance, would now receive an increase in pension, albeit still only a fraction of a living wage. Under the new rates, a totally incapacitated soldier could receive £2/2/0 per week, his wife 18/- and three dependent children a further £1/2/6, making a total family income of £4/2/6. Most soldiers, however, were *not* totally incapacitated but partially incapacitated. This meant that the soldier, his wife and children, each received only a fraction of the full rate.[66] For example, a man assessed as having a 50% incapacity would receive only £1/1/-, his wife 9/- and the three children together 11/6 making a total family income of £2/1/6 which was less than half the cost of living for such a family. (Figure 18) Such computations were foremost in the minds of the Minister and his bureaucrats. As Millen informed Cabinet,

> Although it may involve a somewhat greater immediate cost, it has to be remembered that as a very considerable proportion of the pensions are in the 'indeterminate' category and subject to periodical review, it is obvious that once the maximum is reached there must thereafter be a gradual decline. However, current experience indicates that, in a general review, appreciable savings may be effected through close administration. During the sensitive period which we have just passed through, many supplementary allowances have been paid which the necessities of the individual did not fully warrant, and there is reason to believe that the same may be said in regard to pensions.

While they are explored in greater detail in subsequent chapters, a number of vital issues raised in this paragraph warrant brief comment. Perhaps the most critical is the recognition by Millen and his Department that most War Pensions were 'indeterminate', that is, the conditions they compensated were not fixed, static, unchanging states of health. They needed 'periodical review' by a medical officer. It was also believed that the number receiving such pensions would decline. That is, there is a clear connection between the review and a decrease in numbers. The other issue related to this is the reference to 'close administration'. Until the 1920 Act was passed, pensions were administered by Treasury. Millen clearly believed – and he was to be proven correct – that his bureaucrats would be more economic in their distribution of this particular benefit. Such arguments were helpful in convincing his Cabinet colleagues of the need for the proposed increase.

There were other factors which could be used to justify his proposals. The budgetary allocation required for the new scheme was around £1.25 million, that is twice the Treasury allocation, Millen argued that

> whilst the proposed schedule … represents an increase of 19.2%, the increase in the cost of living (house rent, food and groceries) has been 38% since August 1914 and 19% since the last revision of the War Pensions in 1916, also that the Old Age Pension rate has increased 50% since August 1914.

As noted above, the increase in the cost of living from 1914 as calculated by the Royal Commission was around 70% nationally not the 38% claimed by Millen. That aside, the Minister still needed to assure Cabinet that the new scheme and new rates would contain costs. To cap his arguments in this respect, Millen explained to his colleagues that the new Bill was designed to prevent the Repatriation Commission from granting any additional allowances to supplement the pension.

> I attach much importance to this as it will give finality to the rates affecting those payments which may be continued for indefinite periods. Hence the necessity for a schedule, in the first place, which will appeal to the public mind as adequate to the requirements.

The 'public mind' was accustomed to war propaganda where soldiers who had lost limbs or who were blind became symbols of the returned AIF. When the RSSILA asked for a special pension rate for blinded soldiers just prior to the election campaign, it was difficult for Hughes to refuse. This promise of a special rate, double that of the temporarily incapacitated soldier, once again had to be redeemed after the election. On this occasion, however, the Repatriation Commission were openly hostile. In submitting their draft Schedules to the new Act to Millen, the Commission noted that

> No attempt is made to justify this provision, which has only been included in the suggestions because it is understood that the Government is in some way committed to provide £4 per week for blinded soldiers.
> It is not considered that any satisfactory reason for this particular rate can be put

forward, but it is felt that it is utterly impossible to make such provision for the blinded soldier without doing the same for the 'totally and permanently incapacitated soldier' whose position in life, in the majority of cases, is far worse than that of the blinded soldier.[67]

This was hardly a serious fiscal problem. There were fewer than 100 totally blinded returned soldiers and fewer than 150 totally and permanently incapacitated soldiers in Australia.[68] Yet the Commission objected to the increased rate. It also recommended that wives of these pensioners should receive only 50% of the lower rate for temporarily incapacitated soldiers and that the special allowance then paid for an 'attendant' be dropped, as well as a housing allowance. These recommendations were incorporated in the new Act.[69]

In the same document the Commission also suggested a number of new provisions regarding pensioning including the following suggested Clause for the Act:

The Commissioner of Pensions shall have power to reject a claim for a pension from the dependant of a soldier or to terminate a pension granted to any such dependant in any case where he is of opinion that such person is unworthy of a pension.

An explanatory note was appended to rationalise the inclusion of this clause:

There have been cases where persons have been granted pensions to which they were legally entitled and which the Department has been powerless to terminate, although definite knowledge has been in the Department's possession that the pensioner was utterly unworthy and it was a public disgrace that the pension should have been continued.

The clause was not included in its original form but Section 37 of the new Act allowed that

A [State] Board may reject a claim for a pension by a dependant of a member of the Forces, or may terminate any pension granted to such a dependant, if the Board is satisfied that the grant or continuance of the pension is undesirable.

Cleansed of the language of moral certitude, the discretionary power of this Section still allowed the 'suitable men' of the bureaucracy ample room to manoeuvre.

In the end, Millen's arguments, like those of his bureaucracy, were successful. Treasury finally capitulated under pressure from Hughes, who seems to have been convinced of the safeguards put in place, the minimal net increase and the political necessity of appearing to increase the rates.[70] Debates in the House over this part of the Bill were perfunctory. Who, after all, was prepared to argue publicly against an increase in benefits to Australia's returned soldiers? War Gratuities were another matter.

A 'most odious piece of corruption'[71]

According to Pryor, 'the payment of a war gratuity to returned soldiers was, perhaps, associated with one of the most distasteful developments in the repatriation policy'. For Pryor, the 1919 election was fought mainly on this issue.[72] Opportunistic politicians used the Gratuity to 'bribe' soldiers and many returned men 'spent their gratuities on some wasteful or temporary enjoyment'. The immense sum involved 'could have been devoted to the purposes of civil re-establishment in a much more definite and more profitable manner'.[73]

But within a discourse on the politics of returned soldier organisations, obtaining the Gratuity can be seen as a jewel in the crown, an 'unassailable benchmark' in the history of the RSSILA.[74] It symbolised the concerned efforts of its leaders to obtain for Australian returned soldiers a reward then being paid in New Zealand, South Africa, Great Britain and Canada. From the transcripts of meetings between Hughes and the League Executive, the official historians of the League construct a scenario in which the valiant President 'fought hard' for a cash lump-sum payment against an 'intransigent' and 'irascible' Prime Minister who finally convinced them of the need for a payment in non-negotiable bonds. The League Executive are portrayed as passively agreeing to such a suggestion on the grounds that it was 'against the national financial interest to press for the cash payment'.

More attentive reading of the transcripts reveals a somewhat different picture. At his meeting with the Executive on 16 October, the first meeting at which War Gratuities were discussed at any length and for which transcripts survive, Hughes opened discussion by announcing, in a pot pourri of metaphors,

> I am in favour of a gratuity, but I am not able to make bricks without straw or clay or whatever they make them out of, and I must cut my coat according to my cloth.[75]

After a brief résumé of the costs and benefits of Gratuities overseas, Hughes made it clear to the League that the Australian war debt precluded use of revenue for a cash payment and that loans from Britain were out of the question. In response, Dyett proposed an alternative:

> Have you considered the idea of issuing war loan certificates? That is the way out of it … Supposing you say you will pay so much for the first year and give scrip for the two years, to be presented at the termination of that period, which would not be negotiable in the meantime. Why not make them keep this scrip? Why let them sell?[76]

Hughes was quickly convinced of the 'business-like' nature of this suggestion although he remained unconvinced as to whether it would be satisfactory either to the Government or the soldiers. Still, an amicable agreement was reached and Hughes took the matter to Cabinet.[77]

In Australian federal politics, the Gratuity was clearly an issue on the electoral knife-edge. Hughes announced the bonus whilst on the campaign trail in Brisbane on 22 October. The following day, in the dying hours of Parliament, Watt attempted to pre-empt criticism over the lack of notification or opportunity for debate by assuring the House that the government had taken the 'democratic course' of putting the question to the electorate. The sum of money involved was vast, he argued, and the government required a mandate from the people before it could consider the issue any further. Even the Labor left had to agree with this, albeit reluctantly.[78] As a result, with both sides committed to the principle of a mandate, the election became a tussle over means of payment and over the source of finance. For the conservative government it was important to reassure Australian capital that such a measure would not be funded from revenue nor would it entail more debt. The solution was the non-negotiable bonds proposed by Dyett but funded from anticipated war reparations, estimated to be worth between £7 and £10 million and due by mid 1921.[79]

For Labor the only course open was to promise cash and immediate payment. Indeed one hopeful Senator promised the Gratuity before Christmas.[80] The sources of finance were to be the traditional enemies of labour: the 'war profiteers', the 'Mining King', the shipping companies and the banks.[81] The Nationalists' incessant references to national debt, to Australia's incapacity to pay the Gratuity and the need for 'economy', were labelled 'nonsense and bunkum'. Tudor and others were trenchant in their condemnation of such spurious claims, pointing out that in mid 1918, when the war was expected to last at least another two years, Hughes and the Nationalists were facing an obligation to raise over £100 million in Australia for war purposes on top of the £200 million already raised.[82] War Gratuities were estimated to cost around £25 million and were therefore well within these loan estimates.[83]

For the government, debate on the Bill provided an opportunity to represent *their* War Gratuity as a flower of democracy. Unlike War Pensions, the Bill proposed a flat rate for all ranks, making it unique within the Empire. Hughes was apparently captivated by this strategy, assuring the House that the Gratuity made no distinction between ranks but

> treats all alike, as is, I think, proper in a democratic country like Australia, with its democratic army. Much of the success of the Australian army lay in the fact that its organisation was essentially democratic …The scheme in this Bill rests upon this basis, and the scheme is not only democratic but equitable and liberal.[84]

This 'democratic', 'equitable and liberal' scheme, copied from the New Zealand arrangement, amounted to 1/6 per day of service with numerous qualifications on the definition of 'service' and on who was eligible.[85] An average payout seems to have been anticipated at around £100 to £150, or 5-6 months wages for a family, plus interest.[86] What recipients did with this sum appears to have been of little interest to anyone but the government. In announcing the proposal to seek a mandate in October 1919, Watt alluded to 'arrangements' then being made to allow the use of the bonds to pay Commonwealth loans for land or homes, thus giving Treasury the opportunity to recoup some part of the value of its loans to soldiers or to the states.[87]

The 'suitable men' who staffed the Repatriation bureaucracy, and determined its functional meaning, were quick to see the utility of the Gratuity. From November to March, the Deputy Comptrollers in all states wrote repeatedly to Gilbert as to whether

Gratuities could be used to recoup so-called 'bad debts'.[88] For J. Claude Henderson, DC in Brisbane, the 'deliberate delinquents' who accepted Departmental loans and then failed 'through their own fault', were an obvious target. For the DC in Adelaide, J.W. Bell, there were two problem categories: those who sold Departmental property purchased by way of loan and then 'decamped' without a trace, and those who 'allowed their assets to evaporate ... and are now not in possession of sufficient cash or property to warrant an action by the Department'.[89] A number of 'test cases' were also forwarded to the Comptroller for direction.

The Departmental reaction to this situation was swift. Gilbert asked Treasury under what conditions it would accept Gratuity bonds. In particular he asked whether they could be used to repay Repatriation Department loans. Such a use was also considered by Cabinet prior to the Bill reaching Parliament. Notwithstanding the speed of the Bill's passage through Parliament, on 19 April Gilbert confidently predicted that an amendment was imminent. And so it was. The Amendment to Section 7 of the Act prescribed that 'any amount due to the Commonwealth' by the grantee could be deducted from the Gratuity 'where the indebtedness ... was caused by fraud, deception or mis-appropriation' or where the recipient had 'improperly disposed of property' loaned or otherwise owned by the Department.[90] When the Bill was passed, two days later, Gilbert cabled all the DCs to immediately prepare lists of 'offenders'.

As with War Pensions, Millen's bureaucrats rose to the occasion. While the Bill was being finalised, Tilney (DC Perth) suggested that since around 10% of soldiers in receipt of loans had 'moved from [their] original address leaving no trace of whereabouts', these soldiers had deliberately intended to evade payment and were therefore defrauding the Department. Elvins, the Departmental Accountant, supported this view and advised Gilbert that by giving the wrong address there was a 'case of indebtedness thro' fraud'.[91] Over the next six months these expanded definitions of 'fraud' and 'deception' allowed the Victorian branch of the Department alone to recoup over £20 000.[92]

The authority to make deductions from War Gratuities was contained in Regulation 401a (ii) of Treasury's War Financial Instructions. This Regulation provided that a District Finance Officer of the Department of Defence or the Navy Office needed nothing more than a certificate from a Deputy Comptroller stating that the amount was recoverable from the Gratuity under Section 7 of the Act: the DC's certificate was 'sufficient evidence to warrant action'. By June of 1921, the Departmental use of the Gratuity appears to have roused the indignation of the Central War Gratuity Board who complained to Treasury that the Department was using the Gratuity 'as a line of the least resistance for recovering amounts due to the Department where no case of fraud, deception or mis-appropriation could be proved in a Civil Court'. Treasury conveyed this information to the Chairman (then Semmens) commenting that in their view the existing procedure was satisfactory. Elvins, the Departmental Accountant, had the final word on this matter:

Advise DCs [Deputy Commissioners] it is not proposed to withdraw previous instructions. Deception stands by reason of removal [of soldier from address] but D.C. must prove that the soldier's intention by removing from place to place was deliberate. This could be proved by reason of monthly notices being ignored etc etc.[93]

The 'system' operated efficiently thanks to the careful selection of 'suitable men' to fill key positions, men who could ensure 'close administration'. However, the government had promised a new Commission and that posed a new set of problems for Millen in terms of staffing.

The new Repatriation Commission

From at least late 1918, the RSSILA were urging the formation of a paid Repatriation Commission of three men, with one a nominated representative of the League.[94] This request was revived during Hughes's meetings with the League in October 1919. Hughes claimed he supported the request. Similarly, the existing Commission did not oppose the idea of a paid Commission carrying out the administrative work, indeed Gibson indicated that their current workload was 'something more than any Government would expect men to do in an honorary capacity'. However, while the Commission was 'only too willing and pleased to serve' and not wanting 'any reward in any shape or form', they baulked at a new Commission taking over their advisory role. As Gibson explained to Hughes in words reminiscent of Millen's original proposal, 'we have no jobs to lose and we have no money to gain'.

> If we have ability to advise … then I think we are a great source of strength to the Government in resisting that political pressure which the soldier question must always bring forward … The present commission acts as a buffer.[95]

While the Commission advocated a paid administrative body it also wanted the creation of an Advisory Council which would interpret the Regulations. Gibson asked Hughes to 'consider the advisability of obtaining some of the present Committee on that body'. The Deputy Chairman was adamant that the administrative load he and his colleagues were bearing should go to a paid Commission and equally adamant that the existing Commission, under a new name, should act in a 'legislative' capacity in regard to interpreting Regulations under the Act.

What Gibson was referring to when he spoke of administrative work sufficient to occupy three highly paid Commissioners is not entirely clear. Minutes of meetings of the Commission from its inception in mid 1918 to just prior to its dissolution in early 1920 indicate that the Commission did little else but interpret Regulations. It also indicates who was doing the work. Initially, attendance at Commission meetings by the honorary Commissioners was adequate to the task. For example, from July to November 1918, there were thirty meetings, some of which were held over two days. Gibson was the only member to attend all of these. Other members' attendance was as indicated in Figure 19.

121

Figure 19. Attendance of Commissioners at Meetings of the Repatriation Commission,
July to November 1918 (30 meetings)

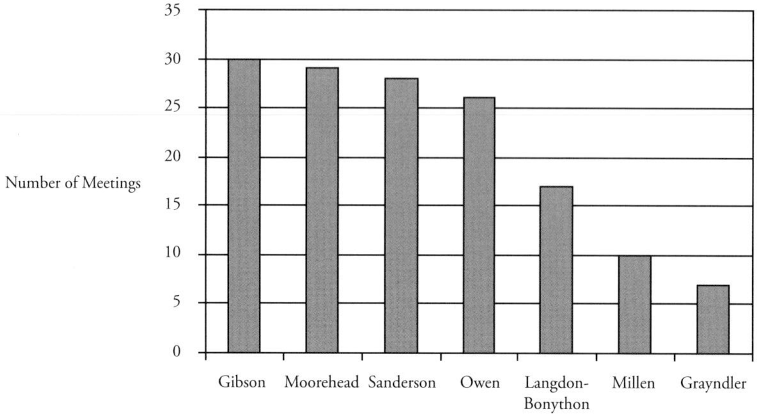

Source: Repatriation Commission, Minutes of Meetings, July to November 1918.

Millen's, Grayndler's, Langdon-Bonython's and Owen's attendance progressively declined over this period while the number of Special Cases referred to the Commission by the States rose from 6 to over 50 per session in the same period. By July of 1919, by which time Semmens had replaced Owen, a core group consisting of Gibson, Semmens and Moorehead were the effective decision-makers. At times Gibson alone *was* the Commission, his decisions on cases being ratified by the remainder of the quorum of three at the following meeting. On many other occasions, two of these three Commissioners were the only attendees.[96]

By December, when the RSSILA and the government were publicly debating the future of the Commission, this pattern had become more or less fixed. Robert Gibson, James Semmens and Harold Moorehead interpreted the Regulations and acted as final arbiters on the welfare of thousands of ex-soldiers. By this date, with the tightening of the Regulations described above, the State Boards made recommendations less frequently, simply forwarding cases for a 'decision' by the Commission. The progressive restriction of eligibility meant more of the cases submitted were refused and increasingly this refusal was made on the basis of a Departmental Medical Officer's report. At the meeting of 11 December 1919, for example, of 42 cases considered, 37 were 'Refused'; at the meeting of 19 December, 22 of 37 cases were 'Refused'. By early 1920, as ex-soldiers were denied assistance, found work or disappeared from the books of the Department, there was a clear decline in the number of cases submitted. In March, for example, there was an average of 20-30 cases per sitting of the Commission.

As well, by this date the Commission was more inclined to over-rule State Board recommendations granting assistance. At the meeting of 11 March 1920, for example, twenty cases were considered and of these only eight were approved. Of the eight, two were for allowances to blind soldiers, two were loans of £42 to Law Clerks for their 'admission fee' to the Bar in Victoria, one was a Gift of £40 for University fees and one a £5 Grant.[97] The remaining two were considered 'Special Cases', one being a small loan to an incapacitated soldier for furniture, the other a Living Allowance equivalent to 15/- per week to a widow with three dependent children, whose health was 'not too good', and who had been forced to give up work to look after a sick father.

Those refused assistance by the Commission also warrant attention. William Scott, for example, a bricklayer out of work for the six months since his return to Australia, applied for sustenance while awaiting employment. In his application he explained that because of the strikes there had been no work and that he was 'up against it during the first strike but refrained from appealing for sustenance'.[98] The Officer in Charge of Employment recommended 'favourable consideration'. The medical report was of a gun shot wound to the buttock with no disability. The State Board simply referred the case to the Commission for decision without recommendation and the Commission refused the application.

Amy Grady was the defacto wife of G.M. Turner, who died on service, with one dependent child. She applied for a Living Allowance to supplement her War Pension of 30/- on the grounds that the Defence Department had paid her a Separation Allowance in addition to Turner's 'allocation' from his Army pay, thereby officially recognising the relationship. The Investigating Officer recommended the granting of the Allowance and the Board referred the case to the Commission who decided they did 'not feel disposed to grant a Living Allowance to [the] applicant on [the] evidence submitted'.

Harvey Gordon, a married man with two children, had been a wool presser and horse breaker prior to the war and claimed he earned £8 per week. Back home, after the war, he found a job as a clerk on £3/15/0 per week and in addition received a pension of £1/1/1½ for war injuries which were still under treatment. His total income was thus £4/16/1½ or approximately 82% of the cost of living. At some unspecified period he had also been paid 'sustenance'. In February 1917 Gordon was loaned £25 by the Department to purchase furniture. By March 1920 he had made no repayments and wrote to Hughes requesting the loan be converted to a gift since, he argued, he lost considerable work time receiving medical treatment. The State Officer in Charge of Assistance recommended against the appeal, the Board referred the case to the Commission without comment. The Commission's decision was recorded as follows:

> It is pointed out that according to the File, applicant has been in receipt of suste-nance, presumably during periods when he was incapacitated from following his ordinary occupation. In addition to this, it is pointed out that applicant is in receipt of a pension of £1/1/1½ per week, which represents more than the lost time indi-cated in the evidence. He is not a totally incapacitated man within the meaning of the Regulations and there would be no more justification in granting him a gift of £25 for the furniture than there would be in hundreds of similar cases. Under the circumstances, the Commission cannot treat it as a special case and the application is refused.

The unremitting efforts of the 'suitable men' in framing and then refining the Regulations allowed the Commission sufficient discretionary power to arbitrarily refuse assistance, as in the case of Amy Grady, without reference to the Regulations. But they also provided legitimated weapons with which to beat off the 'undeserving'. The Regulations were a bulwark against the liberalisation of benefits to those perceived as morally defective or economically unproductive, Gilbert's and Millen's 'residuum'. They allowed the Commission to override the State Boards' 'sympathetic' treatment of ex-soldiers or their dependants by calling on the imperative of staying 'within the Regulations'. The League's demand for representation and for a paid Commission without Ministerial control could therefore be seen as potentially disruptive or, at worst, a source of prodigal expenditure. Bearing in mind that Repatriation expenditure was second only to Defence expenditure at this date, it is not surprising that Hughes refused to contemplate the removal of Ministerial control during his negotiations over this issue with the League.[99]

Yet in effect, by the end of 1919, the Commission of three requested by the League already existed. Semmens's presence ensured AIF representation at sittings and with Gibson representing conservative interests and simultaneously dominating proceedings, the Nationalist government had an ideal working group. Indeed when Hughes cabled Millen in mid October requesting his approval of the new arrangement, Millen was surprised and critical, doubting both the 'wisdom and necessity for [the] proposed change of Commission'. For Millen, the bulk of the work was over and the scheme was 'in working order'.[100] The combination of two 'suitable men' on the Commission and a set of Regulations and Rules that reflected the ideology and the pragmatic economy of a conservative government could hardly have worked better. But Millen was first and foremost a politician. He readily agreed to Cabinet's wishes acknowledging the importance of the issue to the election outcome. After the election, it was a question of maintaining the status quo.

The Bill for the Australian Soldiers' Repatriation Act of 1920, which repealed the previous Act along with the War Pensions Act, was introduced into the Senate by Millen in March. It is clear that he understood the function of the existing Commission very well, despite Gibson's claims about the burden of administrative work. With his usual bluntness, Millen informed his colleagues that 'the present Commission is not an administrative body. It is really a legislative body for the Repatriation Department'.

> It determines the benefits to be allotted and hears appeals from applicants dissatisfied with the Board's decisions.[101]
>
> I desire to say, quite frankly, that I do not think the new Commission, apart from its administrative functions, will discharge the duties now performed by the honorary Commission in a better way, or with a greater measure of success. The soldiers have expressed a very strong desire in favour of the appointment of a paid body, on which they shall have direct representation, and surely their views should be considered ... It seems that by substituting a new body, even if we do not secure better

results, we shall be imparting to the minds of the soldiers confidence in the administration; and if we do that, we shall have achieved something.[102]

In other words, as far as Millen was concerned the new *structure* would make no appreciable difference to the working of the Department. What was of critical importance to Millen, however, was the nature of the office-bearers. Again and again he stressed the need for 'competent men', 'men who are best equipped for the job', 'men with some business knowledge', men with 'merit and ability of no mean order, in addition to the right personality and temperament'. The government needed 'efficiency', particularly in the handling of War Pensions and that required 'suitable men'.[103]

Millen would not be drawn on the precise salary for such men but commented that he 'had always held that the Commonwealth pays insufficient salaries to its chief executive officers'.[104] The *Age* was more specific, predicting £1500 per annum for the Chairman who, it forecast, would be D.J. Gilbert, and the other members Semmens and a Lt Col Wanliss, each on £1000.[105] At this date Gilbert's salary as Comptroller was £900, yet the Principal Medical Officer and the Director of Vocational Training were each receiving £1000. When Tudor raised this anomaly in the House he was told that the government 'could not expect to get a good doctor for a lower salary'.[106]

As it transpired, the *Age* forecasts were only partly correct. The final salaries were £1500 for the Chairman and £1250 for the other members. Gilbert had 'certain business undertakings' and wished to retire as soon as possible.[107] As for the other members of the honorary Commission, Gibson, Sanderson and Langdon-Bonython were hardly likely to give up their financial empires to become full-time public servants. Grayndler's role in the AWU undoubtedly precluded him from selection even if he had shown some interest in the work of the Commission. In 1920 Moorehead was only twenty-seven years of age and although his attendance record at the Commission meetings was admirable, his brief pre-war career as a journalist hardly fitted Millen's criteria for 'suitable men'.[108] That left Semmens, the career public servant, former intelligence officer and committed member of the Commission.

After the passage of the Act, Semmens was duly appointed Chairman. Joining him as co-member appointed by the government was Major James Edward Barrett, another of Lockyer's co-opted bureaucrats who had moved from Deputy Comptroller in Adelaide in 1918 to DC Melbourne the following year and then to departmental Inspector for the Commonwealth in 1920, a position he held when appointed to the new Commission. Barrett had a long association with the militia. He joined the South Australian Mounted Rifles as a private in 1900 aged twenty-six and by 1910 he was a Captain in the 17th Light Horse Regiment. He served on Gallipoli with the 3rd Light Horse but was medically evacuated in November 1915. Prior to the war he is described as an 'Accountant, in business as a general storekeeper'.[109]

The RSSILA nominee was Colonel Chaplain Ashley H. Teece. Teece was with the 6th Light Horse in Egypt from 1915 until he was invalided home in 1917. After his return he became active in the League, filling several official posts including Vice-President of the South Australian branch of the League at about the time Barrett was President and soon after the Presidency of Rev. J.C. McPhee, Secretary to the Commission from 1918 to 1926 and subsequently DC for Victoria until 1939. In 1920 Teece was a member of the Federal Executive.[110] Teece is an unremarkable individual until his connections are examined. In 1907, Teece married Muriel Giblin, daughter of Mr Justice Giblin and brother of L.F. Giblin, sometime Commonwealth Statistician, Director of the Commonwealth Bank, and Ritchie Professor of Economics at Melbourne University. Of perhaps more importance here, L.F. Giblin was also a member of the AIC in Tasmania from 1909 at the same time as E.L. Piesse, one of the major civil intelligence figures of the war years and the ensuing decade. Giblin was seconded to the Intelligence Section of General Staff in 1914 and remained active in intelligence until at least 1923, during the period when he was also Government Statistician for Tasmania and Deputy Commonwealth Statistician.[111]

Yet it was not just Teece's brother-in-law who was notable. His father Richard was the 'master-mind' behind the growth of the AMP Society and of his brothers, both Richard Clive and Roy had outstanding legal careers. Roy has also been described as 'one of the pioneer builders' of the League, being President of the New South Wales Branch from 1918 to 1920.[112] However, the other feature of Roy's career of interest here is his membership of the AIC. He joined the Corps in 1913 becoming temporary Assistant Censor of 2nd Military District in 1914 and like Giblin then joined the Intelligence Section of the General Staff. Also like Giblin he remained attached to the AIF during the early 1920s, in this case as Legal Staff Officer. Ashley Teece's connections could thus be seen as reflecting at least one departmental characteristic.

Historically where does this tangled web of connections lead? There are no categorical statements to be made on the composition of the new Commission. There was no straightforward class basis to the choices and in the case of Teece, there was no career experience. All that can be said of the three is that they had credentials as patriotic gentlemen; all had 'served' as officers. Yet militarism was not *the* defining characteristic of the Commission or the Department, despite 'preference'. What we see is more an expression of a ruling 'culture' than the embodiment of a ruling class, an expression of the values of individualism, pragmatism and traditional political economy. In these appointments, as was the case with Private Eade in 1918, the 'culture' and ideology are manifest, while a discrete ruling class is not.

Millen had clearly been satisfied with the work carried out by Gibson and Semmens and, once forced to accept a new group of 'suitable men', chose those who would least disturb the status quo. Provided the Chairman of the new Commission was a trustworthy man, and powerful enough in concert with the other government appointment to withstand the anticipated demands of the League's representative, there was no cause for concern. Indeed the history of the Department over the next decade provides ample evidence that this was the case. Early evidence of Semmens's power and influence can be gauged by the appointment of H. Gordon Bennett as DC in Sydney in 1920, an appointment 'presented' to Bennett by his old commanding officer.[113]

The power, both fiscal and social, exercised by the new Commission was immense. The addition of War Pensions to the activities of the Department greatly expanded the responsibility placed on the individuals interpreting the Regulations and deciding appeals. The composition of the new Commission made it even better adapted to the government's goals than its predecessor. The outgoing Commission, while conforming to the conservative ideology which governed the Department, had been beyond Millen's control unless he exercised his veto, something he would have undoubtedly been loath to do to a major capitalist like Gibson or Langdon-Bonython. A bureaucrat, on the other hand, was within his control. The new structure and the new office-holders provided the government with a perfect vehicle for the pursuit of its goals. To the government the new Commission's greatest asset was therefore its instrumentality. While it wielded great power and was to attract significant honours for its members, the Commission was always vulnerable to dismissal and its existence predicated on Ministerial approval. One other group in the decision-making hierarchy shared this predicament. That group and its activities during the 1920s forms the subject matter of the following chapters – the former AAMC doctors who staffed the Department's war pensions arm.

CHAPTER 7

War, Medicine and Responsibility for Illness

In order to understand the significance of medical knowledge and medical practitioners to both the Army and the Repatriation Department in the early twentieth century
it is necessary to understand something of the history of medicine. It is particularly
important to understand the changes that occurred in medicine's stature within society
in the period (see Chapter 5), but more important to understand the major shift in
understanding of the world medicine and science inhabited between the late eighteenth
and early twentieth centuries. This is not a discursive philosophical detour but rather a
means to understand the way massive social changes affected an enquiring and burgeoning profession.

To do justice to this subject is impossible here. Instead this chapter starts with a
thumbnail sketch of the main shifts in scientific and medical thought in the century
prior to the Great War.

Medicine and health

In 1835, one year after the passing of the New Poor Law, the Scottish chemist and writer
Andrew Ure remarked that 'when capital enlists science in her service, the refractory
hand of labour will always be taught docility'.[1] Ure's attention was explicitly directed
at the technology which, by its development and application in manufacturing, allowed
greater profits to be made. Yet his comment is equally apposite in describing the function
of the Poor Law. In this case science, in its medical guise, not only intervened in poor
relief, but simultaneously, and for the first time determined that contracts for the care of
the poor were confined to medical men.[2]

By the end of the century, science as medicine was legitimating state intervention in
the health of workers and the health and safety of the workplace. By the 1920s, due in
part to the Great War, medical men (and this was then almost entirely a male enclave)
were firmly ensconced in highly complex medico-legal bodies as mediators of the
relationship between the worker and the state. Workers compensation, invalid pensions
and war pensions had become the doctor's domain.

One part of the reason medicine was able to achieve its new stature was because
historically it was allowed to fashion not simply specific medical knowledge but

definitions of health and disease – and therefore 'life'. Critics would argue that medical knowledge is inadequate and inexact because it is value-laden and far from autonomous, and because it does not address a social being but rather a pathological and biological entity.[3] How then has it become a paradigm?

In the late eighteenth and early nineteenth centuries, when science emerged as the chief bearer of reason in a rationalised cosmology, medicine as the art of healing humanity was slowly transformed into the science of healing the body. Cartesian dualism had described a separation of mind (spirit/God's province) from body (machine) which was ultimately elaborated in the development of bodily science.[4] Initially preoccupied with determination of the animate/inanimate boundary and with the very nature of vitality, the early nineteenth-century physiologists, Müller, Richerand, Bell and others, looked to comparative anatomy for what historian Karl Figlio has described as 'a patient, observing and unintruding science appropriate to the study of life'.[5] Life was inviolable and sacred even if it did reside somewhere in the anatomical components of the body.

By the mid nineteenth century what has been described as an engineering model in the perception and study of the body emerged: that is, a technological approach.[6] The parts and compartments of the body and their individual functions became more important than the individual's purpose and integrity. The search for pure and autonomous knowledge of the body became more important than the idealised enrichment of human life. One of the most important intellectual currents which this mechanistic, engineered model encouraged was the idea of intervention. If the body could be defined as merely a conglomeration of parts and functions and the idea of life could be dispensed with as a metaphysical entity, then vivisection and experimentation were possible.[7]

This conceptual understanding had its clearest expression in the writings of the French physiologist Claude Bernard. In his 1865 treatise, *Introduction to the Study of Experimental Medicine*, Bernard wrote at some length on the meaning of life and the place of vitalism in science. The essence of his writings is expressed in the following exhortation to his readers:

> we must always seek to exclude life entirely from our explanation of physiological phenomena as a whole. Life is nothing but a word …[8]

As Figlio has noted, 'with this identification of knowledge with unlimited intervention, and with the dissociation of means from ends, it became increasingly easy to justify *any* intervention'.[9]

The growth of experimental medicine, of technological intrusion into the body, also meant that norms were rapidly developed. Georges Canguilhem has written that 'between 1759, when the word 'normal' appeared, and 1834 when the word 'normalised' appeared, a normative class had won the power to identify … the function of social norms, whose content it determined, with the use that that class made of them'.[10] Notions of disease, illness and sickness all became deviations from these norms: therapeutics became the intervention which restored normalcy so defined.

Thus, by the 1860s or 1870s, the major conceptual elements of modern medicine were firmly established. What had made this possible was what Foucault has called the 'birth of the clinic': that is, hospital medicine.[11] In Britain, rapid industrialisation with its associated problems created a surplus pool of labour forced to rely on private charity for sustenance. The Poor Law and its subsequent amendments meant that incarceration in one of a growing number of state-funded institutions was often the only alternative to starvation. Sick paupers provided an unprecedented source of material for the taxonomists of disease as much as for the experimenters – whether in physiological theory or therapeutic technique.[12] Simultaneously, the individualism which underwrote bourgeois liberalism found its expression in medicine not only in the corollary to the deserving and undeserving poor – the deserving and undeserving sick – but also in theories of disease aetiology (cause). According to these theories, the hereditary or innate weakness of the individual was responsible for the success of the pathogen in its invasion of the body.[13]

At about the same time, public health measures, inspired by the work of the (medical) social reformers Robert Koch, Rudolf Virchow and others in Germany, found their way into Britain as working conditions in factories were linked to working class morbidity as well as mortality.[14] The underbelly of industrialisation became apparent in a plethora of reports and public inquiries on the conditions of the working class.[15] Consequently, the state stepped in to contain, observe and police the health of workers through the use of medical factory inspectors and school inspectors. In addition, laws were passed seemingly to protect workers from the worst ravages of the factory.[16] The introduction of these measures, which reached a peak in the first decade of the new century both in Britain and Australia, and which saw a corresponding increase in state intervention – defying the tenets of laissez-faire capitalism – was frequently legitimated via science and scientific medicine.[17] The new discipline of epidemiology benefited from these trends and contagion theories appeared which emphasised environmental conditions: housing, sanitation, ventilation and so forth. The possibility that the determinant of such oppressive living conditions was economic was not addressed, but rather scientific medical theory emerged which made the slum demolition, sewerage works, ventilation of factories and other measures appear to be the right and natural correctives. That these same measures dispossessed thousands of workers and their families and made little serious difference to their living or working conditions was the ideological function of medicine: that is, it translated the social or economic into the 'natural' or 'environmental'.

It can be seen that two major and inherently antagonistic aetiological strands developed simultaneously in medical theory: the one blaming the individual; the other, environmental causes. These divergent theoretical paths found their expression within the war pensioning process in the issue of whether an illness or disease was 'war-related', a concept explored at length in Chapter 8.

War and medicine

The relationship between war and medicine is complex. The positivist tradition, which has dominated medicine, would recount the progress made in medical science, the therapeutic advancement and the general expansion of medical knowledge which resulted from the Great War. This argument would go on to detail the mass of diverse experience medical men gathered; the opportunities for technical experimentation on hundreds of thousands of similar injuries in order to find the 'best' treatment; the extraordinary opportunity for de-facto vivisection in examination and treatment of mutilated bodies; the 'discoveries' in pathology and disease aetiology; and, of course, the chance to observe and treat so-called deviant behaviour on an unprecedented scale. There is also the fillip given to the profession by an increase in the demand for services; this led to increasing specialisation and professionalisation.[18] The conclusion to the positivist argument would be that this 'mass of clinical material' and its use as 'evidence' were 'sufficient to eliminate sources of error'.[19]

This argument hinges on at least two important pre-suppositions. First, that published research ('evidence' in this context) guarantees the validity of a proposition; and, second, that the extent of research (the 'mass of clinical material') eliminates error. Both propositions can of course be considered fraught with problems in contemporary scientific discourse yet their persistence bears witness to the longevity of the positivist tradition. The entire tradition is built on the premise of the function of war in and for medicine and therefore begs the question: what was the function of medicine in war?

In a seminal article on the relationship between war and modern medicine, Roger Cooter has noted that 'virtually everything that has been written on the subject of war and medicine stresses that the former, for all its horrors, has brought benefit to the latter'.[20] This premise is reiterated by Cooter and Steve Sturdy in *War, Medicine and Modernity* where the authors rightly point out that 'it is not enough to ask simply whether war is good or bad for medicine. What is needed is an account of the relationship between war and medicine that is sensitive to the role of both in society more generally'.[21] The 'triumphalist reckonings' of the positivist tradition, the 'self-serving narratives of technical and organisational advancement' that dominate the literature they describe, are to be decried in favour of a theoretically sophisticated historical and sociological analysis of the relationship between war, medicine and modernity, the latter being defined in a strictly Weberian sense. While the characteristics of Weber's modernity – rationality, standardisation, organisation, routinisation – are indeed examined at various junctures in this work, notably in relationship to the Repatriation bureaucracy where such phenomena have a heuristic value, this work has sought to look more broadly at what Macpherson has described as a whole of society or ideological framework.[22] And it is within that framework that the relationship between war and medicine is examined here.

Before moving on to an exploration of the function of medicine in war, the 'goodness of war' literature conceals two further benefits to doctors that deserve noting in passing.

Trainee surgeons, those who wanted their Fellowship of the Royal College of Surgeons (FRCS), needed surgical experience. There is no question that conditions on the Western Front provided all the surgical experience any hopeful could ask for and the DMS, Howse, was well known for his patronage. As Tyquin tells us 'promising doctors were transferred to units near the front where they could hone their skills whether surgical, medical, orthopaedic, plastic or neurological'.[23] In 1917, Howse (a surgeon) wrote a discursive confidential letter to the DGMS in Australia, Fetherston (another surgeon), on the state of things in England and France. Howse at this date had three ADMSs assisting him at Headquarters in London: Reginald Millard, Victor Hurley and Donald Mackenzie. (Sir) Victor Hurley became DGMS to the RAAF in World War Two. By the date of Howse's letter (June 1917) Hurley had managed to fit in his first FRCS exam while attached to Howse in London. Howse then posted him as '2nd Operating Surgeon' to the 2nd AGH in France where he could 'could get on with his surgical work, or he will find himself left by a number of younger men'; 'he will be responsible for half the Surgical work …He now intends to go up for his final [FRCS examination] in November … His final should be an easy proposition'.[24] Hurley was awarded a CMG, like Kenneth Smith at the 1st ADH, prior to his departure for France, in other words for administrative work.[25]

The other benefit worth mentioning (yet again) is linked to this, and Howse's own words are worth repeating:

> the whole Personnel [of Headquarters] are very much more pleased with doing service in France, as it is looked upon as the Seat of War, and they get a better opportunity of receiving some reward for their work; in fact D.S.O's and M.C's are only eligible for those in War Zone.[26]

The rewards of war then in this case were membership of an esteemed College and military decorations. A history of the latter in this war is long overdue.

Returning to the question of the functions of medicine in war, the more obvious functions were the maintenance of the army and treatment of the sick and injured. As the war of attrition in France progressed, the military demand for 'effectives', fit or able-bodied soldiers, also increased, the source of replacements being either new recruits or 'reconditioned' invalids. As noted earlier, Australian recruiting numbers declined drastically during the war. Pressure on Army doctors to rehabilitate or, more importantly, re-classify invalids increased correspondingly. At the beginning of the war there were three categories of fitness: 'A' or fit for general service; 'B' or temporarily unfit for general service; and 'C' or permanently unfit for general service. According to Butler,

> the [assessment] procedure was crude. No accurate record was kept of the many men classed 'B'; 'reclassification' was carried out by a medical officer who walked along a line of men on parade and picked out those who looked fit.[27]

Rupert Downes, later DGMS of the Second AIF, was DDMS in Cairo after Howse left for England. In November 1916 Downes issued instructions to his medical staff that 'sentiment' must not enter their assessment of men's fitness for active service.[28] By mid 1917 in the 2nd Australian Division in France, the DDMS was exercising even greater caution. The Divisional medical officers were issued with an instruction that 'all cases of reinforcements considered unfit by their Regimental Medical Officers will be seen by A.D.M.S.'. They were also reminded that 'R.M.O.'s should use great discretion in sending men down to the A.D.M.S. for Boarding':

> Only men who present some physical or mental defect should be sent, the high standard required at the beginning of the war cannot now be maintained & men should be encouraged to carry on despite vague rheumatic pains & similar subjective symptons [sic].[29]

The latter 18 months of the war were even more utilitarian. According to Butler,

> As the war progressed towards the exhaustion of available material and as the material available from convalescents, being picked over and over from R.A.P. [Regimental Aid Post] to Base, became less and less amenable to medical reconditioning, categories were elaborated to fulfil increased refinements of medico-military treatment.[30]

By 1918, the 'ABC' system was elaborated into a ludicrous hierarchy of thirteen categories including such 'conditions' as 'Physically fit, but in need of hardening' (A3) or 'Medically fit, but dentally unfit' (B1a4). (See Appendix 2). The crucial 'B' category, those who could be 'picked over' again, was expanded to seven subdivisions and, according to Butler, after the huge losses of the First Somme, the medical classification of men was carried out on a 'rigidly utilitarian' basis.[31] 'Reconditioning' became a matter of passing a pen over a piece of paper to re-classify a soldier as fit for service.[32]

This 'reconditioning' process, where invalids were re-classified as fit for something, even if not front line service, was only one part of a much larger problem of finding sufficient numbers of 'effective' troops. By early 1918, the problem had resolved itself into a war of wills between Pearce as Minister of Defence and the senior officers of the AAMC, notably Howse. Although Butler claims a victory for his peers in this battle, describing it as 'the first time on record the commander of the military forces of a nation at war was materially influenced in a strictly military decision by his medical adviser', this was only true in relation to the fitness of recruits.[33]

Howse had been Director of Medical Services of the AIF from late 1915. According to one biographer, he viewed the medical service as a 'fundamental of fighting efficiency' and 'no mere humane amenity for soldiers'.[34] This philosophy was clearly expressed in his insistence on an extraordinarily high standard of recruit ('perfect' men according to Fetherston) and his belief in medical reconditioning of experienced soldiers. As far as the recruits were concerned, by the end of 1917 he had sent over 10 000 soldiers back to Australia without their seeing any action. Pearce, on the other hand, seems to have favoured sending 'older, younger and less fit men' and giving them a chance of serving in France while 'risking some breakdowns'.[35] According to Butler, Howse was able to gain the support of Birdwood and in the end Pearce was forced to tighten-up recruiting standards in order to meet the Army demand. Yet while these standards were raised, the process of reclassifying invalids continued apace. From April to September 1918, for example, 51 516 soldiers rejoined their units 'ex "sick and wounded"'.[36] Indeed, Butler acknowledges that this was 'one of the most thorny of the medical problems' of the war.[37]

Doctors were also vitally important to maintaining the appearance of the Army as an effective and efficient machine. For example, in 1919, Butler, then at AIF Headquarters in London, compiled a report for Howse on the question of Australian soldiers being retained 'longer than necessary' in military hospitals during the war.[38] His report on Field Ambulances in France reveals the heart of the problem. Once a soldier was evacuated to a base unit he became 'Army wastage' and could only be returned to the front via a 'complicated and tedious channel of Depots, as a reinforcement'.[39] Army doctors were keeping soldiers in these 'Rest Stations' principally from

> the desire to avoid shewing a large sick evacuation, especially evacuation from conditions the existence of which in considerable numbers was looked on as a reflection on the Division or especially the Corps, e.g. Trench Feet, I.C.T., Scabies.

Butler continued,

> At the beginning of 1917 … the keeping down of the sick rate was a difficult matter and was a subject of very close and strict note by the 4th Army which was administering the corps at the time; and specially on the evacuation for trench foot. It was found by the D.D.M.S. 1st ANZAC that the diagnosis 'I.C.T.' (inflammation of connective tissue), or 'sore feet', were being used to cover up cases of trench foot, and that there was a tendency not to evacuate but to hold these cases in the Rest Stations.

In other words, doctors were falsifying diagnoses in order to make the AIF command appear effective.

Doctors served the Army's purposes in other ways. In 1915 Butler was concerned at the extent to which medical services were used 'to achieve ends not properly the responsibility of the medical service'.

> Officers commanding combatant units and the combatant service in general is constantly endeavouring to use the R.M.O. … for the purpose of getting certain things done which are not possible otherwise, from the getting rid of undesirables, to the procuration of extra-whisky on a medical order. The practice in respect of getting rid of undesirables has grown up in the British Army, in respect of officers whom it is wished to get rid of. It commenced early in the A.I.F.[40]

Doctors also determined whether recruits were fit for Army service. How far this was from being a straightforward assessment of health in the Australian case has already been

134

outlined. The politics of military medicine were even clearer in Canada. The 1918 Report of Australian Surgeon General R.H.J. Fetherston on the fitness of recruits amongst the Allies describes French-Canadian recruits from Quebec as 'practically all antagonistic to serving, many being disloyal ... and as many as 90% appealed when passed as fit'. As well, French-Canadian doctors 'regularly differed' from the doctors of the Canadian Army Medical Corps in their opinion of 'fitness'.[41] In the United States, Fetherston visited recruiting camps and 'arranged to have the smaller and poorer type of soldiers' brought before him:

> They were stripped, so that I might see their physical development. This afforded me opportunities of studying the physique of the poorer type of recruits.[42]

Fetherston was also impressed with the way American authorities dealt with 'minor ailments' amongst recruits. He described procedures whereby

> all men with minor ailments which could be cured, such as hernia, piles, varicose veins, and deformed toes [were passed into the Army]. They were sent into hospitals in camps, and compelled to undergo surgical treatment. Refusal to undergo opera-tion was met with severe punishment and imprisonment. At all camp hospitals there were large numbers of men undergoing treatment to fit them for service.[43]

There were, of course, other secondary functions for medicine such as the ability of the state to claim a share in the identity of the doctor-patient (in this case doctor-soldier) relationship – one traditionally associated with compassion and caring. More important perhaps was the ability of the doctor to observe and medically police individual soldiers on behalf of the state. This latter function will be elaborated in some detail in later sections but it will suffice here to note that there is an important and inextricable relationship between disciplinary infringement, moral judgement, medical treatment and eligibility for benefits under the Repatriation scheme.

War pensions and responsibility for health

War Pensions were available to Australian ex-servicemen (ex-servicewomen only after 1915) under the *War Pensions Act* of 1914, subsequently incorporated into the *Australian Soldiers' Repatriation Act* (1917-20). These Acts legislated that incapacity or death due to war service was compensatable: in other words the state, as employer, was liable to pay compensation to its employees for disabilities arising in the course of employment on active service. Closely modelled on contemporary workers compensation legislation for its detail, itself drawing on the principles of commercial insurance enshrined in other older veteran benefit systems, the pension was paid as compensation for loss of earning capacity: that is, it was assessed on the basis of worker productivity.[44] This requires brief comment.

Historically, ex-soldiers have always been dispersed with some form of gratuity or booty and, not infrequently, with gifts of land. Such handouts have functioned not only to reward service but also to obviate threats to civil order from a discontented or truculent soldiery.[45] In modern times, injury and disability have come increasingly within the scope of charity: in Australia, as in Britain, charity relief funds were established to offer some form of immediate assistance to soldiers returning from the Boer War and a voluntary relief fund (the Australian Soldiers' Repatriation Fund) was established in 1915 by the Federal Government. Yet even as early as 1914, the Fisher Labor Government had argued against the Liberal (Fusion) Party's notion of paying a pension as a reward or unalienable right: instead Labor had fought for and won the principal of compensation. The same (or similar) principle underwrote veteran benefits established in Britain, Canada, the United States and elsewhere around this time.[46]

Irrespective of their form, these compensatory measures undertaken by the state needed to be seen as humane, benevolent and just; as encompassing the social costs of war. In the case of the Australian repatriation process, this legitimation was largely achieved through the instrumentality of medicine. By establishing disability – whether injury or illness – as the yardstick by which loss of productivity was measured and therefore a war pension paid, medicine and medical knowledge were in a position to mediate the relationship between labour – represented by the ex-soldier's claim for a pension – and the state, which both during and after the war was bent on containing costs. It is necessary now to look in more detail at the pensioning procedure as established and subsequently modified in its day to day operation in the AIF and to examine the principles which guided the assessment process.

The body of the soldier was under scrutiny from the moment he enlisted. Height, weight, chest measurement, physical development, pulse, vaccination marks, vision, 'marks indicating congenital peculiarities or previous disease' and 'slight defects, but not sufficient to cause rejection' were all recorded – or at least provision was made for recording – at enlistment.[47] Throughout the period of service, every injury and illness was also recorded, only now the instructions to medical officers were specific: in addition to dates of admission and discharge and name of the disease, doctors were instructed to provide

> remarks bearing on the cause, nature, or treatment of the case, likely to be of interest or of future use. In cases of syphilis, admissions and re-admissions to hospital will be shown. The subsequent progress, including particulars of treatment out of hospital, transfers, etc., will be given in the special syphilis case sheet.[48]

As well as detailed medical or hospital records, each medical incident was recorded as an entry on the soldier's service record card along with movement between units and disciplinary infringements. These cards contained basic information on date, place and institution of medical treatment, disease or complaint. A special annotation was frequently made in cases of venereal disease.

In the event that a soldier was deemed unfit for general service, whether temporarily or permanently, he was subjected first to examination by a local medical board and then to examination by the Permanent AIF Medical Boards, 'Senior' and 'Junior'. If he was returned to Australia as Medically Unfit, then after May 1917 he underwent a final assessment by a Permanent Referee Board at discharge. These last three encounters between the soldier and the army doctor are of critical importance.

Armies are hierarchical and reflect class and social divisions. In the case of the Australian Army Medical Corps this was also true. The first medical assessment for fitness was generally undertaken at the place where treatment was *consolidated* — that is, not a field or front line hospital – and usually by a junior medical officer (commonly a Captain or Major). Instructions for examination and reporting were quite scrupulous and doctors were instructed to read them carefully since

> the object of these questions is, in the event of the man being invalided, to put the authorities of the Military Forces of the Commonwealth in possession of the most reliable information grounded upon the opinion of those best capable of judging, so as to *guide them in deciding upon the man's claim to compensation,* clear and decisive answers must in all cases be given ... In answering the ... questions the Medical Officer will carefully discriminate between the man's unsupported statements on his case, and recorded evidence furnished by his documents, military and medical. He *will also carefully discriminate cases entirely due to venereal disease.* (original emphasis)[49]

A definition of the soldier's health was then formulated by the doctor through answers to twenty standardised questions centred on the date and place of origin of the disease; the nature and cause of the disability (often used interchangeably with disease); whether or not the soldier aggravated the disease through 'intemperance' or 'misconduct'; whether there was evidence of self-infliction; the nature of treatment offered, instituted or refused; and, a recommendation regarding discharge.

The next formal stage in this process was an assessment described by Butler as the 'most difficult art of "medical boarding"'. The findings of this Board, which usually functioned from a Hospital or Depot in England, 'purported to express the sum total of medical knowledge as applied to the condition and case under review'.

> It involved diagnosis, both clinical and pathological, of the condition, and the amount of therapeutic possibilities; together with that *ultima thule* of the medical art, a prognosis. It called for the highest clinical acumen implemented by a wide knowledge of human nature, in particular, of the soldier, young and old.[50]

The Boards were also influential in regard to policies on civil redeployment of invalids. Just prior to the appointment of a Director of Medical Services to the AIF, while the British War Office still formally controlled the Australian Medical Corps, the Medical Boards were instructed to take great care in filling out Army Form B179 since it was considered 'of paramount importance to the national interests for every one to do any useful work of which he is capable'. They continued,

> it is desirable from every point of view that [an invalid] should have full inducement to find regular employment at the earliest moment compatible with the due

progress of his recovery. Medical boards will, therefore, exercise caution in assigning the higher degrees, and especially the total degree, of incapacity.[51]

The personnel of the Senior Board, appointed in 1916, was unchanged throughout the war and consisted of the Australian Consulting Physician, Colonel H.C. Maudsley, and Consulting Surgeon, Colonel (later Major General) C.S. Ryan. Maudsley and Ryan were the final arbiters within the AIF medical assessment system abroad.

Of Maudsley, Butler merely tells us that he turned 'boarding into a science'. One biographer describes an 'extremely modest and self-effacing' man with a 'quiet voice and a friendly, whimsical manner'.[52] Maudsley's professional interest was in psychiatry and neurology. His nosology of cases reviewed by the Board reflected these interests. In his 1918 Report to Howse, cases were divided into two sections, 'war neurosis' and others. In both this and the 1919 Report Maudsley was quick to classify those soldiers of 'poor mentality' or 'poor mental make-up', 'men ready to suffer from neurosis on the slightest provocation'. Even those men classified under some standard medical classification such as 'Diseases of the alimentary canal' did not escape his gaze: in a 'considerable number of cases', he opined, the condition was 'mainly one of neurosis'. Under the heading 'Rheumatism & Myalgia', there was a group 'whose so-called Rheumatism seemed to me to be a manifestation of Neurosis', as were 'some of the cases of Sciatica'. Even 'Gas Poisoning' was not immune: 'some were suffering from Neurosis'. Indeed out of a total of over 19 000 cases reviewed, Maudsley claimed that nearly 19% suffered from nervous conditions. The next largest category was 'premature senility' which constituted just over 18%.[53]

Maudsley's diagnostic decisions on these cases were a reflection of assessment procedures which, in Smith's words, were 'integrated with theories of human action'.[54] In this case and perhaps following in the footsteps of his uncle, the eminent alienist and 'most forceful English writer on insanity', Professor Henry Maudsley, Maudsley's constitution of a nervous disorder was simultaneously a character judgement.[55] While the knowledge content of Maudsley's particular beliefs on the aetiology of neurosis need not detain us here, his diagnoses were nevertheless of great significance to returned soldiers in subsequent years. 'Neurosis' was perilously close to 'malingering' in the nosology of so-called mental illness and the latter diagnosis almost by definition incurred harsh treatment by the Repatriation Department doctors as well as its bureaucrats.[56]

As for the other half of the Senior Board, Charles Ryan, Butler is more forthcoming.

> As Senior Surgeon to the Melbourne Hospital he had a reputation for courage and common sense rather than for more intellectual qualities, and his service as Senior Surgical Boarding Officer was in accord with this. He acquired a reputation, probably not without some justification, for inconsistency ... [being] unduly influenced by the military situation. In this ... he was but a reflex of the war mind.[57]

John Springthorpe was rather more forthcoming on the Senior Consultants. In September 1915 he noted that Maudsley was about to be made Consulting Physician to Field Hospitals of the AIF 'with a trip home!'. He went on

> What has he done? His work as senior physician to No. 1 A.G.H., and a few weeks temporary O/C. Yet what matter! He has influence, he offends none, and he attempts nil.

Personal vitriol aside, Springthorpe reiterated his chief complaints right to the end of hostilities: the Consultants only came to the 3rd AAH to Board ('queer Consultants!' he notes); they did not use the 'available evidence'; 'too rapid work to be fair in all but slight cases', 'no time for others – so unfair – examines heart (in non-heart cases) through jacket – rubbish!'. By November 1917 according to Springthorpe the Consultants were visiting only weekly: 'Ryan finalising 400, Maudsley 200 in one day'. He believed it was 'farcical and unfair', 'a crying injustice':

> Frequent examples in my Histories of men up to 38 months service with only one furlough, kept on until they break down, sent back before they are fit, etc. – what can be done?[58]

While the two Consultants had immense potential power and indeed wielded it, what often seems to have happened in practice is that the first boarding assessment was carried out by the same junior medical officer who undertook the initial history. If the case was straightforward (particularly the case in injuries or woundings), his reporting and decision-making was generally ratified by his senior colleagues. This process was slightly different in England where Australian hospitals were sometimes staffed by older and sometimes more experienced doctors (doctors considered unfit for frontline duty). Indeed the qualifications of the doctors in some Australian hospitals outstripped those of the Consultants. It also varied when the diagnosis was a disease (as opposed to injury) and varied considerably when the diagnosed disease could be construed as 'neurosis'. To what extent the Junior Board anticipated the attitude and demands of the Senior Board requires considerable further research. Springthorpe was clear: 'I'd kick up a row if they didn't [agree]'.

What is of particular interest here is the further refinement of instruction to all Boards, the specificity of information required and the demand for non-medical information. For example, instead of merely reporting refusal of treatment, opinion was requested on whether this refusal was 'unreasonable'. But, for the purposes of this study, one of the most important questions was 'To what extent … capacity for earning a full livelihood in the general labour market [is] lessened at present?' (expressed as a percentage) and, secondarily, the probable duration of this disability (expressed in months).

These instructions, contained in Army Form B179, were continuously revised as the war progressed and by 1918 included further refinements as to the relevance of the assessment to a claim for pension. For example, included amongst explanatory 'Notes' for the examining medical officer were the following:

> The rates of pension vary directly according to whether the disability is (A) caused or aggravated by service in the present war; (B) due to causes not connected with the present war … It is therefore essential when assigning the cause of a disability to differentiate between them.

And

> State whether the disability is clearly attributable to -
>
> (i) Service during the present war;
> (2) Climate;
> (2i) Ordinary military service;
> (iv) Want of proper care on the man's part, e.g., intemperance, misconduct, etc; or
> (v) Whether it is constitutional or hereditary.

At the time of discharge in Australia, the Permanent Board reviewed the recommendations of the Medical Board on these various aspects of a soldier's illness and made final recommendations as to the incapacity of the soldier, the duration of such incapacity and its cause. This recommendation invariably formed the basis for a decision within the Repatriation Department on the eligibility of the soldier for a War Pension. For the first six months or so after granting the Pension it also determined the rate. Thus, the Army doctor determined in the first instance at least whether or not a soldier received a Pension at all and the amount he would receive.

It became increasingly clear as the war went on that the state and its senior medical agents demanded more and more specific detail on a soldier's illness and required more and more decision-making from medical staff on both responsibility for the illness (intemperance, misconduct, venereal disease, refusal of treatment or self-infliction) and its aetiology (climate, active service, heredity and so on). With regard to responsibility, there is a clear directive here to discriminate between the deserving and undeserving sick. The language of nineteenth century poor relief is mingled with the ideological assumptions which permeated medicine and which portrayed 'intemperance', for example, as innate weakness and self-inflicted rather than a response to social conditions – in this case the obscene and terrifying conditions of the front. But it is also more than that.

The rank of the soldier could be extremely significant in the assessment process. Louse infestation, for example, was a perennial problem for all soldiers of all armies in France. The common soldier lived with his lice in a wet trench for weeks at a time with only short breaks behind the lines.[59] After August 1916 treatment for his infestation consisted of disinfection and laundering of clothes and bathing in Corps 'baths'. The 'ideal' arrangement, one put forward at the Inter-allied sanitary conference of 1917, was a bath and change of underwear for men every ten days.[60] Army discipline, as noted in Chapter 3, was used to enforce compliance. However, medical assessment of such infestation seems to have varied with rank. Lieutenant Clarke was diagnosed as suffering from 'debility the result of scabies which is now cured'. The Medical Board who assessed him made no mention of lack of discipline nor did it mention poor hygiene but rather recommended two weeks leave in England as a treatment.[61] Such 'treatments' were common for minor ailments amongst officers. Lieutenant Paull, for example, broke down and required three weeks in England as a result of 'the strain of his work as an Instructor' at a Corps School.[62] Lt Carlisle's disability in April 1918 was 'Age' (he was 41) and 'DAH'. Although 'Disordered Action of the Heart' was considered a 'functional' disorder by this date and one treatable by exercise, Lt Carlisle's condition was considered 'caused by military service' – 'Strain of Infantry Work' – and it was recommended that he was unfit permanently for General Service.

One other group who seem to have received preferential treatment was the members of the Australian Army Nursing Service. Sister Farquhar was diagnosed as suffering from 'Debility, the result of Appendicitis', Sister Langford from 'Debility following an attack of Tonsillitis', Staff Nurse Gibson from 'Debility following inflammation connective tissue of finger', and Staff Nurse Collins from 'Debility following Influenza'. All were considered 'caused by military service' and the Boards all recommended 3 weeks leave in England.[63] This clear discrimination in favour of officers was equally clear – although reversed – in the decisions of the most senior officers of the AAMC against ordinary soldiers. (See Chapters 8 and 9).

The question of responsibility for illness also raises the broader question of responsibility for the troops generally, that is, the function of officers in maintaining the health of soldiers. A number of criticisms were made on this account during the war. At the front, criticisms of officers' behaviour could be savage. This was especially true during the heightened gas warfare of 1918. In October of that year, Major Herbert Wilson, Chemical Adviser of 4th Army, wrote a report to 5th Army Headquarters concerning an incident involving five men of 517 Company and a bombardment of 'Yellow Cross'. Wilson came straight to the point:

> I have seen these men. One of them is still alive but I do not think he will live. I know of no more flagrant case of carelessness and irresponsibility on the part of officers than in this case – where five men were sent to clear a pill-box contaminated with an unknown amount of Yellow Cross.[64]

This was not an isolated incident or a solitary criticism.[65] As noted previously, in an attack on 'excessive evacuation for Trench Foot' in the 5th Australian Division, the DDMS, Colonel C.C. Manifold, reported that the real cause, in his view, was the 'Australian Officer'. Butler's correspondence with relevant senior officers during the 1930s over the issue of Trench Foot reveals, if anything, a singularly united effort by both military and medical officers to maintain the health of the troops. Indeed Butler notes that 'the experience of the Somme winter brought home once and for all the fact that to win the war the preservation of health and maintenance of man-power were vital'.[66] This two-fold imperative, preserving health and maintaining man-power, meant that from late 1916 both officers and Army doctors were being scrutinised by higher command in an attempt to find a cause for the high attrition rate for Trench Foot. 'Effectives' had to be found and if new recruits were not forthcoming then responsibility for this 'wastage' had to be attributed and a solution found. Manifold's comments simply reflect the process of finding a suitable non-medical scapegoat. The army solution was to insist on increased discipline and more medical involvement.

In the end the 'manpower' problem was addressed – though not solved – by improvements in routine hygiene. But, as noted earlier, it was also achieved by the medical re-classification or deliberate misdiagnosis of the condition by some army doctors. Soldiers suffering from Trench Foot were simply re-classified and sent back to the front. Throughout this processing the owner of the Trench Feet somehow lost significance. Indeed the evidence reveals a medico-military definition of the soldier akin to Foucault's bleak comment that he was 'above all a fragment of mobile space'.[67]

Alongside Trench Feet as a cause of 'wastage' in late 1916 and early 1917 was 'shell shock'. By this date there was a military war on the medical diagnosis of this condition. 'Shell shock' was an indeterminate diagnosis from the Army point of view. In the first years of the war it incorporated various physical traumas associated with shell explosions, particularly wounds, concussion and burns. It also included diagnoses where the principal effect was emotional or psychological but there was an additional traumatic effect such as the blowing-in of trenches by the force of a nearby explosion or men being buried. The term also was used to cover the emotional and mental collapse of soldiers who had seen men literally blown to pieces in front of them. The evidence indicates a clear lenience on the part of some doctors in these early years towards the latter two groups, an understandable lenience given the horror of the circumstances. But it was short-lived.

By August 1916, the statistics of evacuation for 'shell shock' attracted the attention of the Allied command. Orders were subsequently issued to all armies to differentiate between severe concussion, or other manifest signs and symptoms caused by a 'specific shell or other explosion', now categorised as 'Shell shock, W [Wounded]' and all other cases, now re-categorised as 'N.Y.D. [not yet diagnosed] ?shell shock or ?neurasthenia'. The diagnosis of 'Shell shock W' was outlawed unless there was evidence from the Officer Commanding 'or other responsible witness' of direct contact with an explosion. Indeed Police Posts were set up to deal with those men excluding officers *not* diagnosed this way.[68] The Adjutant General pointed out that

> It has too often happened that Officers and men who have failed in their duty have used such expressions [as shell shock] to describe their state of noneffectiveness, and Medical Officers without due consideration of the military issues at stake, have accepted such cases as being in the same category as ordinary illness.[69]

By January 1917, the 4th Army Medical Society were recommending that in cases of 'functional nervous disturbance', doctors should not just indicate 'how long the patient has been exposed to shell-fire', but should also 'indicate any weakness of character noticed before the time of the nervous shock'.[70]

Doctors, then, were encouraged to make judgements about responsibility for health in two separate jurisdictions. First, according to Army directions, they were ordered to differentiate between gross physical damage and all other kinds of damage. This was an extremely simple procedure in terms of clinical assessment. A man suffering from grotesque wounds could easily be differentiated from one suffering only bruising. What it masks, however, is the fate of those soldiers *not* suffering from major physical trauma, those who by definition were instantaneously labelled 'neurasthenic' or 'nerve failure'. So, a soldier who had been buried by a shell explosion, had somehow crawled back to his unit and been evacuated to a Field Ambulance, was a 'nerve failure', a subject for military police action, and such behaviour could be recorded on his military record card.

The other judgement, that of 'character', a judgement that was both explicit and implicit in directions from the Allied command *and* the AAMC, was more complex. The shortage of man-power meant finding ways to re-categorise invalids. Shell shock was one of many indeterminate diagnoses: the evidence for the disease was sometimes flimsy, the proof of 'trauma' often inconclusive, the attribution of responsibility easily transferred to the individual soldier. That transferral came about through the doctor's assessment of the soldier according to guidelines laid down by the Army as much as by his peers. As noted earlier, Army Form B179 required doctors to make value judgements on both responsibility and aetiology. This form had been in use, with minor modifications, in the British Army since 1895. When the predominantly lay [War] Pensions Appeal Tribunal was established in Britain in late 1917, presided over by His Honour Judge Parry, it immediately attacked the Form as inadequate, biased and misleading. The Tribunal observed that

> nowhere is there any direction to the Medical Officer in charge, or the Medical Board, to make any enquiry from the man himself, or to set down his statement of how his unfitness came about … it is often possible that a man's unsupported statement may be correct in fact, whilst the evidence recorded in a military medical document may be inaccurate.[71]

With regard to attribution, it commented that 'we do not think that the filling up of Answers to printed questions is the best method of obtaining reliable information'.[72] Indeed, the Tribunal considered certain sections blatantly misleading for the Medical Boards using them. This was evident in the use of the word 'disability' instead of the word 'unfitness' within Form B179. According to then current usage, 'disability' inferred a 'specific injury' and therefore excluded any other damage to health from eligibility for a pension. The Tribunal also pointed out that there was too much emphasis on the 'character' of a disease rather than whether the 'unfitness' was attributed to or aggravated by military service.

Perhaps the most important criticism, however, was that which revealed the structural inequity of the process up to that point. The Tribunal noted that this system of deciding on pensions contained no 'judicial enquiry into facts':

It is indeed a wholly medical enquiry. As far as the man is concerned, the decision upon his claim to a pension is really concluded by the Medical Board. His case or claim to a pension is not really heard at all. It is determined without hearing ... it does not seem to us in accordance with the principles of English justice that the right of a man to a pension should be determined against him until he has had an opportunity of being heard in support of his case by those who are going to determine it.[73]

This reliance on medical opinion without recourse to appeal became enshrined in the Australian war-pensioning system, an appeal tribunal only coming into existence in 1929. Why such a principle was introduced so early in Britain and so late in Australia is a complex question. It has been suggested that the reason may lie in the British legal system being more centralised and stronger in prestige than the Australian system (and before 1920 the High Court took a largely anti-centralist line); alternatively it may be that the federal nature of the Australian system was seen as affording enough protection.[74] The detail in the files examined suggests the answer is also embedded in the history of medico-legal discourse, in the power of the professions concerned vis-à-vis the state, in the political power of organised resistance through veteran organisations and in the sensitivity of the incumbent government to these issues. The subject is vast and largely beyond the scope of this work. Suffice it to say that the relationship between the medical profession and the state in Australia at this date was crucial to the processing of veterans.[75]

One final matter related to responsibility demands attention. It has been noted above that medicine has the capacity to recast problems of health and illness: to make social phenomena appear 'natural'. One such phenomenon in this circumstance is 'Misconduct'. Behaviour indicted as misconduct in the First AIF ranged from being Absent Without Leave, through drunkenness, giving cheek to Officers and stealing to – crucially for this study – refusing medical treatment. Army discipline, like the medical practice to which it was co-joined at this time, functioned through observation of and power over the body of the soldier. In war, one acted to legitimate and reinforce the norms of the other. Just as army discipline was brought to bear on a so-called recalcitrant *patient* by the imposition of fines and other punishments, medicine denied the recalcitrant *soldier* a pension. The following account exemplifies this.

Private Timothy C was evacuated from the trenches at Bapaume with Trench Fever in 1917 and some weeks later he was invalided to London. While there he noticed some symptoms and presented himself to the army doctor for further examination. He was diagnosed as having both syphilis and gonorrhoea. The soldier was given a course of treatment over the next six months involving injections of synthetic arsenic – an early use of chemotherapy in modern medicine – as well as doses of mercury and urethral lavages.[76] The diseases and the fact of his treatment were also recorded on the soldier's service record card. (It is worth noting that this was then perhaps the most brutal and invasive treatment for any disease in the repertoire of medicine). His debilitated state after the treatment, which appears to have been largely caused by the treatment (iatrogenic), resulted in an examination by the Medical Board and on the basis that the disease was considered self-inflicted he was denied a pension and discharged from the army as unfit for further service. (He subsequently developed interstitial keratitis in one eye, possibly as a result of the arsenic treatment, and went blind in that eye. He was never paid a pension.)

Figlio has commented that 'naming transfers the locus of pathology from the society to the individual'.[77] In its broadest sense, this is true of pathological behaviour as well as illness. What was a thoroughly social phenomenon – the emotion associated with trench warfare, death and dying and the accidental result of a sexual liaison – was represented as 'misconduct' and 'disease'.[78] The individual soldier thus became the 'locus of pathology', not war itself. This understanding of trench warfare was underpinned not just by the overwhelmingly ideology of individualism, but also by a profound, unquestioning belief in the morality of war and therefore of the recalcitrance or moral bankruptcy of soldiers who failed in their duty by wantonly contracting disease. In this instance, as in many others, it was not the nature of the pathology or aetiology of the disease that was in question but the issue of responsibility. Venereal disease continued to be a focus for debate and a reason for denying a pension in Australia until the Royal Commission of 1924 recommended the acceptance of war-relatedness.[79]

Aetiology and war-relatedness

Alongside and intimately linked with the notion of responsibility was the notion of aetiology: what had *caused* the injury or disease?[80] War, climate and 'ordinary military service' as causative forces at least removed responsibility for illness away from the individual soldier and re-defined the cause as environmental. In practice the most important question and one always addressed by the individual medical officer and the two Medical Boards was the decision on whether an illness or injury was caused, aggravated by or unrelated to active service. (A pension was only payable for illness due to or aggravated by active service).

Superficially, the question of war-relatedness appears straightforward. It is, after all, difficult to deny the causal relationship between a gunshot wound or shell wound and a resulting fracture or flesh wound. Indeed, the evidence suggests that in cases of traumatic injury, where the disability was severe enough for the soldier to be returned to Australia (or to die) such injuries were invariably classified as war-related. However, the clarity of aetiology stops there. Contemporary medical knowledge and its social construction were necessarily implicated in this decision. A medical officer could only decide the issue of war-relatedness on the basis of his own or his peers' knowledge. As well, such practice assumes a professional disinterest, whereas it has been argued that moral judgement of the behaviour of the soldier was an integral part of the procedure.

Two common conditions of the Western Front provide evidence of the indeterminate nature of medical knowledge and show clearly how such indeterminacy allowed other factors such as ideology or professional interest to dominate the assessment process. The vague and ill-defined boundaries of Trench Fever as a pathological entity and the then unknown pathological effects of gas warfare, both addressed in Chapter 3, meant that the Army medical record of soldiers suffering these conditions was clinically unreliable. Yet soldiers who claimed to have suffered from either condition were frequently treated as hypochondriacs or malingerers on their return to Australia. Both conditions highlight the unreliability of diagnoses as well as the importance of that diagnosis in the Repatriation Department procedures.

With regard to Trench Fever, the range of possible diagnoses with this infection was considerable, anything from headache or muscle pain to a serious cardiac condition. Yet it was only in mid 1918 that this knowledge was beginning to circulate amongst the medical units on the Western Front. The extent of missed diagnosis and misdiagnosis will never be known, but all those suffering in this way had to live with the administrative legacy that it entailed. In years to come the medical records that actually survived the war went uncorrected and became the determining evidence on which war pension claims were adjudicated. (See the case of Private Robert O below, for example).

The other pathological condition to affect vast numbers of the AIF but again a condition not always correctly diagnosed was the effects of gassing. It has already been pointed out that 'gassing' was sometimes unavoidable: troop movement at night, sometimes in response to bombardment, meant gas masks or respirators had to be removed for visibility; at other times exposure was inadvertent, such as sleeping near men whose clothing was impregnated with the chemical. There was also the officer problem as outlined above. Of importance here, however, are the long term effects of gassing. For the post-war period this is especially important in those situations where the exposure was not documented or even recognised by the soldier, such as in cases of exposure to contaminated clothing or soil, or when the exposure was deemed 'slight' but the gas was highly toxic, such as phosgene, or, where the effects of exposure were misdiagnosed. In August 1918, for example, the 3rd Worcestershire Regiment experienced around thirty minutes bombardment. The Officer in command, allegedly an experienced officer, asserted there was no smell except the usual smell of high explosives and so men had not adjusted their respirators. The report on the incident was as follows:

> None of the men had any immediate symptoms – e.g., sneezing, smarting of the eyes and face etc.
> Three days later, about 40 of the Company … began to develop sore throats and huskiness. They were isolated and left under observation of the M.O. who at first was inclined to suspect 'Spanish' influenza as this was at the time epidemic. There seems, however, to have been no change of temperature.
> After a few days, many of the cases recovered but the majority showed signs of stomach trouble, pains in the back and over the chest and were sent to the special

C.C.S. (No.54) at Aire. So far as I can make out, they are allowed back to duty, with the exception of two who were sent to England, evidently because the symptoms were unusual and merited further investigation there.[81]

It is clear from this report that soldiers suffering from gassing were readily misdiagnosed as suffering from influenza. In the post-war period, claims for conditions attributed to gassing, where there was *evidence* of the gassing in the medical record, were generally not refused. 'Influenza', as an entry on a service card, was more problematic.

Clearly, the determination of aetiology – the labelling of cause of illness – was a medical function. It is argued here that that determination was seriously compromised by the values and class interests of senior doctors, by the characteristic indeterminacy of medicine as a body of knowledge and by the social constitution of disease or illness, here so explicit in the activities of doctors working to maintain an efficient fighting machine for the army. Needless to say the shifting boundary between war-related and non war-related illness reflected these influences on medical decision-making.

This procedure is perhaps best clarified by an examination of actual instances. However, before proceeding it should be noted that frequently the decision of the Permanent Board in Australia was at variance with the Medical Board in Britain (or overseas generally) in that there is a marked tendency for the Permanent Board to deny war-relatedness and simultaneously to reduce the degree of disability suffered by the soldier. This is almost invariably so in instances where diagnosis and assessment was not straightforward and in instances involving venereal disease or misconduct.

For example, Private Robert O, who had enlisted in May 1916, was admitted to hospital from the Somme early in 1917 diagnosed as suffering from Trench Fever and 'Disordered Action of the Heart' (DAH). It will be remembered that at this date Trench Fever was thought to be little more than a fever with general malaise. He was discharged the following month suffering from a heart murmur, chest pain, dyspnoea (difficulty of breathing), and pains in his legs. The Medical Board's assessment was of a (probable) pre-existing cardiac disease *aggravated* by active service. The soldier was returned to Australia and was examined by the Permanent Board in November of 1917. The Permanent Board's decision was that this soldier suffered 'old cardiac trouble' which was '*not aggravated* by service'. (emphasis added)[82] It seems entirely possible from the evidence on Trench Fever outlined in Chapter 3 that had this soldier contracted his illness late in 1918 instead of 1917 he may still have been diagnosed as suffering from Trench Fever but, with the advantage of a more complex understanding of the infection and its affects, the symptoms may well have been considered war-related and the Board *may* have agreed.

Private Gerard H enlisted late in 1915. In the following year he was recorded as being Absent Without Leave whilst serving in France. In 1917 he suffered a gunshot wound to the right arm then, later in the same year, a severe flesh wound to the neck as a result of a shell explosion at Ypres. The attending medical officer recorded that a piece of metal had been removed in the field hospital in France and that the metal was 'deeply imbedded behind spine of axis [second joint of spinal cord below skull] '. The doctor noted that movement of the soldier's neck was impaired, but that his condition was slowly improving. In December the Medical Board considered his condition war-related but only temporary and recommended that he be re-examined in three months. One week later the soldier was examined by Charles Ryan who wrote:

> This man states that he cannot move his head, this injury he has received cannot affect the muscles of his neck, he is really quite fit for G.S. [General Service] but as he persists in his present attitude, he should be kept on home service or returned to Australia. Service has in no way injured him.[83]

Private Martin L enlisted early in 1916. Twelve months later he suffered frost bite of the left foot and was in hospital for three weeks. In July he was evacuated from the front line with Myositis (inflammation or infection of muscle) in the left leg and was in and out of hospital for the next six months. The medical record also noted a pre-existing injury to the left leg. In December the Medical Board described his illness as Myalgia and determined that it was pre-existing but 'greatly aggravated' by service and by climate. Back in Australia, the Permanent Board considered there was no war-relatedness and that the fact that the left leg was one and a quarter inches shorter than the right was due to 'old tubercular disease [of the] hip joint'.[84]

What is clear here is the role subjective assessment played in the definition of aetiology. In fact, there is little evidence of consensus in all but the simplest mechanical injuries. It is also apparent that there is a relatively straightforward divergence in opinion between the more senior doctors behind the lines or home in Australia and their colleagues at the front. Some of the reasons for this discrepancy have been addressed in Chapter 5.

However, perhaps the most important aspect of this procedure is the very idea of war-relatedness. The way the image of war was managed was crucial: that is, the mobilisation of nationalist as well as imperialist sentiment along with the legitimation of murder and atrocity on these and other grounds. In essence, war was defined to the civilian soldiers of the First AIF as necessary for the protection and defence of Britain, her allies and indeed Australia. Such powerful ideological weapons along with economic conscription and the propaganda which seductively portrayed a veritable 'Boy's Own' war were successful in persuading over 400,000 Australian men (and a small number of women) to swap their civil identity for that of a soldiery bent on adventure as much as honour, duty and the protection of women and children. This mythological image of war also served to conceal the antagonistic economic forces which were the concrete reality of war.

Thus, at one level, the concentration in the boarding process on war-relatedness insidiously diverted all responsibility for injury and illness away from its real cause and laid blame at the door of 'duty', 'defence' and other reified notions. Injury or illness became the 'natural' consequence of war so defined. Yet there is another more subtle dimension to this process, this time involving medicine.

The way war was depicted simultaneously and logically defined the nature of its effects. It is no accident that extant photographs taken during the war are so sanitised: the war of the myth could hardly be seen to produce such a devastating legacy.[85] Gross disfigurement featured as illustrations only in specialised medical texts. Similarly, profound psychological disturbance was typically the subject of incarceration. More problematic still is the hazy psychosomatic region of 'neurasthenia' and 'hysteria'. The very real alienation which resulted from death, killing and mutilation and which found its expression in differing forms of ill health, was defined variously as hysteria, cowardice, malingering, neurasthenia or debility. All of these descriptions relocated aetiology back to the 'constitution', hereditary predisposition or innate weakness of the individual and were therefore considered not-war-related. Thus, the range of disabilities attributable to war was partly determined by the way war itself had been defined.

For these medical and army arbiters of health, war-relatedness tended to reduce to a fixed set of well-defined injuries and illnesses. The literalness of such definitions and the overwhelming concentration on observable physical phenomena also meant that secondary health problems, arising months or years after service, were located in a grey aetiological area indeed. What was considered a war-related injury at the time of discharge frequently lost that stature in the following decade through either the re-definition of the nature or cause of the illness or through re-assessment of the deservedness or undeservedness of the individual. More commonly these processes went hand in hand.

The notion of war-relatedness thus became a most powerful tool in the hands of the state. Prior to World War Two, the cost of War Pensions paid to veterans of the Great War was both the largest single cost to the Repatriation Department and the largest single expense in the welfare or social services arena.[86] Such seemingly extravagant expenditure could be readily interpreted contemporaneously as generous, or, more recently, as preferential treatment on behalf of the state for a sexually and occupationally differentiated social group.[87] The idea of war pensioners as an economic 'elite' analogous to workers compensation beneficiaries is touted by Peter Bartrip.[88] Garton has described a 'welfare "apartheid"' and a 'privileged class of welfare recipients'.[89] Such interpretations reveal a serious misunderstanding of the contemporary monetary value of the 'pension', the extent of health damage that the pension supposedly compensated and, most importantly, the labour relationship which underpins the principle of compensation. Such interpretations serve to reveal the strength of an ideology whose role in reality was to contain such costs through the instrumentality of medicine and medical knowledge.

CHAPTER 8

War Pensions: The 'Clinical Toss Up' and the 'National Purse'[1]

Medical diagnoses and pronouncements on war-relatedness, both during and after the war, had an instrumental value that was often in accord with the requirements of the state. In some respects there was a natural affinity, for example in the labelling of certain signs, symptoms or behaviours as 'neuroses', as the product of 'nerve failure', 'fatigue' or mental instability, all of which diagnosed the cause of the problem as inherent failure of the individual to cope with the pressure of war. Labelled in this way, the soldier was considered inadequate, inefficient and/or personally defective. But this constitution of neuroses was imbued with the ideology of its practitioners. This was an ideology which promoted national economic efficiency and productivity far more than any naive humanitarianism. At war the military mind of the senior members of the AAMC kept the army efficient, quickly disposing of such neurasthenics or subjecting them to rigorous, sometimes brutal treatment: 'uneducated' soldiers suffering from so-called 'reflex nervous disorders' were treated with electrical shocks while their 'cultivated' (officer) counterparts were treated with 'moral persuasion'.[2] Back home, while out of army uniform, the mentality and the discipline were maintained by many of these officers in the uniform of the white coat.

Yet, despite the usefulness of doctors and medical knowledge to the state, there were persistent and serious tensions. These tensions are clearly revealed by examining the relationship between doctors and senior bureaucrats in the repatriation process. At the same time it is possible to trace the careers of a small number of ex-AAMC doctors and to observe the growing strength of the profession.

Accounts of the establishment of the Repatriation Department's medical service are few and, with the partial exception of Butler, they are uncritical narratives.[3] As with the appointment of Repatriation bureaucrats in 1918, the medical service did not and could not simply come into being by the sudden appearance of perfectly qualified men for these newly invented jobs. The process of determining what kind of service was necessary, who was eligible for treatment and who should staff the operation was contested by all those with an interest – the Department of Defence, the AAMC, Millen, senior Repatriation bureaucrats and the medical profession. The full history of that process is too complex to treat here. Instead an analysis of two aspects of that history – the creation of new structures of power and the appointment of Departmental doctors – is used to reveal the often difficult relationship between the profession and the state. The effects of this relationship on former members of the AIF are pursued later.

Expert opinions and honorary services

The medical treatment of former members of the AIF underwent a profound change between 1915 and 1921. This change is associated with two events: the substitution of a paid medical staff for Honorary medical advisers and the transfer of War Pensions administration from Treasury to the Repatriation Department. Superficially, these changes may not seem especially significant. Medical treatment passed from one group of doctors to another and political control from one bureaucracy to another. But a real transformation occurred, with a devastating impact on ex-members of the AIF. By careful examination of the sources, it is possible to trace the death of colonial liberalism within this key 'welfare' bureaucracy of the early twentieth century and its rapid domination by the forces of conservative liberalism.

The principal involvement of medicine in repatriation before April 1918 was in the assessment of War Pensions for Treasury and in the Honorary positions on State War Councils. As has been seen, a harsh rationalism emerged within Treasury when James Collins took over the position of Commissioner of Pensions and Secretary of Treasury in 1916. However, Collins's treatment of soldiers and their claims for War Pensions was rather different. An uncharacteristic sympathy appears in Treasury Rulings and it is worth noting that despite overall control of the Pension budget and Pension rates, Treasury seems to have resisted pressure from Defence and Repatriation to decrease or refuse War Pensions.[4] For example, in October 1918, the Deputy DGMS, Dr G.W. Cuscaden, wrote to Gilbert complaining of Treasury's lenience towards former soldiers who, he alleged, were not following medical orders after their discharge from hospital:

> up to the present the Department of Pensions has refused to bring pressure to bear on invalids by with-holding all or part of the pension. The Department of Repatriation however may not feel bound to the same procedure.[5]

On a superficial reading, there was a parallel softening of attitude in Lockyer's efforts to appoint the first group of Departmental doctors, those attached to the Vocational Training Committees. In April 1918, he advised all Deputy Comptrollers that he was having difficulty obtaining expert advice as to 'the particular type of medical man' suitable for the job. Departmental experience provided some guidance, as he explained

> A great many of our men returning from the severe hardships and terrific experiences in the trenches are naturally suffering from mental excitement which it will take some time to subdue.
> There is a grave danger of many of these men being misunderstood, and of their being treated as malingerers. They are unsettled, it is extremely difficult for them to settle down in any quiet continuous occupation, and to ensure any success in

dealing with them it is absolutely necessary they must be treated, not only with sympathetic firmness and generous consideration, but be submitted to close medical examination.[6]

The tone of Lockyer's letter suggests a genuine interest in the welfare of former soldiers. However, his basic concerns were apparent in his advice to Millen that 'from the time a man is damaged his possible future, not only in his own personal interests, but for the economic benefit of his country, should be steadfastly kept in view'.[7]

As far as the Departmental appointments were concerned, the ideal arrangement according to Lockyer was a combination of young, salaried, ex-AAMC doctors in the capital cities, with a collection of honorary specialists available to advise as required. This arrangement was in fact instituted on an unofficial basis until late 1918, when the Department proposed formally appointing three honorary doctors in each state to advise the DMO. In many instances the Honorary Medical Officers had been those who had advised the State War Councils. However, during 1919, DCs in several states experienced difficulties obtaining such honorary service. The DC for South Australia advised Gilbert that there were no medical consultants available 'to accept appointments in honorary capacity, but [they were] available and willing to act as special referees if remunerated'.[8] The DMO for Queensland, Dr Donald Cameron was outraged:

> Personally I strongly disapprove of the appointment of Honorary Medical Consultants. Why should medical men, who have already given their services with the A.I.F., be asked on their return to Australia to give honorary advice to the Commonwealth? No other profession is thus exploited.[9]

Possibly in response to this situation, Millen established a federal Medical Advisory Committee (MAC) in February. The Committee's functions were 'to advise on questions of present and future Medical policy as may be submitted [to the Commission]' and on 'matters relative to Medical services both ethical and practical'. Initially concerned with advising on policies and procedures, the MAC quickly became an ex-officio appellate body for War Pensions and eligibility for medical treatment generally. Accounts of the MAC, such that exist, have portrayed it as a body which established precedents, rather like Treasury's Rulings which gave rise to precedents for decisions on Invalid Pensions and provided the basis for its policies.[10] As shown in previous chapters, precedent was also the system used by the Repatriation Commission for the establishment of Departmental policy. Bureaucratic decision-making, freed from real democratic or at least parliamentary control by virtue of the sheer mass or cases dealt with, created policies which affected hundreds of thousands of people. Yet this process was antithetical to one of the keystones of medical professionalism – the indeterminacy of medical knowledge and the need for one or more experts to interpret the evidence on an individual basis. And in practice, it was on the latter basis that the MAC exercised its functions.

This Committee was a group of medical specialists. For them, at this juncture in the history of the profession, there was no room for rationalisation of the indeterminacy of medicine, for prescribing unequivocal criteria by which individual cases could be adjudicated. Each case needed to be assessed on its merits in order for medical knowledge to be shown to be necessary to the process. From a DMO's point of view, however, this was far from ideal. Professionally, DMOs at this date stood somewhere between general practitioners, reliant on their capitation fees and a few private patients, and specialists commanding £2/2/0 or more per consultation.[11] However, the power if not the salary of the PDMO placed him closer to these specialist advisers than to his underlings, the SMOs and LMOs. There is little professional or personal collegiality in evidence between these groups in the period under study. On the contrary, the PDMO, Agnew, showed little support for the newly appointed DMOs during his tenure and his successor, Charles Courtney, even less.[12] The state-based SMOs and, later, the doctors appointed to assess War Pensions, dealt with thousands of individual cases. Their decisions on entitlement and on assessment of war disability were closely aligned with Departmental objectives and Departmental rulings. This was increasingly evident from 1920 onwards once the new Repatriation Commission was appointed and Semmens became Chairman. But such opinions were not infrequently overruled by the MAC.[13]

When Graham Butler was writing the final Volume of the Official History of the AAMC, he corresponded at length with the then retired Courtney and with other senior DMOs on the history of medical repatriation and the problems associated with War Pensions. Butler had sat in on MAC meetings in the late 1920s and early 1930s and this experience together with his interviews with members of the Committee, forged a rosy impression of the body and its workings. He therefore found it something of a 'bombshell' when Dr Hastings Willis, a Departmental doctor in Sydney from at least 1922 until his retirement as SMO in 1955, a President of the New South Wales Branch of the BMA and Alderman of Willoughby Council[14], wrote the following in response to his inquiries:

> Your paean of praise for the M.A.C. is not deserved. It was really a very inefficient body and no one within or without the Department, except its immediate entourage, lamented its passing as an Appeal Board. Its delays were as bad as the Laws (*sic*) delays, and its refusal to establish precedents, but to deal with each case on its merits led to endless confusion from glaring inconsistencies in its decisions … [by the time of its demise] it had so magnified its job as to place it beyond its capacity, just as the frog in the fable blew himself out until he burst.[15]

What Hastings Willis describes here is a clear intra-professional division between the Specialists who were mobilising to control the practice of medicine, and salaried doctors who worked within bureaucratic structures and espoused a bureaucratic ideology, whether that of Treasury or Repatriation. The professional power of the specialists was considerable. As noted above, they could withhold honorary services and to an extent dictate fees. On this latter issue, Millen initially declined the MAC's recommendation on payment of fees to Honorary Medical Officers (HMOs), but when honorary services became unobtainable he was forced to approve a fee of £1/1/- per consultation, approximately half the standard specialist fee for private patients. This fee was soon declared 'inadequate' by some specialists. Dr R. Scot Skirving, for example, a prominent Sydney physician and surgeon, considered that a fee of £5/5/- was 'not too much' for the examination of 'malingerers' by a 'Board' of two specialists, including himself, and that a fee of £2/2/- was a more appropriate amount for his services alone.[16] The DC supported Scot Skirving's claim and Semmens ultimately approved the new standard fee of £2/2/- but directed that in future, if more than one specialist was required, the case should be sent to Randwick Hospital.[17]

Claims of this kind, together with the inconsistencies in decision-making that Hastings Willis described and which, in the early years, tended to favour soldiers, ultimately led to the demise of the MAC and its substitution by quasi-legal appellate bodies. The decisions and the demands of the specialists were beyond bureaucratic control, yet such control was mandatory in a state body as fiscally important as the Repatriation Department.

Departmental doctors were altogether different.

'Nice kind doctors' and 'wounded warriors'

In April 1919, Treasury advertised positions for nine temporary full-time and eight temporary part-time medical officers in its War Pensions Department. Over 60 applications were received. The Deputy Commissioners of Pensions in each state made recommendations on the applications and the guiding criteria seem to have been age (recent graduates, it was argued, would leave to set up their own practices and lacked experience) and service in the AIF.[18] Of the applications that have survived, most had held positions as either Commonwealth Medical Referees for Invalid and/or Old Age Pensions or had been members of the PMRBs.

In the previous month Agnew had written to the PMO of New South Wales, Col E. Sinclair, requesting a report on the work of the Pensions Review Board in that state for the six months ending 31 December 1918. The Report of Lt Col W. H. Read reached Agnew in late March. The Board, he recounted, had examined nearly 7000 soldiers in that period and there were many difficulties encountered. His chief concerns were with soldiers' exaggeration of their disabilities, about over-assessment of disability, about determination of 'how much' of a disability was war-related, about pre-enlistment disabilities, about Treasury's insistence on ignoring earning capacity, about the economic usefulness of invalids and 'over sympathetic hospital treatment' ('In some such cases it would be the kindest thing for the man himself to reduce the pension and thus compel him to seek some remunerative employment'), and about the positive deterrent effect of threatened hospitalisation on pension claims. Read identified other issues as problematic and in particular criticised the workings of the (Treasury) Pensions Department because it was subject to a final decision by lay opinion.[19]

For Agnew, these issues were critical. In a personal letter to Sinclair, Read's superior, Agnew stressed that he too had experienced 'every difficulty' mentioned by Read. He had experienced all the men who had 'lied at enlistment to get away overseas';

> they lied again overseas when there was serious work ahead and wanted to dodge it and, finally, they assumed the part of the injured innocent and disappointed 'warrior' when before the Pensions Board.

He had also seen men 'who had been twelve months and more loafing about, nursing their injured limbs and parading the city day after day doing the wounded warrior stunt, extracting sympathy and liquid "refreshments" from stupid admirers'.[20]

From Agnew's point of view, Treasury control of War Pensions was unacceptable for many reasons, not least of which was the lack of 'military discipline' brought to bear on former soldiers. He also objected to lay interference, indeed he wrote to Sinclair in late July that he had 'stopped the Pensions Department making the appointments advertised'.

> The Commissioner of Pensions was very wroth at my 'interference', as he termed it, but I said I objected to a layman making any medical appointments and, if he carried out his intention, I would not take over his Boards, irrespective of the personnel.

He informed Collins that if he made appointments on the basis of his advertisements he (Agnew) would re-advertise the positions when Repatriation took over war pensions. Agnew was clear that he personally would 'appoint men considered best qualified and experienced to do the work'. To this end, he informed Sinclair, he had 'induced the Minister to interfere with the result that the Military Boards are still working'. Agnew then asked the PMOs of all the states for similar reports. Extant reports in the files indicate similar 'difficulties' as those recounted by Read: fraud abounded, exaggeration of disabilities was 'very frequent', 'senility' and 'natural degenerative changes' and not war service accounted for too many illnesses, and many claimants had incomplete war records – sometimes no Board papers at all.

It is clear that the other chief reasons Treasury control was unacceptable were to do with money and with the selection of suitable men. The PMRBs of all the states recommended that payment 'be sufficient to attract the best men available'.[21] The Boards also recommended that 'great care' was needed 'to select a firm, tactful man, who will convince the pensioner that he is getting a "fair deal", even though the pension awarded does not come up to his expectations'.[22] They also argued for full-time positions and not part-time positions since the work of doctors was often 'slurred', or was not careful or thorough when dividing their time between private practice and pensioning.

Willis was rather more blunt in his description of DMOs. His description of his and his colleagues' work, their hearty contempt for supplicant ex-soldiers, their recognition and acceptance of the economic rationalism of Departmental objectives and their cynicism about the role of medicine in that process staggered Graham Butler. All Butler's interpretations of the medical aspects of repatriation, Willis wrote, were 'tinged by the "nice kind doctor" attitude towards the "wounded heroes"'.

> Of course a departmental M.O. cannot be a 'nice kind doctor' by giving away public monies, he has to be like all Public Servants 'a careful custodian of the public excheq-uer' ... Moreover the majority of the departmental clients were not 'heroes' but plain men and many of them not as much 'wounded' as they wished to be.[23]

In this brief space, Willis spelt out explicitly the bureaucratic values that have been examined in detail in previous chapters. 'Economy' ruled and fraud was endemic; notions of 'kindness' had no place in the system. While the older career bureaucrats like Lock-yer and Collins attempted to understand the experience of war vicariously, and tended towards generosity in the establishment of the medical service, the incumbents of the 1920s tolerated no such romanticism. For the Repatriation Commissioners as much as the senior doctors, experience of war seems to have brought forth a hardening of attitude that re-invigorated the values of classical liberalism in dealing with their 'deserving' and 'undeserving' supplicants, and a pervasive adherence to military ways and military values. In the interwar years this mentality was manifested most clearly in the pensioning proc-ess, one largely under the control of the Departmental doctors.

The transfer of pensioning from Treasury to Repatriation

In 1920 there were over 90 000 war damaged veterans receiving a payment from Treas-ury as compensation. Eligibility for that payment and the amount paid to those deemed eligible was largely determined by medical bureaucrats. Contrary to the well entrenched public image of the medical profession as caring and patient-centred, and to the simi-lar image conveyed by one relatively recent official history of repatriation, it is abun-dantly clear Departmental doctors frequently put the interests of the state before those of veterans.[24]

War pensions became the terrain over which a protracted civil war was fought.[25] On one side were the veterans, their families, their lobby groups, some politicians and some-times the press. On the other was a formidable state apparatus. In Chapter 9 the broad social consequences of this other war are examined. In this chapter the pensioning proc-ess itself is analysed: how loss of bodily parts or functions was compensated, the mecha-nisms and procedures used to determine eligibility and percentage incapacity, and how such mechanisms and procedures were controlled in order to contain costs. It is a study of the power of a bureaucracy both to rationalise the individualism that underpinned medical practice and to deploy individualism's ideological arsenal as a defence against criticisms of punitive policy. In practice it is an examination of the imperative that medi-cal assessments be standardised within the system, marginalising individual assessments, while retaining the vocabulary of individualism so that judgements could still be based on a soldier's 'failings'.

Generally, it is a study of the power wielded by a conservative liberal state over a damaged and dependent population. The division of labour within the bureaucracy meant that a handful of men trained in the militia, the army and in intelligence organisations, and saturated with the values of Australian bourgeois society, controlled the administration of war pensions. It will be argued that the values of these key figures – both administrative and medical – shaped practices, procedures and an institutional culture which survive to the present.

Commonwealth Treasury administered war pensions from the time the War Pensions Act 1914 commenced operations until June 1920 when pensions were finally transferred to the Repatriation Department. Treasury policy and rulings on war pensions were shown in Chapter 5 to have been relatively lenient compared with those on invalid pensions. This is not to say that Treasury officials were generous. Pensions were regularly cancelled or reduced, but the Commissioner's rulings on pensions for incapacitated soldiers tended to favour the veteran, often overruling the (Pensions) Deputy Commissioners in the states and/or the opinions of the Commonwealth Medical Referees. This approach was not simply confined to the senior bureaucrats of Treasury but was evident even at ministerial level: in 1916 Pearce (Minister of Defence) asked Treasurer Higgs to rule that pensions should be cancelled if a soldier refused medical treatment, but Higgs refused.[26] Commissioner Collins advised Higgs subsequently of his difficulty in determining the percentage of incapacity and of the need for a liberal and sympathetic understanding of the soldier's plight:

> It is not merely the visible injury which has to be taken into account, but the nature of the man's previous occupation, his intelligence, his opportunities, his general physical condition, and other things. It must not be forgotten either, that few of the soldiers will suffer only from visible injuries. All of them have been through very trying experiences, and it is only reasonable to expect that their health throughout life will suffer from the shocks and the horrors of war.[27]

He also encouraged Higgs to ignore a soldier's earnings in the assessment process. Higgs agreed to all his recommendations.

Other Rulings which highlight the relative benevolence of Collins towards former soldiers were, for example, his objection to the use of police reports to determine the health of a veteran. While such reports were commonly used in assessments of invalid pensions (see Chapter 5), Collins directed the Deputy Commissioner in Melbourne to discontinue the practice immediately in regard to war pensions and to 'tear up any forms on which the typed request already appears'.[28] Of greater importance here were his repeated but unsuccessful attempts to establish the principle that enlistment and service abroad were proof of the good health of a soldier prior to enlistment, thus helping to establish the cause of a presenting illness as war-related.[29]

There is a striking contrast between this view and the Repatriation Department's (and, earlier, the AAMC's) remorseless search for evidence of pre-war illnesses to counter pension claims. It was therefore possible for a senior, economy-minded Treasury bureaucrat to envisage and enforce a relatively generous policy on war pensions, and to rationalise this in terms of the special status of soldier-citizens and the horrors of their wartime experience. The very different approach which was to be adopted by Semmens's Repatriation Department was thus clearly not the only conceivable one for conscientious servants of the Crown to take at the time. It was rather a product of the conjunction between political decisions concerning the economic limits of state 'generosity' and the specific values and priorities of the men who had been recruited to control the repatriation process.

Collins and his Pensions Deputy Commissioners were civilians. Collins had no military training and no association with intelligence organisations. He had rigorously enforced controls over the granting of Invalid Pensions, directly through Rulings and Opinions and indirectly through his use of the Commonwealth Medical Referees. Yet these same mechanisms of control were applied far less systematically to soldiers, and indeed the opinions of the CMRs were often ignored when they conflicted with his own generous interpretation of particular cases. It is likely that this softening of policy was directly linked to a highly emotive 'civilian' view of war and its devastating effects on veterans. The language of militarism, which characterises the AAMC and the Repatriation Department administrators, is absent from Treasury correspondence and Rulings. 'Discipline', so dear to the military mind, is not mentioned.

The first step towards a new form of control over war pensions was the establishment in early 1917 of the Permanent Medical Referee Boards. From April, these Boards took over the functions of the civilian Commonwealth Medical Referees scattered throughout Australia. In principle, all war pensions were based henceforth on the percentage incapacity specified by the army doctors who comprised the Boards.[30] This introduction of military values into the pensioning system was initially a source of conflict between the Boards and Collins. The Boards saw Treasury as lenient, while Collins in particular interpreted the Boards' decisions as harsh. This tension was resolved in 1920 when administration of the entire war pensioning system was transferred to Repatriation, thus ending direct Treasury control. Coincidentally, when war pensions were transferred to Repatriation, Collins was made the financial representative of Australia at the first meeting of the Assembly of the League of Nations at Geneva. He was awarded a CMG in the same year.[31]

During the process of transferring pensioning to Repatriation, and after protracted and sometimes bitter inter-departmental negotiations, it was decided to transfer 'en-bloc' Treasury officers who had been dealing solely with war pensions to the staff of the Repatriation Department.[32] In effect, this meant the transferral of 66 permanent staff and an unknown number of temporary staff. Heading up the 'Central' Branch on a salary of £560 per annum was Collins's other long-time colleague, C.J. Cornell, then Assistant Commissioner of Pensions.[33] This transfer of Cornell and other experienced pensions staff was at Millen's request with the stated aim of ensuring the 'smooth running' of pensioning after the transfer.[34] With them also went the Treasury pensioning mentality, the poor law values that readily put moral judgement of deservedness ahead of other considerations. If there was any residual effect of Collins's generosity to ex-soldiers, it did not survive for long.

Treasury officials and repatriation bureaucrats, the latter mostly returned soldiers, made up the bulk of the administrative staff of the Repatriation Department. Less significant in number, but wielding enormous power, was a third group of civil servants, the Repatriation doctors. In October 1920 the Permanent Medical Referee Boards were disbanded. By this date the medical staffing of Repatriation consisted of over 20 full-time temporary doctors working in the capital cities and without evidence to the contrary, it can be assumed these doctors were appointed by Agnew. In Melbourne the Senior Medical Officer was Charles Courtney. In Sydney, in addition to the Senior DMO Vivian Benjafield, the DMOs were doctors Appleyard, Cowlishaw, Lawson-Kerr, Parkinson, Reiach[35], Roth, Rutledge, Willis and Smith, all on a salary of £750 per annum. All were former members of the AAMC.[36] The role these doctors played in war pension assessments and the values they brought to bear on the process are discussed at length in the following chapter through a series of case studies. First, however, it is worth noting something of the careers and credentials of the more important members of this group, particularly those in 'command' positions as either PDMOs or state SMOs.

Sydney Vere Appleyard was born in Middlesex England in 1882. He had both an MRCS and LRCP from London when he enlisted in Australia in March 1916, and he joined the 9th Field Ambulance when he was nearly 34 years of age and single. He had prior military experience as a Transport Officer in South Africa (1902), with the British Red Cross in the Balkan War (1912-13), and as a Captain in the AAMC 18th Infantry. He served in France in the 2nd and 3rd Field Ambulances, and the 9th and 10th Battalions as RMO until mid 1917 when he developed 'Severe' Trench Fever and was a convalescent for several months. Between March and September 1918 he served in the 2nd AGH and the 5th Field Ambulance but was diagnosed as 'seriously ill' with nephritis in September and returned to Australia in December 1918. His final boarding in January 1919 records that 'the indications are that he has chronic nephritis with marked cardiovascular changes and is permanently unfitted for the strenuous life of a general practitioner'. His nephritis was also noted as Due to War Service.[37] Appleyard died in 1926.

Leslie Cowlishaw was born in 1877 and graduated from Sydney University in 1906. At the time of his enlistment in March 1915, he was a general practitioner in Cooma, a small rural town in southern NSW. Cowlishaw, like his future boss Courtney, actually enlisted as a combatant in the 12th Light Horse Regiment, not as a doctor. He had been a member of the volunteer CMF for 12 months prior to enlistment. He embarked from Sydney in June 1915 but in September he was transferred to the AAMC to replace a RMO on Gallipoli. Later that month he was evacuated to hospital with an apparent case of 'scarlet fever'. However, his Medical Boarding papers state that on 1 March 1916 he was suffering the end results of 'an attack of dysentery at Lemnos, followed by a recurrence of an old fistula in ano ... now healed'. One of the members of the Medical Board on this occasion was Captain E.H. Rutledge (see below), the other Lt Col Flashman. Cowlishaw returned to Australia with his War Related disability in May 1916 as SMO on the *Themistocles* but then returned to Europe in October. He served at AAMC HQ in London as Acting Adjutant and Acting Registrar of Parkhouse Hospital in November, was then promoted to Major in December and proceeded to the 1st Field Ambulance. He served there until transferred to the 4th Australian Divisional Base Depot at Etaples in March 1917, then, once again, to HQ London in August and was returned to Australia in October 1917 and struck off strength.

Cowlishaw's life is not known for his war service, such as it was. Rather he is known internationally as a 'physician and bibliophile' and 'doyen of medical historians in his lifetime', who collected over 2000 rare and historic books now in the possession of the Royal Australian College of Surgeons. Most of this collection was put together between 1906 and 1914.[38]

George Lawson Kerr was born in Edinburgh, Scotland in 1869 and received his medical degree from the University of Glasgow. From 1912 to November 1915 he was the medical officer in charge of a small rural Hospital at Raleigh on the north coast of NSW. In November 1915 he joined the Reserve AMC and became Registrar and Senior Resident Medical Office of the Garrison Hospital in Sydney. He remained in this position until July 1918 when he enlisted in the AAMC and was attached to the No. 6 Sea Transport Section. He made one trip to London and returned in October. His appointment was terminated in August 1919.[39]

Charles Kingsley Parkinson was born in Tamworth (NSW) and graduated from Sydney University in 1914, in the same cohort as Hastings Willis. Unlike some of his more senior peers, Parkinson had extensive frontline medical experience. He enlisted in May 1915 and served in Gallipoli, Egypt and France. He was promoted to the rank of Major in June 1917 and appointed DADMS to the 5th Division of the AIF, that commanded by McCay (see Chapter 6), at the end of 1918. He was awarded the Military Cross when attached to the 14th Field Ambulance for bringing 'several stretcher-bearers into the dressing station under very heavy fire' at the end of 1916. In 1920 he was aged 29.[40] Parkinson transferred to the AAMC Reserve in 1925 and was mobilised for duty with the Second AIF in 1941 as Physician to the Standing Medical Boards with the rank of Lt Col. He contracted dysentery in the Middle East but was evacuated in April 1942 with a 'carbuncle of neck' and was returned to Australia. He was appointed President of the Medical Boards in NSW in January 1944 but admitted to the 113 AGH in February with 'Ligamentatious injuries' of his left knee and elbow. In December, after many hospital admissions, he relinquished this appointment.

Parkinson was a career bureaucrat with both Repatriation and Defence who became SMO for Repatriation in New South Wales in 1934. In 1935, then living in 'a quiet corner' of Double Bay, Parkinson wrote to A.G. Butler suggesting that if he was serious about his medical history he should talk to him or to his boss, the PDMO Ken Smith, in Melbourne. Parkinson advised Butler that 'many extraordinary things are written and said and commonly accepted concerning the late effects of war service on the human male' and suggested he should 'billet' with him in Sydney for a confidential chat.[41] A 'Note by Doctor Parkinson' in Butler's files for 1935 gives a clear indication of Parkinson's views on the effects of war service:

> It is my belief that apart from actual woundings and exposure to certain infections, army training and service conditions generally, were on balance, favourable to the fitness and health of soldiers. I do not believe that exposure to wet, cold, and heat, infection and 'stress and strain' in general, produced serious ill effects. My experience over the past 20 years has been such as to prove beyond all possible doubt that the propagation of statements as to early death and the incidence of disease in ex-soldiers has a most serious and widespread effect in increasing invalidity, incapacity, and unhappiness among ex-soldiers.[42]

Colonel (later Brigadier-General) Reuter Emerich Roth, a 'virile and very attractive character' and 'expert fencer' according to Butler, was a veteran of South Africa, Gallipoli and France and was President of the PMRB in New South Wales from 1917 to 1919. He was also a 'leading exponent' of 'physical therapy and training', the basis of modern physiotherapy. In April 1919, aware of the imminent demise of the Boards, he wrote to DC (Colonel) Farr asking for a position in Repatriation. His letter states his qualifications as being the organisation of the Boards and the instruction of 'subordinates' in disability assessment and 'the detection of malingerers etc. etc.'. He suggested meeting Farr at 'the Club'. Roth, like Cowlishaw and Lawson Kerr, had applied to Treasury for one of its positions advertised in April at a salary of £600 per annum. However, late in 1919 a new position of Assistant DMO was created in the Sydney office and Roth was appointed at a salary of £700 per annum. The creation of this unique position may be explained by the fact that Agnew and the Sydney SMO Benjafield had a less than harmonious relationship since Benjafield did not 'fit' the profile of other DMOs.[43] Roth retired in 1923 to his house and 'large garden' in Tusculum Street, Potts Point, and died the following year aged 66.[44]

Edward Hamilton Rutledge was born in 1882 and graduated from Sydney University in 1908 in the same year as Kenneth Smith but, unlike Smith, he had no prior military experience when he enlisted in May 1915. From this date until until June, 1917, he worked in various administrative positions in the UK (AAMC HQ, Registrar at Harefield Hospital and AIF Depots). He was then sent to No. 2 AGH at Wimereux and joined the 3rd Australian Field Ambulance in August 1917. He was CO of the Field Ambulance from December 1918 until March 1919. He remained attached to the AAMC after the war rising to the rank of Lt Col and CO of the 8th Field Ambulance. By 1929 he was Medical Superintendent of the Prince of Wales Hospital at Randwick[45].

Working with Reuter Roth on the PMRB during 1917 and 1918 was Major Vivian

Benjafield. Benjafield was born in Hobart, Tasmania, in 1879 and was a graduate of Sydney University. He was a surgeon, but unlike most of his peers, he had no previous military experience. He served at Gallipoli, in Egypt and in London but was invalided back to Australia in October 1917 due to varicose veins. Ryan and Maudsley, the Boarding Officers, pronounced him permanently unfit for General Service, but fit for Light Duty at Home for three months. His condition was considered 'Due to War Service' and the cause was listed as 'infection'. Benjafield was appointed DMO in 1919 and remained SMO in Sydney until he left the Department in 1928 and was replaced by Kenneth Smith.[46] He became a prominent Macquarie Street surgeon who, it is said, 'continued to visit his repat patients on a regular basis even after he had retired'. He was 94 when he died. Benjafield was something of an anomaly in the Department both for his lack of military ties and his apparent concern for his patients. He had a very strained relationship with Agnew.[47] He is also oddly invisible in the day-to-day clinical workings of the medical section in Sydney, something that would radically change after his departure.[48]

Henry Hastings Willis was born in Sydney in 1890 and graduated MB ChM and BSc (winning the University Medal) in 1914. He had been in the University Scouts for 7 years, including a period as Adjutant, and joined the Reserve AMC 9 months prior to his enlistment in April 1916. He embarked in August as a Captain in the No. 3 Field Ambulance. Between this date and late 1917 he was constantly on the move, with many temporary postings including brief tenure as DDMS to 1st Anzac Corps. In September 1917 he was promoted Major and at that date was CO of the 3rd Field Ambulance, working alongside Rutledge, and he remained in this position until December 1918 when he moved to the 2nd AAH and Rutledge took over his position. Willis was mentioned in Despatches of March 1919. The Recommendation states that on 20 September 1917 he showed 'coolness, courage, energy and determination under conditions of great difficulty and danger'.[49]

However, by far the most important DMOs throughout the 1920s and early 1930s were doctors Smith and Courtney. Courtney retired as PDMO in 1935 when Smith took over the position until his retirement in 1949.[50] He had been the SMO of New South Wales since 1927. Smith is an elusive character. When Charles Bean wrote to him in 1941 requesting biographical information he provided his date and place of birth and his address. He was also guarded in his occasional correspondence with Butler. His biography is outlined in Chapter 5 in the account of the 1st ADH. He remained on the AAMC Reserve as a Colonel.[51] The classic faceless bureaucrat, Smith was careful not to commit his views or opinions to paper, or only on very rare occasions. His harsh treatment of returned soldiers remains hidden from public scrutiny, locked in the personal case files of veterans.

Unlike Smith, Lt Col Charles Arthur Courtney was a prolific correspondent and a highly opinionated individual whose medical career was undistinguished but whose military background and administrative approach won him the position of PDMO from

1922 to 1935. His passion for military life gives him a natural affinity with Smith, but only in this respect. Born in 1869 and a graduate of Melbourne University, he worked as a general practitioner in rural Victoria prior to the war. Of more importance, he had served in the Victorian Voluntary Infantry, the Junior Cadets, the Garrison Artillery Rifle Club (8 years), and the Victorian Rifles and Australian Light Horse (11 years). He was promoted to Captain in 1906, but twice failed his military examinations for promotion to Major, a rank he only achieved after enlistment. Indeed, when he enlisted and was sent abroad in 1914 it was not as a member of the Medical Corps but as the Officer Commanding 'C' Squadron of the 4th Light Horse, a position he retained until he was invalided out in March 1916. Two of Courtney's brothers became Generals and a third a Colonel, while his father is described in terms of his 'intense patriotism and long military service'. His two sons became doctors, one enjoying a distinguished career in the 2nd AIF, the other serving in the Navy.[52]

Courtney served in the 4th Light Horse at Gallipoli. He was recommended for (but did not receive) an Honour by his Commanding Officer on the basis of his action at Lone Pine in August 1915. The CO's recommendation is intriguing. It begins 'Being Senior Officer in the firing line showed wonderful coolness under and in directing fire'. All but the last six words are then crossed out. The final summary reads 'For consistently good work – He has shown himself to be a cool and resourceful leader'. 'Coolness' was also an attribute displayed by Hastings Willis (see above).

Courtney had the first of many Medical Boardings in October 1915 in London. His disability is recorded on this occasion as 'Shell Shock'. On subsequent occasions it was reported as either 'debility' or 'neurasthenia'. The Board reported that 'at Gallipoli on 24th September 1915, he reported sick with debility. Four days before as the result of shell explosion he had concussion, deafness, headache and insomnia'. Five Boardings later, and with many statements on the instability of his 'nerves', he was examined by McWhae who pronounced him unfit for General Service. He returned to Australia to take command of a new fighting unit but ended up in command of the No. 5 Australian General Hospital in Melbourne. He then became a member of the PMRB and in 1919 became Senior Medical Officer of the Victorian Branch of the Repatriation Department.[53] He corresponded earnestly with Defence during the early 1920s to retain his post-service temporary rank of Lt Col and in 1924 was finally allowed to hold such an Honorary rank and 'to wear the prescribed uniform'.

According to his anonymous but well-disposed biographer, 'it was never Dr Courtney's attitude to beg anyone's pardon in soldiering. Just as in Repatriation it has been his way to say what he thinks and say so fearlessly'. And indeed this was true of his thoughts on every aspect of war pensioning. His views on the 'weak-kneed' Commission and on 'scheming politicians and pension wanglers' are reiterated in his correspondence with Butler over a period of nearly twenty years.[54] In the eyes of returned soldiers, however, Courtney was 'the petty country practitioner, utterly unexperienced, elevated by some odious mischance to a position of the highest responsibility', he was the man who 'by an extraordinary freak of officialdom – was kicked upstairs' and who 'always jumped eagerly at any disclosure of a pre-war disability to cancel a man's natural claim'.[55]

What did these medical bureaucrats have in common? To begin with, all were former members of the AIF and all were men of means.[56] With regard to the first qualification, giving preference to returned soldier doctors was at least superficially consistent with the overall 'preference' policy of both federal and state governments. Further, it was argued that such doctors were supposed to understand the illnesses and injuries caused by war better than civilian doctors. This was not just an argument put forward by former AIF doctors but also by governments and returned soldier organisations. Indeed it is an argument that is sometimes borne out in the medical records of returned soldiers in their dealings with non-departmental veteran doctors. But in the case of Smith and Courtney in particular, we are not dealing with run-of-the-mill service in the AAMC. Courtney's pre-war 'recreation' is described as 'soldiering' and his service abroad was not in the capacity of medical officer but as Commanding Officer in the Light Horse. Smith, similarly, had extensive pre-war military experience. He was overseas with the AAMC from 1915 to 1919 but largely in senior administrative positions ending up as assistant to Monash. Both remained members of the reserve army. Military life and values clearly appealed to both men and to many of their colleagues.

As far as the second qualification is concerned, the upper middle class orientation of the Repatriation doctors is also clear even if their £750 a year Departmental incomes did not quite support their inclinations. In practice these doctors can be differentiated from 'Lodge' doctors and from rural and suburban general practitioners by virtue of their greater salaries and the orientation of their careers towards serving the interests of the state. They were also quite distinct economically and socially from their 'specialist' colleagues who commanded many times their salary in private practice.[57] They had even less in common with the men and women they examined for war pensions.

However, the Repatriation doctors appear to have been hand-picked for their jobs on the basis of other common 'qualifications'. Doctors working for the Department had to possess the qualities deemed valuable by Agnew and his AIF colleagues: belief in the therapeutic value of discipline and self-discipline, in moral 'worth' as a criterion for pensioning, in individual responsibility for health or illness and, importantly, in cognisance of the public purse, the same values as those espoused by the senior bureaucrats of the Department. This affinity of interests and values was brought to bear on every aspect of war pensioning. It becomes transparent in the meanings assigned to the pivotal concepts underpinning the pensioning process, concepts examined in the following sections.

Constructing meanings

Damaged soldiers, those whose lungs were like cheese, those who had metal fragments in their heads or who had lifelong nightmares, had a legitimate claim for compensation from their employer, the Australian state. If we accept the immense power of the nationalist and imperialist ideology that propelled Australia's involvement in World War One, and the weight of that ideology in mobilising recruits, and if we also accept the importance of economic imperatives in recruiting, in the maintenance of the AIF and in its demobilisation, then it seems the barest justice that the often naive victims of the war, with its revived and intensified nationalism, should be given full compensation. The political arm of the Australian state accepted the idea of compensation in principle, but with a conservative ideology shaping the institutions of war and a poor law mentality directing what was presented as compensation within the administrative arm, pivotal concepts such as incapacity, war-relatedness and aggravation were defined and applied to the pensioning process in a way that reflected the values of its members.

It took several years for the senior bureaucrats of the Department to define the conceptual basis of war pensioning. As late as 1922, a senior official in Western Australia wrote confidentially to the DC in Perth seeking clarification of what was clearly a crucial point: was a pension paid as a reward or as compensation for lost earning capacity? The startled reaction of the upper levels of the bureaucracy suggests that a fundamental problem had been raised which demanded immediate and definitive resolution. The DC forwarded the letter to the Secretary of the Commission who forwarded it as a matter of urgency to Cornell, then head of pensions within the Department, who forwarded it to Senior Clerk W. Keays. Keays' reply, which formed the basis of the official reply, laid down emphatically that a pension had nothing to do with compensation for lost earning capacity. Semmens added that it was not and never had been 'an appreciation of services rendered' because clearly not all returned soldiers received one. The basis of pensioning, according to the official response, was indeed compensation but compensation for *incapacity* not loss of earnings.[58] This was despite the fact that the earning capacity of the returned soldier had been a significant factor in assessment for pensions since the Act of 1914 was proclaimed.

Regulations of the Acts of both 1914 and 1920 defined 'Incapacity' as an infirmity which 'wholly or in part prevents the earning of a livelihood'. The medical certificate (Form K) of the 1914 Act, filled in by hundreds of doctors for thousands of soldiers during and after the war, specifically asked for the percentage 'earning power' that was lost and this percentage formed the basis of the war pension. Pensions were regularly cancelled if a soldier was employed on 'Home Service' by the Department of Defence. In other cases arbitrary income limits were used to cancel or reduce pensions, or wages paid by government departments were fixed in relation to the amount of pension being paid. In some cases where a soldier was employed particular disabilities were accepted arbitrarily as pensionable over others.[59]

The relationship of war pensions to earning capacity proved to be a minefield for the Repatriation Department as it attempted to get veterans back to work. Soldiers who wanted work knew that their war pension would be based directly on their earning capacity. The application for a pension asked for specific detail on earnings since discharge, on dependants' earnings or other means of support and on any other income or payment 'by way of compensation, pension, retiring allowance, superannuation, or gratuity'.[60] Employment details continued to be of vital importance to assessment during the period under study. How then was Keays able to deny the relationship? The answer is complex. From 1921 to 1923, senior Repatriation bureaucrats and doctors tried to change the definition of incapacity contained in the Regulations from an assessment of lost earning capacity to an assessment of incapacity or disability; that is, from an assessment of ability to work (or not work) to a medical assessment of physical or mental incapacitation. Arguments about inconsistency and, more importantly, about the Department's vulnerability to criticism were repeatedly raised.[61]

Clearly, from the bureaucrats' point of view, if a war pension was associated with earning capacity the overall pension debt would be lowered: most soldiers did some kind of work, however unrelated it was to pre-war employment or to their skills, experience or training. But the problem of inconsistency remained. A soldier who had lost an arm or a leg was written into the Regulations of the Acts as eligible for compensation at a particular percentage of a full war pension *in addition to and irrespective of* his earnings. The 'value' of these parts of the human body changed over time.[62] On the other hand, the percentage loss to a soldier who suffered from recurrent pain or bronchitis or mental disturbance as a result of trench foot or gassing or warfare generally was not written into the Act and was therefore subject to assessment by a DMO. The majority of Australian soldiers fell into this latter category. Assessments of these soldiers were entirely dependent on the opinion of an individual doctor, on that doctor's knowledge, and on his attitude towards the soldier. The efforts of the bureaucrats to change the statutory basis of assessment were in effect an attempt to displace responsibility for pension assessment from the Department to the medical profession and this is precisely what happened. Until the Medical Advisory Committee's authority was superseded by lay Tribunals in 1929, doctors were established within the Department as the principal determining authorities, and medically decided percentage incapacity rather than loss of earning power was the basis of pensioning.

In theory, their determinations were based on a purportedly scientific calculation of the extent of incapacity suffered by an ex-soldier. Such assessments continue to shape the outcome of workers compensation claims in Australia and elsewhere today, and their scientific validity remains a subject of vigorous dispute.[63] In practice, as the Departmental files of the 1920s show, doctors regularly if inconsistently used the veteran's capacity to work as a tool for measuring that incapacity. The argument was frequently used that an ex-soldier's incapacity could not be as bad as he claimed if the man was able to work. So while 'science' was called on, along with notions of 'expertise' and 'professionalism', to testify publicly to the validity of the percentage incapacity, and thus percentage war pension paid, the confidential medical records prove the arbitrariness and the inconsistencies of the assessments along with the overriding importance of the individual doctor's values, doctors Butler describes as the soldiers' 'natural enemies'.[64] Throughout the period under study, the problem of deciding percentage incapacity remained problematic. Senior bureaucrats might decree earning capacity to be irrelevant, but doctors faced with the day-to-day decisions involving quantification of the unquantifiable effects of war regularly fell back on it as a rough guide. And this rough guide was rough indeed. There was no way in which a doctor supposedly deciding percentage incapacity 'scientifically' could avoid making personal judgements as to the relative importance of ability and willingness to work in a soldier's post-war employment history.

Two other basic concepts which shaped the pensioning process were equally problematic: war-relatedness (or attribution) and aggravation.

War-relatedness

If an incapacity could be medically established, it also had to be proven as due to war service. Disease aetiology in general is far from straightforward. What *causes* a common cold, for example, remains questionable. Causation can be variously constituted as a function of a virus entering the body, as a result of environmental degradation (pollution, cold, damp, etc), as a result of biological weakness (innate or inherited predisposition), as due to social factors (low income, poor nutrition, inadequate housing and health services, etc), as due to previous injury or disease (trauma to the respiratory system or damage to the immune system) or to any combination of these. The inexact, constantly changing nature of medical knowledge, and the reliance (usually) on one fallible individual's interpretation of that knowledge, will always leave room for legitimate dissent and conflict over aetiology. In the pensioning process, however, doctors were asked to be quite definite in specifying the cause of an illness or set of symptoms. There had to be an unequivocal attribution to war service or no pension was forthcoming. A set of signs and symptoms, whose aetiology even in peacetime civilian life was often difficult to pin down, had to be matched with a soldier's experience in the AIF to find a 'cause'.

In practice, medical assessments of war-relatedness relied largely on the soldier's records. Therein lay another problem, which Butler describes as a 'tragedy'. According to Butler, 'at the end of the war the Australian statistical records constituted a body of accurate statistical material which can never have been equalled in the history of the world'.[65] Butler indicates that the records were held in the British Museum, but 'due to the fact that the combatant branches concerned despise and loathe the idea of mucking about with statistics and figures, and historical trash of that and any other sort', no official agreement was reached over their fate and they were burned.[66] A.J. Withers, who assisted Butler in compiling statistics on the AIF, provided him with the following information for his official account of the remaining records.

> The inadequacy of the records was freely mentioned at the Commission and was undoubted a factor in men obtaining pensions who should not have received them

but it is not less probable that some men were at a disadvantage in their claims through the absence of records. The A.F. B103 appears to have been the best record that the Repatriation Department had to deal with but that only covered the period that the man was on 'active service' … and [it] was defective … The A.F.B178 and A.F.B179 were the other forms that the Department had. The former was not always kept up to date and often went astray, and the latter (which the Department state they pay particular attention to) contains and is based on the man's statement which is given to accord with his immediate desire; i.e. in the case of men repatriated they stated they were fit, to get freedom, whereas during the war many exaggerated their case to get home.[67]

If a soldier was 'invalided' home his medical history sheets were sometimes available, but the vast majority of pensioners were not 'invalided' home. In a draft of his chapter on pensioning, Butler goes so far as to call the medical assessment of attribution a decision based on 'some form of intuition'. A staunch defender of his own profession, he describes the process as one of making 'bricks without straw'.[68] Departmental doctors frequently complained of the lack of medical evidence available to them and of the incomplete nature of what did exist. In these circumstances, it was at least as difficult to make informed, professional decisions, let alone scientific ones, as it was with the determination of percentage incapacity.

Some indication of how decisions were reached on this extraordinarily complicated question can be obtained from the following letter from the DC Tasmania to the Commission in 1918. The DC sought clarification as to the nature of the 'record' that should be used in assessing attribution,

> Certain information, such as length of service, medical history, reason for discharge, and physical condition at time of discharge may be obtained from Defence records and the Deputy-Comptroller has a confidential record of punishments awarded to certain men, but beyond these there is no general record of a man's service.
> … the question was raised as to whether the [State] Board should take into consideration the fact that a man may never have reached the firing line and his service may have been such as to be only an expense to the country, without any corresponding benefit; the individual may never have had any honest intention of rendering effective service.

The Commission's response directed that the 'record' should indeed include the military record, 'information on the Departmental file' and 'other available information'.[69]

In practice, the lack of medical records combined with the inclinations of the Departmental doctors proved a formidable barrier to establishing proof of war-relatedness. The responsibility of providing such 'proof' was placed on the shoulders of the veteran, an individual often poorly educated, sometimes illiterate, frequently unemployed or only intermittently employed, and often suffering some kind of physical or mental damage. The 'burden of proof' that a condition was *not* war-related was only legally assigned to the Commission in 1935.[70] Proof of war-relatedness, during the 1920s and early 1930s, therefore rested on the outcome of a contest between two far from equal parties over incomplete and indeterminate information. It is no wonder soldiers were denied access to their medical and pension records within the Department. This issue was raised by the RSSILA in 1924 but the Departmental response was quick:

> It should be realised that statements contained in files concerning a soldier's service have been compiled from accurate and reliable authorities and that opinions expressed therein, principally in regard to the incidence and effect of medical disabilities, have been made by medical practitioners of standing as the result of an honest study of the case. It is upon the evidence of such documents that decisions by the Commission are arrived at. To allow the parties concerned to peruse their files would interfere with the proper administration of the Department and, therefore, cannot be permitted.[71]

Some years later, when the matter was again raised, the principles of ex-soldiers' privacy and the confidentiality of doctors' records were also wheeled out as a defence. Cornell argued that 'doctors have actually refused to set down their full opinions unless assured that their reports will be treated confidentially'.

> Files contain information concerning complaints, such as venereal disease, etc. from which pensioners may have suffered; also reports re alcoholism, imprisonment etc., which, if made available, might cause the pensioner great trouble and anxiety. Other instances cover concubinage, illegitimacy of children, etc.[72]

Departmental doctors argued that disclosing the information constituted a breach of their Hippocratic oath. The Secretary to the Commission also claimed in a confidential note to Semmens that the police would 'cease to report' on ex-soldiers and that physical violence could be expected. In addition, the correspondence on this issue repeatedly raised the concern that ex-soldiers might find out what was wrong with them. Giving evidence at the Royal Commission into War Service Disabilities, E.J. Didbin, General Secretary of the RSSILA, argued that

> If I am suffering to-day because of something, surely I am entitled to know what it is … If the department say it is not through war service, and I say that it is, surely I am entitled to be shown how it could not possibly be due to war service and that it is due to something entirely different. How can the Commissioners be satisfied that a disability is not due to war service if they do not know what it is due to.[73]

'War-relatedness' was thus the outcome of a complex decision-making process which rested on highly questionable aetiology and scant medical records. The 'conduct' of the soldier, his employment, information put together from surveillance measures, including the use of the police, and other *non-medical* factors were treated as equally important. Some of these factors are documented in Departmental files. Proof of war-relatedness, however, was required of the least powerful person in the system, the ex-soldier, and that individual had no access to the files.

'Aggravation'

If attribution of war-relatedness was a thorny issue then 'Aggravation' was a festering sore. In 1920 the word was used to describe the effect of war service on 'any condition which the soldier was pre-disposed to prior to or during his period of service and which has become intensified during such service', the onus of proof being on the soldier.[74] In the same year war pensions paid to incapacitated soldiers peaked at 90 389, a figure not exceeded until 1944. In 1921 this figure dropped by over 10 000 and by 1925 reached 72 128. Part of the reason for this reduction was an Amendment to the Act in 1921 which, following the lead of the British Ministry of Pensions, set a time limit of six months from the date of commencement of the Act for claims based on aggravation. In effect this meant a claim had to be made prior to 17 June 1921.[75]

It seems clear that the number of pensions being paid far exceeded Treasury's expectations. This explains the Departmental concentration on proof of war relatedness and the value of the Departmental doctors who refused, cancelled or decreased pensions which depleted the 'national purse'. Still the pension bill burgeoned. Part of the explanation can be found outside the cities, that is outside the immediate reach of Departmental doctors in places where local doctors could sometimes 'stretch' aetiology to define both visible and invisible conditions as war-related or aggravated by war. There were more than 680 Local Medical Officers assessing tens of thousands of ex-soldiers in 1921. The senior bureaucrats saw a need to control these doctors' assessments, but the method of control was a subject of bitter dispute between doctors and administrators.[76] The Amendment to the Act, on the other hand, provided a seemingly foolproof remedy to one problem at least by imposing a time limit on applications for aggravation to pre-existing disabilities.

Even prior to the Amendment, the Departmental doctors had met in conference and recommended to the Commission that limitations needed to be placed on aggravation and that the percentage assessment needed to be reviewed annually 'with regard to reduction only'.[77] The outcome of the Amendment, however, was unexpected. It was also, in Skerman's words, 'an unhappy episode in the Department's history'.[78] Whilst placing a time limit on claims for Aggravation of a pre-existing disorder, another section of the Act provided that an incapacity was pensionable if it 'resulted from any occurrence happening during the period he was a member of the Forces'.[79] So, a soldier with a pre-existing disability, say rheumatism, whose rheumatism was made worse by the cold and mud of the Western Front, was entitled to a pension for the *additional degree* of incapacity brought about by war service. This became the working definition of Aggravation until the Act was amended and the distinction between Aggravation and War-related Incapacity was removed altogether in 1943. Departmental doctors, without the benefit of pre-war medical histories and without adequate war records, that is without any substantial comparative documentary or other evidence of a soldier's pre- and post-war fitness or health, determined in precise percentages to what extent war service aggravated a pre-existing condition. Skerman notes, the 'correspondence of the period certainly indicates that the Department feared an immense increase in expenditure if the relevant provisions were liberalised' and that there was 'other evidence of some hardening of attitude towards the ex-serviceman generally as the First World War receded rapidly into the past'.[80]

These various concepts and their application in the daily workings of the Department will next be explored through a variety of case studies and specific 'conditions'.

What an Australian is Worth by Cut and by Kilogram[1]: A Leg, An Eye and Other Case Studies in the War Pensioning Process

A pension payment was largely based on the result of a medical examination, but the examination process, it has been argued, was seriously flawed. Many pensions were granted: as noted previously, over 90 000 War Pensions were being paid to partially incapacitated ex-soldiers in 1920. What this figure conceals, however, is the percentage paid and the way it was determined. In the following case studies, the determination process is analysed. This is not a quantitative analysis of the outcomes of pension claims or of trends in the medical determination of percentage incapacities, although undoubtedly the latter would prove interesting. Neither is it a representation of 'typical' cases insofar as a particular health problem or its assessment is concerned. Rather, it is an examination of the factors which mediated the pensioning process. Whether a hundred or a thousand files are examined, that process and those mediating factors remained the same. Each factor – the values of the doctor, the state of medical knowledge, the survival of a soldier's war records, the degree of bureaucratic intervention, the soldier's 'conduct', the advocacy of ex-soldier organisations or politicians – could and did shape the pensioning process. There is no one single 'scientific' or 'medical' activity involved here. Rather, there is a highly complex social process with a corresponding socially determined outcome. The randomly selected personal files[2] used here illuminate the process and its outcomes in an historically specific manner. The importance of these mediating factors and not others and their association with major social changes in Australia and elsewhere after World War One, suggests an intimate link with broader social and economic problems.[3]

In 1920, Australia, like the other combatant nations, was in a recession. Unemployment was rising, as was the cost of living, and the Harvester equivalent was only 50% of this.[4] The political strength of the labour movement was slowly eroded. Similarly, the unlikely coalition governments that were forged in the economic crisis of war now became unstuck as conservative business interests brought pressure to bear on like-minded politicians.[5] The highly centralised power structure which was rapidly built-up during the war years facilitated a conservative hegemony at federal level reflected by the institutional framework of the Repatriation Department. As well, war nurtured a world view that cherished discipline, sacrifice and utility. This militarism, along with belief in the values of instrumentalism and individualism, characterised Departmental activity. In the pensioning process this becomes abundantly clear.

'Mental' health, 'malingering', and 'neurasthenia'

The constitution of various human conditions as 'medical' entities has received considerable attention in the past two decades from sociologists and social historians of medicine. This is particularly true in the case of so-called 'mental illnesses'. The critical literature points out that such a nosological classification of mental/physical illness is based on the Cartesian dualism of mind/body. Further, it has highlighted the potential for social control inherent in such a distinction. More recently this dualism has been attacked on the basis of the 'enmeshment' of intellectual or theoretical approaches with practice and the ideology contained within such practice.[6] In pension assessments of 'mental' disorders all three critiques find justification.

Medical opinion on the cause of mental disorders during or after the war was divided. In essence there were two camps: a humanitarian view – by far the minority view – which saw mind problems as a direct result of the horrors of war; and a classical liberal view, which placed responsibility for the manifest signs and symptoms squarely on the shoulders of the individual. Published academic medical opinion included influential examples of the latter genre. In 1922, when Departmental doctors had the opportunity to establish a medical library, around 15% of the books ordered were on mental disorders. In these texts, such disorders were classified variously as 'nervous diseases', 'war neuroses', 'functional nervous diseases' and 'malingering'. One text singled out as important to the doctors was 'Jones and Llewellyn on Malingering'.[7] Figlio notes the appearance of this work in Britain in 1917 as a response to the introduction of workers compensation legislation in 1897; there is a clear connection in the text with the principles and practice associated with that legislation.[8] The concept of 'malingering' ('feigned disorder') in this and other texts is a judgement on an individual's behaviour which presupposes 'fraud', 'imposture' and 'deception' and equates the presumed fraud with an 'imposition' on the state.[9] The work of detecting these 'parasites of society', it was argued, was a 'service' to society and 'very often this service can only be rendered by a medical man'.[10] In war, this function was even more important. Jones and Llewellyn argued that

> the military surgeon cannot be too alive to the dodges of the malingerer; for it has been remarked that the incidence of malingering varies with the astuteness of the military surgeon.[11]

In Britain, one outspoken critic of this approach, Sir Philip Gibbs, the war correspondent, novelist and editor of *Review of Reviews*, wrote passionately of the many thousand 'wounded souls' who suffered 'hidden wounds':

Not all of them have recovered. Not all of them were conscious of mental illness until after the War – perhaps several years afterwards. They were 'nervy'. Their friends and relatives wondered at their quietude, or their ill-temper, or their restlessness and indecision. They had no sympathy from people eager to help the cripple[d] ex-Soldier men or the blinded soldiers and sailors. These others showed no wounds. It was only in their minds that they suffered, until some of them committed suicide and others were sent into pauper asylums, and others still – thousands of them – fell into a hopeless condition of neurasthenia, unable to earn their own livelihood, afraid of the world and themselves, with few friends to understand their misery or give a helping hand. The worst cases of shell-shock received some kind of pension. Other cases, to whom mental distress came gradually, were not entitled to any pension, or made no claim for one. They were among the 'heroes' of the War. They had done their duty with the best of them, but now in the time of forgetfulness they were forgotten, and the busy, joyous, selfish world passed them by …

In many cases it was the aftermath of war – unemployment, the competition of the younger crowd, bad housing conditions and overcrowded homes, the rattle and racket of city life and slum life, which gradually snapped the last thread, as it were, in the nervous system of men who had been through the long ordeal of war and were already overstrained.[12]

Graham Butler, preparing his chapter on mental disorders during war, read Gibbs and after lengthy correspondence with Courtney on the subject annotated this particular article as ' "Bulsh" of the most unpleasant kind', as 'Appalling muck', and added 'I never thought much of Gibbs'.[13] For Courtney as much as Butler, there was no room for sentiment where the nation's purse was concerned.

How, then, were these ideas, these values, brought to bear on individual cases?

Private Richard V[14]

Private Richard V was raised in Western Australia by adoptive parents. His father and mother died when he was in his teens. He 'ran away to sea' and worked on coastal boats for a time, then got a job in Sydney as a drink waiter. Uncertain of his real age – he thought he was either 17 or 20 – he enlisted in late 1915. In 1916 at Ypres he lay down in a trench to sleep when a shell exploded near him. He remembered nothing until he awoke with a sore throat in a Canadian hospital, 'bad with stammering and shaking'. He was subsequently hospitalised for over three months in France and England and medically 'boarded' in October 1917 as suffering from 'shell shock'. His incapacity to earn a living was assessed at 100%, the cause being recorded as 'Explosion of shell … superimposed on a pre-existing neurotic temperament'. His classification at this date was 'CI', that is, 'Permanent Military [incapacity] with no civil incapacity'. Early in 1918 he returned to Australia. For six months of that year he was an inmate of Broughton Hall psychiatric hospital. In July, the PMR Board assessed him as still 100% incapacity but now classified as 'E' -'Permanent Military incapacity with *temporary* civil incapacity which may reasonably be expected to disappear or be decreased by treatment' – and Reuter Roth, then President, noted that he required further treatment.

Richard was granted a 100% War Pension on application to the Department in 1918. On re-assessment in 1919 this was reduced to 50%, in 1920 to 25% and in 1922 his pension was cancelled. After his formal discharge from the AIF in late 1918, he returned to work as a drink waiter with his former employer and lasted 5–6 years. He then worked as a cleaner for 3–4 years and tried working at a rural sawmill but had to leave because 'he was afraid of the saws'. He was then unemployed until late in 1930 when he again applied for a War Pension. When examined by Parkinson he complained of 'pain in the spine which passes up into the top of his head':

> He suffers headache (almost every day) across forehead and behind the eyes. If he gets excited he stammers and can hardly speak at all. With any excitement or with strangers he gets a frightened feeling and his hands shake and he gets a strange sensation in the stomach. His wife says he moans at night. He has noticed these troubles particularly for 3 years. Before that he used to suffer headaches and was 'nervous' always after the war. He used to give satisfaction at [previous employment] but used to stammer so that members would not have patience to hear him out. He does not remember stammering before the war.

This was the selective account of Richard's problems recorded by Parkinson. Parkinson's own judgement on the account and the man was somewhat different. He noted Richard's 'small head', his 'tremor' and a stammer. He went on to add that 'he is obviously congenitally subnormal, and I have no doubt that … he stammered and was "nervous" before the war. The overseas records show that he was unable to stand field service and exhibited symptoms then'. His final 'Opinion' was that his condition was 'Neurosis (is a Moron)'.

> There is no practical disablement for his usual occupation as a cleaner or waiter. His condition is, in my opinion, not in any degree attributable to WS [War Service], his constitution, unemployment and domestic responsibilities being the source of his present complaints.

Hastings Willis agreed and commented as follows:

> On perusal of files I agree … that the aggravation of this man's neurotic temperament by WS passed away and that present Neurosis is not attributable to W.S.

Parkinson's medical history of Richard quotes him as being educated at a Convent School and then a Catholic brothers' school until he was 15 years old. He quotes Richard as saying he was 'too fond of sport' and 'would not learn'. These 'facts', gathered at one examination in 1930 together with observation of a stammer and a tremor of the hands, are then coupled with highly selective use of the records as evidence that Richard was a 'moron'. Parkinson does not mention the three-and-a-half months in hospitals in France or England in his summary, nor the time spent in Broughton Hall, nor the diagnosis of 'Shell shock' by the medical board and the PMRB. All this information is contained in the files but forms no part of Parkinson's written assessment and recommendation to the State Board. What we have instead is a highly tendentious attempt at a moral and intellectual characterisation of Richard. All the evidence that might explain his behaviour is ignored in favour of a diagnosis of subnormality on the basis of unexplained criteria.

Sergeant Ian B[15]

The case of Sergeant Ian B is somewhat different because it involved the classic war injury, an amputation. Ian enlisted in January 1916 aged twenty. Prior to the war he had worked as a clerk in a country town in western New South Wales. In the AIF he served in Egypt and in France. In early 1917 he received a severe wound mainly to his left leg but with many small explosive fragments lodging in the lower third of his left arm and around his thigh and pelvis. He developed gas gangrene in the leg, which was subsequently amputated and re-amputated high on the left thigh. He spent a period of around 5 months in hospital in France and England and in late 1917 was medically boarded as permanently unfit with 100% incapacity. His surviving AIF records were few. He arrived back in Australia in January 1918 and was admitted to hospital for fitting of an artificial leg. The hospital records in his Repatriation file state he had an amputation of the *right* leg. He was discharged from the AIF in June while still in hospital waiting for an artificial leg. In the same year he was granted a full War Pension (100%).

Ian returned to the country in 1918 and lived with his family, apparently doing some work in a family business. A Police Report of 1919, one of the standard Departmental investigations, described him as suffering from 'nervous trouble'. In 1920 he applied for a Special Rate of Pension (for totally incapacitated soldiers) on the basis of his amputation and the effects of gas, but was refused. In 1922, he was hospitalised in Sydney for five months due to an abdominal condition which resulted in surgery. That surgery necessitated removal of a portion of his ribs. The condition was accepted as war-related yet on discharge from hospital his pension was inexplicably reduced to 75%.

Departmental files reveal that throughout the 1920s and 1930s he complained of increasing pain in his right side associated with the surgery and accompanied by headaches. He also consistently complained of acute pain in his stump which was also accompanied by headache. In 1927 he suffered inflamed testicles and, according to a specialist's report, he blamed his amputation for this. This same specialist noted that there was a record of a 'stump neuroma' (a lesion of the nerve in the stump) but that nothing had ever been done for this. He went on to add that

> such neuromata can be excruciatingly painful and are particularly liable to irritation from the bucket of an artificial limb. He complains that he has gripping pains in the stump, is powerless to lift it at times and it becomes blue and cold.

Ian worked for the Repatriation Department as a bootmaker from around 1923 until 1929. The specialist noted that 'the work at bootmaking was always a drag and he often got around on crutches. He suffered from terrific headaches when the stump was painful'. He then had two other jobs until 1937 when, aged 41, he became an invalid, in and out of hospital until his death in 1943.

The files reveal an initial diagnosis of 'neurosis' in 1928. From 1934 his medical record discloses increasingly frequent diagnoses of 'exaggerated' complaints, 'neurasthenia' and 'malingering'. In 1937 he appealed his 75% pension on the grounds that he had not been able to wear his artificial leg for over twelve months due to pain and that his right leg, especially the knee, was 'a source of trouble … and very often fails me'. He complained of 'continual pain' and 'continual nerve storms caused by amp[utation]'. Over the next three years he was repeatedly examined by Departmental doctors, or specialists nominated by them, for complaints of pain. These doctors consistently labelled his complaints as 'functional'. Yet these same files reveal medical evidence that was largely ignored or trivialised.

For example, in 1938 Ian applied for an increase in pension on the basis that his general ill health was due to war service. He was examined in a Sydney Repatriation hospital. The examining doctor, with whom he had had an altercation, reported as follows:

> He states that he does not have one night's sleep in ten. 'His head is bursting and it all comes from the stump'. He gets 'terrific pain' in the right ankle, knee and hips.

The doctor's own examination report stated that 'he jumps when an area at the posterior end of the stump is touched but he can press the same area himself quite firmly without pain'.

> The right ankle is oedematous [swollen] and he states painful to touch … When I pressed the ankle and knee he asked me not to press so hard as it hurt but he dug his fingers into the ankle quite firmly himself without pain …I tried to flex the knee but he said it hurt too much. He smells of C_2H_5OH and admits 3 drinks.

A surgeon's report three days later, requested by the Department, states 'I can find no abnormality in either region to account for his symptoms and consider the condition largely functional. He is very neurasthenic. Looks anaemic'. The Radiologist's report indicated the proliferation of foreign bodies in and around the hips and thigh as well as 'osteo-arthritic changes' in both hips and the right knee. One week later the hospital Departmental doctor reported that according to the 'night report' he was ' under the influence of alcohol. [He was] noisy and disturbed the other patients. Vomited twice on the floor'. The doctor commented that

> when told that he had been drinking and that a half of a half of a bottle of whisky had been found in his locker he was most surprised and denied both statements. He said he vomited on the floor because he was upset. There is no doubt that he was under the influence of C_2H_5OH and was noisy and disturbed other patients. Discharge for disciplinary reasons.

Ian had only one leg and had continuing difficulty with using an artificial leg. His remaining leg thus took much of the weight of his body in an abnormal fashion. He had a swollen right ankle, fragments of metal in his pelvis, thigh and arm. He had consistently reported pain in his stump and in the weight-bearing joints. His X-rays confirmed osteo-arthritis. His symptoms, however, were medically defined as 'neurasthenia' and 'malingering'. Hastings Willis's statement of the case and his recommendation to the State Board was as follows:

> Investigation at … Hospital … resulted in his symptoms being attributed to Generalised Osteo-arthritis and Neurasthenia. Neither of these is considered related to his accepted WD [War Disabilities] and their relationship to WS [War Service] is not established.

After perusing the scant AIF records available on Ian, Willis concluded that he saw 'no reason to regard WS as a factor in the causation of his Generalised Osteo-arthritis or Neurasthenia'. The Application was refused by the State Board.

The following year he went through another series of examinations. The tests revealed that he was anaemic and had lung problems which the radiologist reported were 'probably tuberculous' or 'partially resolved simple pneumonia'. The consultant physician denied there was any significance in the tests and stated in his report that he 'got the impression that he was grossly exaggerating'.

In January 1940, by which time he was bed-ridden, the State Board informed Ian that not only was his lung condition and testicular inflammation considered not war-related but that he was 'not considered eligible for a Wheel Chair'. The RSSILA took on his case in February 1940 and applied for a Special Rate Pension. The League Pension Officer reported that the disablement was so severe 'that he cannot walk even a few yards without assistance'. The League then arranged for a specialist report, as did the Department. The League doctor noted a painful stump, the swollen right ankle and various 'aches and pains in different parts of the body'. These latter he considered functional. But the symptoms overall were described as 'a neurasthenia' and, he argued, 'it seems reasonable to assume that this is the result of the continual pain and discomfort he has suffered with the amputation stump'.

> As far back as 1919 we have a record of a report, by a lay person certainly, that he had 'nervous trouble'. This it seems to me rather strengthens his case than otherwise because it proves that his condition must have been rather obvious for a sergeant of police to have noticed it. There can be no doubt that a painful stump can be productive of such distress as to cause the ultimate development of a neurosis. The length of time taken before it is fully developed depends, of course, on the resistance of the person and his ability to stand up to mental stress and physical discomfort … I believe that over a period of years this man's endurance has been gradually broken down until at the present time he has a fully developed neurasthenia. It can therefore he concluded that it is directly related to his original war injury and arises from it.

178

The Departmental specialist had a different opinion. With regards to his alleged nervous complaint, this doctor considered neurasthenia 'a wide term, covering anything from complaints about symptoms which do not exist, to frank insanity'.

> In this case, giving [Ian] the benefit of every doubt, it seems to cover tremor, sleeplessness, headache, and many complaints for which no organic cause can be found.
>
> These symptoms could arise irrespective of War Service …I saw him … [and] he then would not assist in the examination at all, and gave the impression of malingering or gross exaggeration.
>
> In view of the fact that the alleged neurasthenia did not become obvious until after 1929, more than 10 years after his discharge from the A.I.F., I do not consider that this neurasthenia is related to War Service.

The Departmental specialist considered he should be referred to a psychiatrist. This psychiatric opinion, however, was difficult for the Department to obtain because Ian's 'serious state of health' precluded bringing him to the Department for examination. The Department tried to organise an 'alienist' accompanied by a physician to see him in his home but the 'alienist' demanded two-and-a-half times the standard fee. Ian died in Callan Park psychiatric hospital within three years of this debacle, aged 47. His death was considered not war-related.

Clearly Ian's chief complaint over most of his post-war life was one of pain. He had a stump neuroma, a condition known to be 'excruciatingly painful', yet nothing was done to relieve it. He had explosive fragments scattered around his pelvis and thigh and arm, and yet this was not acknowledged as a possible cause of pain. He had major abdominal surgery for a war-related condition and at least one specialist suggested it was possible he had adhesions causing his abdominal pain and tenderness, but this was ignored. Various doctors claimed that there was no organic basis for his complaints despite evidence to the contrary. Instead, his use of alcohol on two occasions over 25 years was seized upon as though it proved something about his condition.

'Neurasthenia' was a frequent diagnosis yet no-one really knew what it meant or, if they did, one doctor's understanding was different from the next. In some cases it was seen as a legitimate condition and therefore pensionable, in others it was lumped together with 'malingering', a fraudulent non-pensionable condition. An obsession with medical taxonomy, which seems to characterise this period, may provide a partial explanation yet it is highly significant that the specialist hired by the League accepted its legitimacy while the Departmental doctors did not. On the one occasion a Departmental specialist accepted neurasthenia as a possible explanation for Ian's symptoms its war-relatedness was denied. Perhaps it is no coincidence that renewed interest in medical classification of 'mental' and other illnesses occurred at a time when workers compensation claims and soldiers' pension claims represented a huge drain on state revenue in all the combatant nations.

In summary, it was impossible for the Department to refuse Ian a pension: he had, after all, lost a leg as well as having a war-related abdominal condition. Beyond these two straightforward conditions, however, there was room to manoeuvre. By classifying his signs and symptoms as due to his temperament ('nerves' or 'malingering'), it was possible to deny war-relatedness and any additional benefit, even a wheel chair.

Gas

It has been established previously that gassing of soldiers was widespread, often una-voidable and sometimes accidental. It was noxious, symptoms were often insidious in onset, and it had long-term health effects. In many cases it was not documented, or misdiagnosed when it was. There was also the unrecognised problem of toxic formalin fumes breathed by soldiers wearing the 'PH' gas helmet or Large Box Respirator in 1916 and 1917. Finally, there was the diagnosis of 'neurosis' which Maudsley applied in his inventive reclassification of 'gas poisoning' in the medical boarding of soldiers. Here was a classic post-war pensioning dilemma both for the ex-soldier and for the doctors. What was 'genuine' gassing and what was a 'neurosis'? What was an appropriate diagnosis when there was no record of gassing? What did a 'whiff' of gas do compared with gas-sing that caused death or at least evacuation? Did that 'whiff' cause post-war disabilities? These were important questions for the Department, for the medical profession, which was divided on the issues involved, and for the soldiers who suffered from the effects.

An important and very clear indication of the way the issue remained unresolved medically can be found in the following case studies. It is also apparent in Butler's corre-spondence between 1932 and 1934 with Dr O.S. Hirschfeld, who was on the staff of the Brisbane Hospital and whom Butler describes as 'an intelligent and I think ingenuous young fellow'. Hirschfeld was the son of Dr Eugen Hirschfeld, a German-born pioneer in public health medicine and tuberculosis research and sometime honorary bacteriolo-gist to Brisbane Hospital, who was interned in 1916 and subsequently deported in this xenophobic period. He finally returned in 1927 thanks in part to the representations of Monash.[16] The younger Hirschfeld wrote to the medical historian in 1932 asking whether Butler had any 'figures or discussion' on post war effects of gas. He went on,

> I have been horrified with the enormous number of men I see at the General who have been gassed and are now definite invalids without any very definite symptom complex – they have a good deal of struggle to get pensions.

The historian replied that gas was 'the devil to understand – more debated even than "Shell Shock"'. Butler had previously interviewed Stawell, one of the members of the Medical Advisory Committee, on this and other issues and Stawell's classification of gas-related 'pathology' is evident in his reply to Hirschfeld.[17] He wrote that there were three post-war effects that were 'pension issues': tuberculosis, 'Fibrosis' and 'Neuroses':

> In the war the psychic element in gassing was so general and important that M/O's were not allowed to diagnose gassing toward the end but were marked N:Y:D. Gas

– 'Not Yet Diagnosed – Gas' corresponding to N.Y.D.N. [Not Yet Diagnosed – Neurosis] – which explains itself! …

The first thing is – what is the evidence that they *were* 'gassed' – or were even in a position that they might have been gassed. In the second place – are there any physical signs indicative that the condition is not wholly psychic – the reaction to the fear motif – in this instance economic hardship that has replaced the fear motif of return to the front line.

Hirshfeld replied that he was not referring to 'neurotics' and that he was concerned with

decent, typically casual Australians who would rather get on with their job than seem to complain and so they didn't both[er] about the 'touch of gas' – they seem to have poor expansion of the chest and poor breath sounds and low grade bronchitis and no pensions – 'not due to war injuries'. It is a constant worry to me at the hospital.

He also noted the 'lack of resistance to any disease and the gross disability caused by comparatively minor disorders'.

Butler was not convinced. He referred to the 'concensus [*sic*] of opinion in all countries' that there was 'no evidence' that this was a pathological condition. His chief argument was that if exposure to gas did not warrant evacuation at the time, it did not constitute a condition which would continue to develop. Such a condition, he argued, did 'not accord with the known facts of pathology'. Apparently concerned that this scientific judgement may have appeared harsh he added

I hope you will understand that I am in no way unsympathetic to the claims of these cases: but I am wholly convinced of this that pension claims and so forth must be based definitely on facts and exact principles. Sentiment and gratitude of course have their place in the policy and setting out of the action of the country in respect of the Returned Soldiers: but once laid down it ought to be administered with the strictest impartiality and in accord with the terms of the legislation: that is of medical principles. Any other policy will result in chaos.

Hirschfeld wrote again arguing on the basis of X-ray reports that the damage done to lungs by gassing made the lungs vulnerable to later infections and other conditions, a supposition that would now be accepted as legitimate. Butler, however, simply cited the opinions of the men of the Medical Advisory Committee, 'men of the highest ability and unquestionable honesty and sympathy with the Returned Soldier', who denied the possibility of such a relationship and who also considered X-ray evidence as 'very questionable'.[18]

Butler sent copies of this correspondence to Courtney in 1934 asking for comment. Courtney replied that such cases as mentioned by Hirschfeld were indeed common and that the investigations of 'Syme, Stawell and Co' usually resulted in a diagnosis of chronic infection, a 'previously undisclosed or ? forgotten lung trouble' or a new reading of the X-ray evidence which defined the condition seen as 'within normal limits'. In other words, the conditions could be shown to be due to causes other than gassing. As Courtney noted, 'it is not possible for X-Ray to distinguish between gas-fibrosis and that due to other causes'.[19] Hirschfeld rates one dismissive footnote in Volume III of the Medical History.

There are a number of important points to be made here. First, as established earlier, the incomplete nature of the medical records of the AIF has been established. Yet, there was a tendency for senior Departmental doctors to deny that gassing had occurred unless there was proof in the records that a soldier had been evacuated for a gas-related condition. Second, some doctors argued that certain doses of gas could be scientifically proven to have no continuing effects on an individual. But the measure, or quantification, of that dose was whether the soldier had been evacuated. Third, X-ray evidence provided proof of lung damage that was impossible to deny, but diagnosis of the aetiology of that damage was a matter of individual interpretation: it could be used to argue for or against a gas-related condition, depending on the interests and values of the medical practitioner concerned. All three factors intersected in the assessment of whether a particular lung condition was war-related. In other words, medical knowledge was available to accept or deny the occurrence of gassing, its after-effects and the war-relatedness of a post-war condition.

Private Mathew B[20]

Private Mathew B was born in Ireland. When he enlisted in August he was twenty-five years old, and he was a member of the AIF for four years and eight months. After Gallipoli, he was invalided back to Australia with enteric fever but he returned to France in 1916 via Malta. He was at Passchendaele in September 1917, where he received a gunshot wound to the right thigh, and was at Villers-Brettoneux on 9-11 August 1918, where he received a second gunshot wound to the right leg. Mathew's own account of Villers-Brettoneux is worth quoting:

> [At] Villers Brettoneux on the 9th and 10th of August 1918 ...I distinguished myself by carrying on after I had been wounded, for which I was awarded the MM [Military Medal] ... I maintain I inhaled enough gas on those dates to destroy any human lungs ... [a person was] acting as a Stretcher bearer on the 9th of August 1918, when he was wounded in that never to be forgotten big push and the turning point of the war; I dressed him, carried him to safety although I was spitting up blood myself at the time. I returned and carried on with the advance until I was again wounded.

Mathew's army record shows that during his long service in the AIF he also received additional treatment for enteric fever, had influenza in late 1918, had inflamed gums on two occasions and had venereal disease on two occasions. His record also shows that he was Absent Without Leave (AWL) on more than ten occasions during that period, usually from parades. In a sense Mathew was the archetypal larrikin digger, the embodiment of the ANZAC legend.

Back in Australia Mathew was unemployed for around twelve months despite his own and the Repatriation Department's efforts to obtain work for him. He then had numerous jobs around Australia and New Zealand including work as a 'horse driver', as a 'miner' for twelve months for the Broken Hill Proprietary Company (BHP) at Broken Hill, as a 'farmer' working for a relative and as an employee of the state government railways for twelve months. Throughout this period his War Pension was fixed at 10% on account of the 'wasting' of his right leg. In his 1928 pension review the Repatriation doctor at a Sydney hospital noted that he had 'not lost work from illness [but had] lost much work owing to shortage of work at Broken Hill'. In 1929, aged 41 and having just married, he applied to have his pension commuted to a lump sum. The Departmental doctor noted in his physical examination of Mathew that his breath sounds were 'harsh' and his chest expansion only 'fair' but suggested he was otherwise in good health and recommended a commutation rate of 5-10%. Kenneth Smith agreed and set the rate at 5%. As a result Mathew received £86, that is, the equivalent of about 20 weeks wages for a railway fitter in that year.

In 1932 Mathew applied again for a pension for compensation for pulmonary fibrosis. He reported pains in the chest, shortness of breath and a noticeable loss of weight in 1931. There is evidence that a chest X-ray had found a lung problem. The Departmental medical examination, however, declared his lungs clear. Various tests, including the routine tests for venereal disease, were carried out and the radiologist's report stated that he had a 'Fibroid type of Tuberculosis [in] both upper [lung] lobes'. This was the same year that Hirshfeld noted increasing numbers of soldiers suffering pulmonary fibrosis as a result of gassing.

There were other complicating factors present. Two days after the medical examination on 22 September, Mathew wrote complaining about the nature of the examination. His letter to the Department is an eloquent description of the complex outcomes that resulted from using incomplete and partial records:

> On 22.9.32 I was examined at the medical section of the Repatriation Chambers, it appeared to me somebody's history had been getting mixed up with mine. I was aksed by the Officer who examined me if my name had ever been so & so. On arrival home I got out my little diary and I might state what I saw there didn't make me feel flattered at being asked that question. At one particular time during the big arguement and the hun was making it a bit hot around Streezels throwing a few foundrys around we were in the third line trenches the order came to reinforce the front line and this late reinforcement to our Battalion cacked himself went back instead of going forward for which he was afterwards court marshalled for cowardice in facing the enemy, now I dont want my history getting mixed up with his so I am forwarding my Birth Certificate, its the one and only name that I have ever had and it may be placed with my military history whatever my other failings were the huns or military police never put the breeze up me.

Mathew's application was rejected on the grounds that the condition was not war-related.

In 1934 Mathew appealed against this decision. He wrote to the Commission as follows:

> I wish to appeal against the unfair decision of the State Repatriation Board of N.S.W. When I made my application for a pension I was ordered into hospital, I did not go to hospital, although I did not refuse treatment. The next I heard from them I was not entitled to treatment or a pension as my complaint was not caused through war service. Now how a Repatriation Board can reach that decision baffles me. My condition of Pulmonary Fibrosis is gradually getting worse year by year, and I have good reason to believe that it is attributable to war service and no other cause. At Villiers [*sic*] Brettoneux … I consumed enough gas to destroy a million lungs, if a man had been possessed with that many, where I carried on 8 hours after I was wounded all I get was a Military Medal.

The State Board recommended the appeal be disallowed. Courtney recommended rejection and the Commission disallowed the appeal. Mathew then applied to the War Pensions Entitlement Appeal Tribunal, established in 1929, which asked for another medical opinion from a designated doctor. The specialist reported that since there was no 'active' pulmonary disease he considered that there was 'no evidence connecting his present disability with his war service'. The Tribunal disallowed the appeal.

In 1936, now with four dependent children, Mathew tried again for a pension based on his gunshot wounds but since his pension for these wounds had been commuted he was ineligible. In 1937 his application for treatment of his tuberculosis, now recognised, was also rejected. Frustrated with the system, Mathew wrote to Hughes, then Minister for Health. After outlining his war service and how he had 'battled on' for many post-war years, he wrote of his sick wife and the children he had supported on the 'miserable pittance of a Service pension'. [By this time he didn't have a war pension].

> I am now unemployable, and the gentlemen on the Tribunal Board can only make the excuse that they cannot link up my medical history since I was discharged, and find that the cause of my Pulmonary Tuberculosis is due to War Service.
>
> Am I to be put on a par with those who were not long enough on Active Service to get lowsy [*sic*], or am I to be punished because I did not have money to give to doctors and keep running to them with my coughs, colds and complaints, so that the Military authorities could lunk [*sic*] up my medical history.

Mathew's letters and appeals were in vain and his lung condition was never recognised as due to war service.

Private Albert C[21]

The case of Private Albert C is somewhat more complicated. Albert was 32 years of age when he enlisted in late 1915. Having migrated from England, he worked in coal mines around Newcastle until he enlisted. He disembarked in Plymouth in mid 1916 and immediately went AWL for nearly a month. He finally proceeded to France in mid

1917 and after two months was admitted to hospital with 'Debility'. Discharged from hospital after approximately two months, he rejoined his Battalion but after another two months was again admitted to hospital, this time with a diagnosis of 'Diarrhoea'. After around six weeks in hospital he was sent to England but the diagnosis was now 'Myalgia'. Hospitalised in England for another three weeks he was ultimately returned to Australia in June 1918 suffering from 'Myalgia and Debility'.

Albert's medical army record discloses complaints of pain in nearly all of his joints in early 1918 and marked loss of weight. In March, a history of pre-war rheumatic fever was recorded. The Medical Board considered his condition was 'constitutional' but that his disability was Aggravated by War Service. His disability was assessed at 100%. He returned to Australia in August and during nearly two months in hospital gained weight and 'improved considerably'. In October he was discharged, the PMRB finding him 'one quarter' incapacitated.

On his discharge from the AIF and from hospital, Albert applied for a pension and was granted 25% of the full rate. He also applied for and briefly received a sustenance payment from the Department. Returning immediately to his wife in the vicinity of Newcastle, he obtained some temporary light work but was dismissed prior to Christmas because of his inability to 'attend regularly'. Labor MP Mathew Charlton, acting as advocate, wrote to the Department stating that 'there are very few jobs which he can do owing to his incapacity'. In January, the Secretary of the Local Committee wrote to the Department reporting on Albert's use of his sustenance money as follows:

> The Landlord … tells me that he has seen this man coming home under the influence of liquor and he considered that if he could find money for drink it was up to him to pay the rent. Having explained the condition of the Soldier's wife he has consented to take no action for a few weeks towards removing him from the house.
> Confidential information from a most reliable source has been given me as follows. [Albert] is a perfect Devil at home, his wife is a good economical woman if given a fair chance, she is near confinement, and has neither money or clothes for the event. If money is given [Albert] it will be drunk, but if it or even a portion could be given his wife it would be put to good use and fill a long felt want.

By March, with Albert's sustenance payment cancelled, the Secretary appears to have had a change of heart. Having consulted a local doctor who had attended Albert, the Secretary complained to the Sydney Head Office that his pension was under-assessed since he was not only suffering from myalgia but 'suffering mentally, possibly brought about by warlike operations'. The Secretary pleaded with Head Office to pay some sustenance if only to his wife. Charlton also wrote the following month, stating the family was 'practically starving' and days later the Secretary wrote again noting that he had been 'compelled to take up a hurried collection and purchase a small supply of food for his wife and family'. He continued,

I understand sustenance was stopped some time ago on the strength of a Newcastle Medical gentleman's certificate. I would remind you that [another] clever Medical gentleman … is of opinion that this man's trouble which is mental, as well as physical, was brought about by warlike operations.

The Repatriation Local Medical Officer, however, considered that 'he can, and ought to do light work … It will keep his mind occupied'. One week later this opinion was overruled by the Principal Medical Officer of the 2nd Military District and, as a result, Albert's pension was increased briefly to 50%.

At his regular re-assessment in late 1921 the examining doctor noted that the 'applicant claims that he was gassed near Armentières in December 1917'.

[He] now feels weak and giddy, unable to work, lost 1 stone in weight last 3 months, also occasional haemoptysis [coughing up of blood].
On examination I find that chest shows signs suspicious of early tuberculosis, no signs of DAH [Disordered Action of the Heart], or symptoms which can be directly ascribed to gas … Recommended that his present disability is not the direct result of War Service.

Reuter Roth agreed that it was not war-related and an increased war pension was not recommended. His pension was then decreased to 25%.

At his 1922 examination, Parkinson recorded that he was 'very thin and debilitated', that he had had pneumonia, had an indefinite lung condition on the right side which he suggested was 'probably anthracosis' [a lung condition resulting from inhaling coal dust over long periods]. He was subsequently admitted to hospital in Sydney for three months for investigation. Towards the end of that period he left the ward 'although ordered to remain in bed'. He 'returned under the influence of C_2H_5OH and became abusive'. He was discharged that day for 'alcoholism' and his new diagnosis recorded by Parkinson was 'Chronic arthritis and alcoholism' with 'alcoholism aggravating disease'. His pension was continued at 25%. In a final assessment of Albert's case in 1933, Smith opined that

After weighing up the evidence of this case – pre-war, war service and post war history, I … recommend continuance of 25% indefinitely for Chr[onic] Rheumatism. Any other disability which might be present would not be attributable to War Service.

Albert's lung condition was never accepted as war-related. He appears to have suffered from chronic pain until his death, aged 80, from 'Bronchitis'.

What emerges most clearly from these case studies, and also from Butler's correspondence with Hirshfeld, is the indeterminate nature of medical knowledge and the purpose this indeterminacy could serve. Hirshfeld and various other non-Departmental doctors considered the X-ray evidence proof of a war-related injury. Departmental doctors tended to ignore the radiological evidence and focus on other 'facts' in the soldiers' histories. This tendency seems hard to explain until we look at the outcome of the 1924

Royal Commission on War Service Disabilities. The facile nature of the Commission itself is discussed in the following chapter, but of interest here is its recommendation that former soldiers suffering from war-related tuberculosis should be paid permanent pensions. This recommendation was acted on and from 1 July 1925 soldiers so diagnosed became eligible for a 100% pension. Yet, as we have seen, a soldier had to first prove his lung condition was war related and that proof rested largely on his service record and its medical interpretation. More importantly, if Departmental doctors chose to ignore the radiological evidence that the condition existed at all then there was nothing for the soldier to prove.

Departmental historians have accounted for the acknowledged inconsistencies and arbitrariness of TB pensioning with remarkable consistency. Lloyd and Rees are unequivocal:

> While the majority of cases were not contracted on active service the medical officers accepted as beyond doubt that military privations had stimulated the latent disease.[22]

Not only was medical opinion favourable to the ex-soldier, they suggest, but 'for several reasons, the tubercular under Repat's care was more fortunate than his civilian counterpart. The tubercular civilian had to earn a living while the tubercular war veteran was supported'.[23] Skerman is somewhat more circumspect, commenting that 'in view of the lack of medical precision which prevailed at the time where diagnosis of tuberculosis was involved, the course decided upon when considering [the] recommendation … represented a new and bold departure even though based on the best medical opinions available'.[24]

But Skerman's description of the 'repercussions' of the recommendation – a description quoted without comment by Lloyd and Rees – suggests that many former soldiers benefited from the new regime, indeed benefited 'out of all proportion to the degree of incapacity suffered over a period of many years'.[25]

These accounts are an extension of the reformist liberal welfare discourse. Underpinning both is a positivist interpretation of the system: this argument maintains that mistakes were made and sometimes soldiers benefited from them; others slipped through the safety net but then the scheme was progressively liberalised and look at how many ex-soldiers receive pensions now. Such accounts assume a benevolent state handing out increasingly generous payments to ex-soldiers. But implicit in the interpretation is the ideology of the liberal democratic state, one which is always primarily cognisant of the need to protect the public purse from the claims of the undeserving, and bureaucratic responsibility in that regard. This dominant ideology is often neglected in welfare discourse which glosses over concepts like relations of class and power and the state's role in helping to regulate Australian capitalism, by making war if necessary, in favour of a focus on concepts of individual citizen's (soldier's) rights, professionally certified identification of individual needs and amelioration of those needs, or other benefits, by cash.[26]

War pensions represented the largest welfare expense to the pre-World War Two Australian state. This expenditure was tightly controlled. The 'public purse' and the 'national economy' were familiar concepts to politicians and bureaucrats alike. Both concepts are concerned with preventing the unproductive use of state revenue. The political pressure from ex-soldier organisations and from within Parliament, which resulted in approval of modifications to the regulations and compensation for war-related tuberculosis at full pension rate, was a direct result of vehement public criticism of Departmental pension policy. Publicly the response appeared generous and fair. Yet it is clear from the case studies examined so far that practice did not match the rhetoric and that medical knowledge and medical bureaucrats were instruments by which the national purse strings were continually tightened.

Pre-existing illnesses or injuries, use of alcohol, 'constitutional' weakness, physiognomy, 'nervous' habits, could all be used medically to discredit the war-relatedness of a condition. As well, there is ample proof that medical evidence supporting war-relatedness could be disregarded. As argued above, the practice of pension determination was not a rigid, scientific, consistent procedure. It was open to a range of influences which undoubtedly varied from case to case, but the fact that it was so imprecise, was so subject to interpretation and the arbitrary deployment of evidence, made it ideally suited to the imperative of cost-containment. The divergence of medical opinion between Departmental and non-Departmental doctors highlights this.

What is an eye worth?

Private William O [27]

Private William O, a self-employed painter from a working class inner city suburb of Sydney, enlisted in 1916. At the Somme, in the winter of 1916/1917, he received a severe gunshot wound to the left side of his face and lost his left eye. He was hospitalised in France and England for nearly six months, returned to Australia and was discharged as Medically Unfit in late 1917. On discharge he was assessed as suffering from three medically defined problems: loss of the left eye, infection of the socket of left eye and 'nerves'. The PMRB assessed 'incapacity to earn a living' at 50% and the duration was classified as 'Permanent'. On discharge, William applied for a pension of 50% and was granted one on the basis of the loss of his left eye. He appealed against this amount in 1917 and again in January 1918 on the grounds that his right eye was weak and that he suffered from 'nerves' and 'severe pains in the head'. He continued,

> I was a Painter before enlisting, earning £3.10.0d p.w., but it is impossible for me to take on that class of work now – I have been unable to take on any work since discharge, nor have I felt fit to seek any. I could not do any work at present owing to the state of my health.

The Deputy Commissioner of New South Wales rejected his 1917 appeal but the 1918 appeal resulted in examination by three doctors. The first opinion by a Departmental specialist was that the incapacity was purely loss of the eye and therefore assessed at 50%. The second, by Lawson Kerr, a Departmental doctor, was as follows:

> [He] states that he is suffering from shooting pains in front of head, cannot wear his glass eye on account of discharge from socket. Feels nervous on exertion.
> My examination shows – loss of left eye. Artificial eye causes irritation of socket … Has tremor of hands when unbuttoning and buttoning coat.

Lawson Kerr assessed the incapacity at two-thirds (66.6%). The third opinion, by another specialist also noted tremors and increased heart rate and gave the opinion that he was 'not fit for full hard work'.

As a result of these examinations, William's pension was increased to 66.6% for a period of six months. Six-monthly re-assessments confirmed the percentage incapacity until 1921, when Dr Cowlishaw re-assessed the incapacity at 50%. The State Board, however, considered his condition 'underassesed' and recommended 80% based on 50% for the loss of the eye, 10% for the discharging eye socket and 20% for defects in his right eye which they considered could be war-related. Cowlishaw re-considered his assessment and an 80% pension was granted.

Now on annual re-assessments, William was next examined in July 1922 by Dr Reiach who noted that the left socket was chronically infected and was constantly discharging pus so that he was unable to wear a glass eye. He thought it likely that there was a 'septic focus' – a fragment of bone, shrapnel or some other foreign body – in the socket and questioned the likelihood of my future improvement. The following year Smith concurred with this assessment adding that there was 'slight neurasthenia' and that the gradual deterioration in vision in his right eye was a normal ageing process but one 'no doubt accentuated by loss of the left eye'. William remained on 80% pension until 1931.

In 1931 William was assessed by doctors Hasting Willis and Allen. Their report was as follows:

> In addition to loss of left eye this man is suffering from Refractive Error and Arteriosclerosis with High Blood Pressure, and possibly Renal impairment. His total incapacity is 100%.
> … we do not regard his present Refractive Error Rt. Eye to have been adversely affected by his W.S. or the loss of vision left eye. His Arteriosclerosis with raised Blood Pressure and possible Renal impairment has arisen since W.S., and evidence is insufficient to warrant regarding it as influenced by W.S.

Smith, then SMO in Sydney, and adjudicating the assessment, wrote that

> In the years 1921 to about 1926 it was thought that the loss of one eye had an aggravating effect on a refractive error in the remaining eye, but this view is now held to be quite erroneous.
> … He now complains of severe headaches, mainly on the left side. Investigation

Figure 20. History of assessment of incapacity, Private William O, 1917-1935

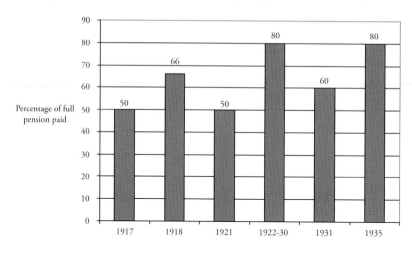

Source: AA(NSW): ST2817/1, Box 888

has shown that the most probable explanation is Arteriosclerosis with High Blood Pressure, and possible Renal Inefficiency.

There is a history of [syphilis] since W.S., but the Blood Wassermann [test for venereal disease] is negative.

Smith's final assessment was 60% based on 'loss L. eye with tender socket and slight Neurasthenia'. In 1935, William was restored to an 80% pension but he died the following year. Since his death was not considered due to war service, no funeral benefits were paid. (Figure 20)

An Aboriginal veteran and his wife

Private Harry P [28]

Private Harry P enlisted in 1916 aged 21. Prior to enlistment he worked as a shearer and labourer in the central west of New South Wales. He was a member of the AIF for 19 months and served in France, where he received a gunshot wound to the right wrist. He was subsequently discharged as Medically Unfit. His AIF records were scant.

On his discharge, Harry was assessed at having 25% incapacity and this incapacity was considered permanent. He returned to a small country town and in 1918 married Molly. His stiff arm restricted the kind of work he could do. He got a couple of casual jobs but only for a few months in each case and ended up trapping and skinning rabbits to earn some money. His pension was increased briefly to 50% but in 1923 it was suddenly suspended. Harry was illiterate but his wife was not. In June she wrote to the Department to find out why. (During these years they had moved a short distance to a larger town). Her letter reads as follows:

I am writing this short letter to find out why No.[pension number] pension was stopped. The Post Master could not let me know so I thought I would write. I think that it must be about not attending the Doctor it is the reason it is he never got no card sent to him to attend. I was thinking it must have been sent to [previous town] and someone got it and was not good enough to send it on to [present town]. I think that they would have sent it here, they know that he is drawing his Pension here … So kindly write and let me know before next Pension Day.

The file shows Molly's letter as 'acknowledged' and Harry's pension was reinstated but at only 10% of the full rate. Molly wrote again, this time more assertively:

My Husband asked me to write to you about his pension as he is a very poor one at writing. He wants to know could not you have his pension rise again as what he is getting he has to keep his family on. As he cannot do any hard work and imagine keeping four on 13/9 a fortnight. It is cruel to think that he went to the war to fight for his country and then to think that he cannot get enough food from it to feed his body. It is cruel on his family. I his wife went to a charity fund to get some food and what they said to me was Is not your Husband getting a pension. Just imagine how I would feel if another war broke out and I had some grown up sons. What would I say to other people. I would not let my sons go. Look how they treated their father. So trusting that you will help me and my husband. I will be very much obliged. They did not give a reason why they lowered my Husband's and family pension so you might let me know.

I have one little girl 1 year and 6 mths but I have not put in for her pension.

The Department's response was twofold: there was a note by Smith to the effect that Harry was to be examined in Sydney and a form letter sent to Molly stating 'Please give reason for not applying for pension on behalf of [child] within six months of the date of her birth'. The following month doctors Lawson-Kerr and Appleyard examined Harry in Sydney. They reported as follows:

States age 29 yrs – P.W.O. [Pre War Occupation] Shearer. Does rabbitting now.

C.O. _[Complains Of]_ pains and stiffness about Rt Shoulder after any heavy work and in wet weather – Rt hand aches at times and he has to knock off work for a bit. Has no other disability.

O.E. _[On Examination]_ Ht 5ft 9in Wt (1/2 stripped) 8st 8lbs. Aboriginal. General health good. Heart-Lungs-Urine: NAD [No Abnormality Detected].

Two small scars in front of lower third of Rt forearm – slight reduction in wrist movement only. Grip is good. There are no physical signs of any disability about Rt shoulder and no reason to connect any trouble there with his WD [War Disability] of GSW [Gun Shot Wound] Rt wrist.

We consider _10%_ an adequate assessment and recommend that the same rate be continued _indefinitely_.

Unemployed and destitute, Harry's pension was fixed at 10%. As for Molly, she replied to the Department's inquiry as follows:

The reason I did not apply for [child's name]'s Pension is because … my Husband's Pension was lowered. I expected it to be knocked right off as they lowered it down so little. And he did not expect it to last long. The thought that that is why they lowered it so they could knock it off [is the reason I did not apply]. And when it still went on I wrote to try and get it rose higher. And then I was going to apply. I did not know that you have to apply when they were six months old. So that is the only reason.

Nothing more is heard of Harry or Molly until 1930, a significant year, when, still on a 10% pension, Molly wrote again to the department trying to find out why one pension payment had not been made.

The pay master at the post Office said he did not know the reason it was marked off, that I would have to inquire to you. So will you kindly let me know. We have no other means of living now only trusting to the little pension we get. We cannot even get the dole that is handed out to the poor just because we get a pension. When my Husband went to the police station the Sergent said you get a War Pension what more do you want. So you can see how we treasure the little pension. It seems very hard that one pay was cut off. But perhaps it was a mistake and you will let us know.

Four years later Molly wrote again.

I am writing to ask you why is it that I cannot receive my Pension. Is it because I will not live with my husband. I am staying with my Mother where my two children are. I help to care for them by washing and cooking for them. My Husband has his meals at my Mothers but he stays on his own. He does not give me any money to keep me. When he took the Pension book from me he told me I could not receive any more pension. So trusting you will explain if I can receive a pension or not.

During the period they were together, Harry and Molly had five children. Only two survived infancy. The pension amount they finally received separately was never varied from 10%. Harry died eight years later from a heart attack and a funeral benefit was paid.

It seems unlikely that Harry was a member of a returned soldier organisation or of any union. He had no Ministerial advocate acting for him – he could not write a letter. He had no 'classic' war injury – no amputation or loss of an eye – yet clearly he had been wounded and that wound, if nothing else, prevented him from returning to work as a shearer. It is clear that his chronic unemployment had a devastating effect on his family. Harry's case is a moving statement about what it is like to be powerless, to be an Aborigine living in an Australian country town in the 1920s and 1930s. But his file reveals something else. When Molly wrote in 1930 that the local Police Sergeant said 'you get a War Pension what more do you want', she describes the social divisiveness which characterised working class Australians in the inter-war period. In particular this retort underlines the bitterness that grew amongst non-veterans over the benefits, however small, which were gained from a war pension.

At a time when most Australian workers found it difficult to survive, here was a group perceived to be benefiting from a state handout and the only apparent qualification for the handout was war service. It can be argued that even 13/9 per fortnight, the sum paid to Harry and Molly, was better than nothing. This sum was enough to buy bread and sugar to last one week for an average family.[29] But even bread and sugar were something when many others had nothing. The payment obscured the fact that war-service was just another form of employment contract, but one with huge health risks. Miners and water-side workers, the classical high-risk occupations, had unionised and fought collectively with some success for conditions and wages appropriate to the risks involved. Miners were the first occupational group written into workers compensation legislation in Australia as deserving special benefits, however inadequate they may have been. Soldiers had no such militant labour organisations. They had the RSSILA, a bourgeois controlled organisation which lost most of its membership in the early 1920s[30] and, from the evidence examined in this study, was largely ineffective. In any event, such a comparison of 'compensation' payments does not appear in contemporary dialogue as an important issue. Instead soldiers and their attempts to gain compensation could easily be seen as anti-labour. That a wife or widow received a compensation sum that sentenced her to penury could be dismissed in a society where war service was celebrated as 'voluntary'. The labour relationship between the soldier and the state was largely ignored.

CHAPTER 10

Epilogue

The long wait Australian war veterans have had to suffer over recognition of the links between their illnesses and Agent Orange was an unfortunate but inevitable consequence of medical science.[1]

In each case [of appeal for recognition] the Government has taken the stand right from the word go that they would fight like mad to avoid paying compensation … The common denominator is the unaccountability of the bureaucracy.[2]

They accepted that I should have compensation and then they paid me that [$55 per week]. If they call that compensation they can shove it.[3]

In October 1994, the Australian Federal government announced that it accepted a report which found exposure to herbicides sprayed in Vietnam caused cancers in veterans, thus ending (perhaps) a 15 year battle for official recognition of this relationship.[4] The medical defence is familiar: 'only over time could doctors and statisticians gather the evidence necessary to make concrete links'.[5] So too is the bitterness of the veteran towards the 'unaccountability' of the bureaucracy and the contempt of some defenders of the bureaucratic position towards the claims of the soldiers.[6] There are other similarities with the practices, the language, the organisational ideology of the post-World War One situation which are worth mention.

According to the Department of Veterans' Affairs' historians, throughout the so-called Agent Orange debate veterans claimed a relationship between exposure to chemicals and certain illnesses which the Department, 'on the weight of [medical] evidence', denied. The Department and the then Liberal government used Defence records to 'prove' that most veterans could not have been 'exposed' to chemicals. The Evatt Royal Commission into Agent Orange (1983–85) qualified this even further, insisting that those few who were directly exposed could not have received 'toxic' doses.[7]

What constitutes a 'toxic' dose of a chemical has been the subject of a vehement and scientifically informed debate in occupational health and safety research.[8] Leaving that inflammatory issue aside, there remains a remarkable similarity here between the response of the Repatriation Department to alleged gassing in the 1920s and that of the DVA to the alleged effects of chemicals in the 1980s and 1990s. In both instances Departmental responsibility was denied on the basis of medical evidence and of Army records. In both cases selective medical knowledge has been instrumental in denying compensation.

Another significant similarity is the experience and attitude of Departmental doctors. According to the Department's historians, the Vietnam Veterans Association (VVAA) complained that Departmental doctors did not understand the conditions in Vietnam. Yet, the Departmental historians assure us, the 'directors of repatriation medical services in both Victoria and Queensland were Vietnam veterans and there were several departmental doctors and officers who had served in Vietnam'. The historians single out the opinion of one former Army and repatriation doctor on the issue of Agent Orange: for Dr Sol Rose the VVAA's claims were a search for 'mythical diseases' and due to 'gain motivation'.[9] The similarity of attitude with the pronouncements of Parkinson, Willis, Agnew and Courtney is undeniable.

A further area of comparison, albeit with a contemporary twist to the terminology, is in the interpretation and treatment of signs and symptoms not considered 'physical'. In the aftermath of World War One, such disorders would probably have been classified as 'mental'. In 1920 veterans suffering these symptoms were either incarcerated or, at worst, denied a pension on the basis of moral weakness. In 1980 they were counselled for 'stress'. In both cases it seems the presenting symptoms were indeterminate and in the absence of a clear, well-recognised aetiology there were in 1920 and, it appears, again in the 1980s and 1990s, labels readily available: 'neurasthenia' in 1920; 'Post-Traumatic Stress Disorder' in 1980. The difference in 1980 was that there was clear (though not officially accepted) scientific evidence that the defoliant herbicides used were indeed toxic and therefore there was the possibility that behavioural problems in veterans had a physiological basis. In 1920, there was comparatively little known about the action of chemicals on the human body, as seen in the case of the PH Gas helmet which gave off allegedly 'harmless' formalin fumes which were breathed by the wearer. (See Chapter 3).

Two final points of comparison should he made. The press coverage of Agent Orange and the VVAA's claim were consistently criticised by the Department, by politicians from both parties and by various 'experts' as partisan and distorted.[10] Headlines such as 'Spraying to Kill', 'Veterans Tell of Illness and Deformity' and 'Agent Orange Veteran Faces Life of Agony' were listed by the Evatt Commission and are represented as 'lurid' examples by the Departmental historians.[11] Yet, by October 1994, it was clear the claims made in these headlines were tragically and penetratingly accurate. The Evatt Commission appears to have been appointed partly as a measure of control to defuse this kind of adverse publicity.

In 1921 and early 1922, *Smith's Weekly*, a populist periodical, conducted a protracted and hostile campaign against the Repatriation Department, labelling it the 'Cyanide Gang'. Headlines such as 'Sentenced to Death: consumptive banished from hospital to die', 'Four Useless Inches of Leg: another ruling of the Cyanide Gang' and 'Forsaken by his country: strong man who is now a hopeless invalid' appeared nearly every week.[12] Even the conservative *Sydney Morning Herald* joined in with 'Keeping him Down: how the Digger and his Dependents are Penalised' plus a series of 'Letters' about soldiers begging in Sydney streets.[13] The *Smith's Weekly* campaign was based on leaked Departmental correspondence and files and appears to have been conducted while the Editor-in-Chief, Claude McCay, was overseas.[14] It also occurred at the height of a campaign conducted from Repatriation Headquarters against the administration of Deputy Commissioner A.G. Farr. Farr's transferral to Perth and subsequent disappearance to South Africa in 1923 may be linked to this.[15] Certainly the vituperative attacks on the Department were moderated early in 1922.

Begging in the streets by maimed and limbless soldiers required another kind of control. This activity, carried out both by individual veterans and by uniformed street musicians, was clearly a source of embarrassment to the Department as well as state and federal governments. Correspondence on the issue together with press reporting ranges over the period 1921 to 1924 when the problem was finally solved. In 1922 the Department approached the Inspector General of Police in New South Wales asking him to obtain names and addresses of these veterans and suggested use of the Traffic Act to control their behaviour. The Minister of Public Health was also approached but decided to 'defer action in the matter'. In 1924, however, the New South Wales Chief Secretary announced that 'in the interests of city traffic', begging in the streets would be prohibited. One paper reported the prohibition with regret:

> Gone from Sydney are the voice of the cornet, the twang of the banjo, and the rattling of the collection-box. Uniformed street musicians have disappeared.
>
> A decree, recommended by the Returned Soldiers' League, ordered by the Chief Secretary, and enforced by the police, yesterday banished the vendors of music to the suburbs.[16]

When the Nationalist Premier of New South Wales, Sir George Fuller, was subsequently approached by a deputation acting on behalf of maimed soldiers claiming that the men needed the money to supplement inadequate pensions, he referred the matter to Prime Minister Bruce, who wrote back reassuringly that the matter had been dealt with effectively by the Repatriation Commission. Indeed, the Commission had assured him that 'all possible steps' had been taken.[17]

It has been argued throughout this work that entrenched assumptions and patterns of thinking shaped the medical and bureaucratic practices and procedures that were established initially in the Invalid Pensions Office of Treasury and then greatly refined and expanded in the Repatriation Department, creating a large part of the infrastructure of the modern welfare state. It seems clear that medical knowledge remains instrumental to the process, that some medical bureaucrats still align themselves with the interests of the state and that 'economy' governs compensation: Departmental officers continue to defend their roles as custodians of the public purse. But the procedures themselves, the mechanisms of control and surveillance and the political emphasis within a broad liberal framework are historically specific. In the following sections these themes are explored in the context of the 1920s.

Instrumentality

The medicalisation of Honour

War Memorials, Rolls of Honour and headstones commemorate the dead. Religious or secular in nature, they also have a significance to national histories that extends far beyond that simple act of commemoration. In recent years, scholarship on the subject has flourished. These 'silent cities' have been examined using post-modern discourse analysis, cultural theory and comparative historical analysis, adding immeasurably to our understanding of war and its international social significance.[18] Even the traditional reverent genuflections towards nationalism still appear.[19] Yet while the memorials are indeed iconic and often monumental representations of society at a particular time, for soldiers and their families they had and have a very personal significance. For the wives and children of departed soldiers, the names of husbands and fathers engraved on plinths, on walls or headstones could be interpreted as a gesture by a grateful state to honour its dead. Looked at another way, these lists distinguished the 'honourable' death from 'other' deaths. For those who died on the battlefields this is hard to refute. In Australia, for the thousands who died after discharge, the situation is more complicated.[20]

In 1922, the Department of Defence announced it would pay for headstones of soldiers *if that death was war-related*. That decision on war-relatedness was one made by the doctors of the Repatriation Department. No funeral benefit was paid by the Department and no headstone was forthcoming unless war-relatedness was established. It has been shown that the lack of medical records combined with the inclination of Departmental doctors was a formidable barrier to establishing war-relatedness and that a variety of non-medical factors, such as 'conduct', could be used to deny such a connection. In this context, the lists of honoured dead take on a new meaning and one with far-reaching consequences.

In 1928, the Chairman of the Repatriation Commission, James Semmens, wrote to the Deputy Commissioner of New South Wales informing him that it was 'proposed to record in the Hall of Memory in the Australian War Memorial ... the names of all those who died, and will die in the future, as a result of Service in the Great War.[21] Semmens pointed out the pivotal role the Commission would play in compiling this list. In fact he advised the Deputy Commissioner to compile three lists: one of deaths accepted as war-related; one of deaths not accepted; and one where the question of attribution of cause had 'not been raised'. In August, after considerable correspondence within the Department over the clerical difficulties entailed in compiling such lists, it was decided that they would simply comprise names of soldiers who had received pensions or those whose families had qualified for pensions.[22]

In this decision, the complexities of the assessment system for war pensions paid to soldiers, their wives and families becomes once again a determining factor, defining the meaning of their lives and that of future generations. Medicine, in its bureaucratic guise, was the principal instrument by which the cost of a war pension, a headstone or a funeral benefit could be displaced back to society, thus saving the 'public purse'. As shown here, it also inadvertently defined 'honour'. Of the many roles medicine had for the state, this last is perhaps the least visible. A Royal Commission, however, was a different matter.

The Royal Commission of 1924

Prime Minister S.M. Bruce was fond of Royal Commissions.[23] The 1924 Commission on the Assessment of War Service Disabilities must rank as one of the shortest. Appointed on 27 August 1924, the Commission was asked

> Is the present method of determining whether an ex-soldier's disability is due to or aggravated by war service adequate to decide the origin or the degree to which it is aggravated, and what portion of his present incapacity can be regarded as having resulted from his war service?

The Commission's final report was on 22 December and, unlike the eight-volume Evatt Commission into Agent Orange, it consisted of a mere five pages.

The Commission consisted of five doctors, one from each state, and was chaired by Dr (later Sir) C. Bickerton Blackburn O.B.E. All were former members of the AIF.[24] The doctors appear to have been selected by the Treasurer, former AIF Captain, Dr (later Sir) Earle Page, a man who, according to his biographer, had 'arranged his war carefully so as not to interfere unduly with his political and business affairs'.[25] The Commission was also established with little consultation with the Repatriation Department or its Commission.[26] Letters were sent out to the doctors on 1 July and Bruce announced the appointment of the Commission on 3 July. Such a Royal Commission, he suggested, will 'result in a general feeling of satisfaction to the soldier and to the public generally'. In response to a question by Matthew Charlton, leader of the ALP in the House, on returned soldier representation on the Commission, Bruce simply retorted that 'every Member of it will be a returned soldier'. When David O'Keefe, Labor Member for Denison, asked whether the Commission would only sit in Melbourne, Bruce assured him that 'the Government will afford the commission every facility desired by it to fully investigate the subject of reference'. Bruce was also at pains to point out that this was not a commission for 'laymen': such men would not 'have the requisite knowledge to deal with the matters to be inquired into'.[27]

As they arrived, Bruce directed the replies from the chosen doctors to Page. All of the responses asked that the Commission be *brief*. Repatriation Commissioner Ashley Teece had the task of drafting a reply to the proposed Chairman, Blackburn, and suggested that about ten days would be sufficient. This letter was then sent out from Bruce's office to the doctors concerned.[28] Bruce also approved a payment of four guineas per day for the Chairman and three guineas for other Members for sittings in the capital city of their residence and a scale of five guineas per day for the Chairman and four guineas for

Members away from home. The Commission only sat in Melbourne so the total bill was twenty guineas per day.[29]

The Commission heard evidence from representatives of three federal returned soldier organisations and five Melbourne-based organisations.[30] In addition to these eight soldier representatives, there were Departmental doctors, members of the Medical Advisory Committee, the members of the Repatriation Commission, senior bureaucrats and representatives of the State Boards, including Semmens's old friend, Gordon Bennett, then Chairman of the New South Wales Board. In all there were 416 pages of evidence.[31] With a weighting of witnesses favouring the Department and the medical profession generally, the Commissioners' recommendations were hardly surprising, finding, as they did, in favour of the status quo. The Report commences:

> [the] Commissioners unanimously agree that, in the majority of cases, the present machinery for determining disability and assessing pensions is sufficient.

All the relatively minor procedural and policy adjustments recommended were subsequently rationalised as unnecessary by the Repatriation Commission, to whom Bruce had sent the Report for comment. Sir Neville Howse, the former head of the AAMC and then Acting Minister for Repatriation, concurred, advising Cabinet that no changes in the 'present system' were necessary.[32]

Years of discontent, of press outrage and agitation by returned soldiers' organisations were dismissed. Even the Department's own historians have expressed dissatisfaction with the outcome.[33] A perfunctory inquiry into doctors by their peers, with a built-in brevity and certainty of outcome, was passed to the body it was investigating for appraisal and their comments accepted without demur.

Surveillance and control

The problem with widows

Confidential investigations of pensioners formed part of Treasury's routine in the case of invalid and old age pensions. Such investigations were simply expanded for war pensions. Standard inquiries were those made of police, previous employers, current employers, the Registrar General's Office, Defence records, Local Committees, attending doctors and the Australian War Memorial's records. In March 1923, one month after the Hughes government resigned and Country Party Leader, Dr Earle Page, became Treasurer, the Repatriation Department commenced a massive re-investigation of the 236 000 war pensions then in force. In a Circular Letter to all states, Semmens wrote that

> The investigation is desired to detect cases where pension is being improperly paid after the death of a pensioner or where a female dependant remarried or where a pension is being paid through fraud.[34]

All soldiers, their dependants or trustees receiving a pension were to be investigated. Two new forms were created for the purpose and were sent to the states in April. In metropolitan areas, all pensioners had to attend Departmental offices and 'give evidence'. Outside the cities, the local Paying Officer was supplied with forms and names of pensioners. A witnessed declaration by the pensioner had to be returned to the state office within four weeks. If not returned, a second notice was issued and if there was no response to that the pension could be suspended. Clearly such a procedure disadvantaged itinerant workers such as the Aboriginal veteran Harry P, his wife and children, described in the previous chapter.

Once the forms were completed, a comparison was made with the pensioner's original claim form in regard to name, regimental details, dates and places of birth, relationship to the veteran and signatures. If there were discrepancies, the Commission ordered 'suitable enquiries' to be undertaken by 'the Investigation Officer or through Local Committees [in the case of non-metropolitan pensioners], Police, Registrars, Postmasters or Postmistresses'. Semmens added that in some cases it might also be necessary to check registers of deaths and marriages 'where the information furnished in the declaration is not of a sufficiently convincing nature'.[35] The entire investigation was to be completed within twelve months. But by July 1927 the Sydney office had completed only half its investigations. During that period one particular group of pensioners was singled out as deserving close scrutiny: 'Marriageable females'.

The problem with these women, from the Departmental point of view, was that they could marry (or re-marry). If they did not notify the Department then they could continue to receive a pension indefinitely. The question of how to detect such fraud exercised the minds of the bureaucrats throughout the 1920s and into the 1930s. In 1923, for example, the New South Wales office asked the state branch of the Commonwealth Electoral Office to supply it with cards giving particulars of marriages in the state. The Office readily agreed and the Department was subsequently swamped with cards from all the Electoral Districts of New South Wales showing 'practically all the marriages in the state'. However, by 1926, a workable system of surveillance was starting to take shape. An alphabetical index of widows and widowed mothers was established and every quarter approximately 5000 cards, compiled by the Registrar General's Office and then processed by the Electoral Office, were checked by Repatriation officers against their alphabetical index. The Deputy Commissioner of Repatriation in New South Wales was keen to commence a retrospective check to 1915 but Semmens wanted 'a progressive and prospective check' and approval was not forthcoming.[36]

Early in 1927, however, a Pensions Clerk discovered that the alphabetical list was not 'complete': the cards only represented females who in addition to receiving a war pension were also receiving medical benefits. It did not include those women who received a pension but had not applied for such benefits and, the Clerk added, 'there are quite a number of these cases'. So, a new investigation of the files was made and this time *all* 'marriageable females' were included and a 'practically water-tight' system established.[37] In the same year, approval was also given for the commencement of a retrospective investigation to 1915. By January 1928, 1644 out of a total of around 6000 'cases' in this latter category had been checked, but no unnotified marriages were discovered. The overall war pension review was more successful. By mid 1927, with the investigation of nearly half the 60 000 pensions in New South Wales complete, the Deputy Commissioner wrote enthusiastically to Semmens on the outcome:

> … how very necessary this check is can be judged from the fact that since the inception of this check in 1923, six cases of fraud have been detected where the dependant has married or remarried without notifying this Department.[38]

Six years intensive labour had produced six cases of fraud. At the same time a sophisticated surveillance system was established and refined and made part of standard Departmental procedures. As with pension assessments, an entire generation of bureaucrats were trained in this system, one that was founded on controlling public expenditure. Indeed this process adds a new meaning to the Departmental historians' description of officers engaged in the Agent Orange dispute:

> Although the generation of World War II officers had largely passed from the DVA before the controversy erupted, the younger officers accepted and were deeply imbued with the repatriation ethos.[39]

Medical surveillance

There were other forms of official surveillance established in the post-war years. Not least in importance was medical surveillance. This took various forms. For example, there were several kinds of institutions which provided medical treatment to soldiers after their discharge. Among these were the so-called Anzac Hostels, established to care for the totally and permanently incapacitated veteran. As one historian of the repatriation process describes it, they were established for 'men whose lives had been permanently warped and whose bodies had been irreparably shattered'.

> it was to these men that the Department had to acknowledge its most solemn responsibility. Though they were rendered helpless, it became a duty to make the remainder of their lives as happy as possible.[40]

In New South Wales there were two such hostels: Graythwaite and Canonbury. Both were administered by the Red Cross although the soldiers were maintained at Departmental expense. In 1926 an inmate of Graythwaite wrote to Howse, as the Minister responsible for repatriation, complaining of the drinking habits of another inmate. The letter was passed to Commissioner Semmens who sent it to the DC in Sydney with a confidential memorandum which noted that if the complaint was reliable it was 'another evidence of the fact that there are some disadvantages connected with the placing of our men in Red Cross Institutions'.[41] He went on to direct that a 'tactful and reliable officer' should interview the matron of Graythwaite and that her verbal and written comments were to be obtained.

The Deputy Commissioner, Barrett, duly carried out these instructions and simultaneously wrote a terse letter to the Superintendent of the Red Cross Society complaining that Red Cross 'officers' were not reporting 'cases of misconduct among Departmental patients'. He continued:

> I desire now to emphasise the importance of informing me at once of any act of misconduct in order that I may take such action as I may deem necessary. Will you kindly instruct the Matron at each of your Homes to telephone such information (where practicable) and to confirm such a telephonic communication by a full report in writing.[42]

The Superintendent duly replied that Departmental wishes would be respected and that instructions had been issued to the Matrons. Yet it seems the Matrons were not as rigorous in their reporting as Departmental bureaucrats would have liked: the discipline so central to repatriation medicine could not be imposed readily on an outside institution. In April of the following year, an inmate tried to commit suicide by slashing his throat and wrists. He was transferred to the Prince of Wales Hospital and some days later when Dr Kenneth Smith investigated the incident the ex-soldier was still in a 'very serious condition'. Smith's report to the State Repatriation Board authoritatively and unequivocally attributed the attempted suicide to 'alcoholism'. He continued,

> I also discovered that several of the inpatients have alcoholic habits and have been repeatedly warned by the Matron ... I spoke to these men personally and informed them that any further bad reports would result in their immediate discharge. The Matron [and others] were asked to report any bad behaviour of the patients to the Dept. & I pointed out that unless we had this information we could not properly adjudicate on any request from these patients.[43]

Barrett immediately wrote again to the Superintendent, this time requesting that their 'management' should 'promptly advise' the Department of the next occasion 'that any of the Departmental patients are guilty of indulgence in alcoholic habits'. This was necessary, it was argued,

> so that prompt action can be taken to safeguard the comfort, health, and possibly lives of all the patients in the Institution by removing therefrom those who will not or cannot control their indulgences and who consequently are a nuisance, possibly a danger, to the other patients.[44]

These soldiers were deemed totally and permanently incapacitated by war service. One man's attempted suicide – one which nearly succeeded – was diagnosed as 'alcoholism'. There is no mention of the state of his mind or his body, factors which may have explained his habits and the attempted suicide. Instead, the consumption of alcohol by these grossly injured soldiers was constituted as a 'disciplinary infringement' and one that posed a 'threat' to other inmates despite the absence of any evidence to support such a claim.

This was not an isolated incident. Use of alcohol was often labelled 'alcoholism' and in the case studies examined it was invariably a cause for a medicalised disciplinary response.[45] In the case of Stewart M, a miner who enlisted in 1915 and was discharged Medically Unfit in 1918, and whose Departmental medical history reads like an encyclopaedia of illness, it was his use of alcohol that was repeatedly used to deny an increase or reduce his pension. Indeed in 1924 Bickerton Blackburn considered that ' "generosity" [had] been stretched to its extreme limits in granting this man a pension'.[46] In the case of Richard B, a pre-existing illness (rheumatic fever) was considered to have been greatly aggravated by war and in 1931 he was assessed as totally and permanently incapacitated by a junior Departmental doctor. Following this assessment, SMO Dr Kenneth Smith ordered an immediate re-investigation of the case. His full report reads as follows:

> Perusal of the collected evidence forces the conclusion that the [War Service] had no material influence on the [Valvular Disorder of the Heart]. There seems reason to review the admitted degree of aggravation. Alcoholism is noted in *September 1917*. [original emphasis]
>
> The Wasserman [test for venereal disease] was +++ in December, 1923 on two occasions but is now negative, and there seems no reason to review the opinion given by Dr Blackburn in January, 1924.
>
> The [heart disorder] was due to the Rheumatic Fever prior to enlistment.[47]

The 'alcoholism' of 1917 was an assessment based on a Police report of 1917 which simply noted that Richard was a married man living with his family, that he had not worked since his return from the front, that this may have been owing to some disease contracted at the front, and that he was a 'fairly constant drinker' and 'a frequent visitor to Hotels'. For Smith, this one isolated report immediately after the soldier's return home, became 'alcoholism'. His second medical reference in his report is to venereal disease in 1923. The 'opinion' of Blackburn referred to was on the question of whether syphilis was 'a factor in his disability'. Blackburn's comment was that Richard was 'extremely fortunate to be drawing a pension at all'.[48]

In the case studies examined in this work, Kline and Wasserman tests for venereal disease were carried out routinely on all soldiers admitted as in-patients or when they required other tests. The evidence so gathered could then be used against them, as it was against Richard B.

Smith's third piece of medical evidence was that Richard's heart condition existed prior to service. There is no other evidence in his report to the State Board and hence to the Repatriation Commission. All the evidence of Richard's illness is ignored in favour of these three 'facts'. As a result, the Commission cancelled his pension. Richard appealed in January the following year, but Charles Courtney, then Principal Departmental Medical Officer, convinced the Commission that the original pension had been granted by a Treasury official 'contrary to medical recommendations'. He argued as follows:

It is clear that his enlistment was malafides; it could be said that he was one of those who 'imputed to himself the possession of good health and by his cunning he imposed this erroneous belief upon the examining physician' … His mode of living was not helpful to him – alcoholism was definite in 1917 and syphilis was diagnosed in 1923 … After discharge (despite unhealthy habits) he was able to work for many years. These facts when taken in conjunction with the serious pre-war illnesses lead me to the conclusion that service was but an incident in his health career and not a lasting deteriorating influence … That this soldier obtained pension at all was due to the unsound methods of administration, e.g. the Treasury official who granted the pension … The medical opinion on the file was unanimous, and was based on clinical facts and on accurate knowledge of the conditions under which they arose.[49]

There is no way of knowing whether Richard's case is 'typical'. No study has been undertaken to date that could provide a quantitatively significant and therefore 'typical' picture of the way pensions were assessed in this period, of the factors influencing that assessment, of the fluctuation in the percentage of pension paid, or of the role of medical or bureaucratic surveillance in the process. But SMO Willis's words to Graeme Butler, that Departmental medical officers were not 'nice kind doctors' resonate throughout these files. In their alignment with the interests of the state, the Departmental doctors were first and foremost bureaucrats. They did not treat patients, they quantified liability in precisely the same fashion as an assessment for workers compensation, but in this case it was the liability of the state. The surveillance and control measures outlined here were instrumental to achieving 'economy'.

Economy

In June of 1919, the Commonwealth liability for welfare payments and war pensions was comprised as follows: £0.6 million (M) for Maternity Allowances; £1M for Invalid Pension; £3M for Old Age Pension; and £5.5M for War Pension. Numerically this consisted of 871 000 recipients of the Maternity Allowance; 32 000 Invalid Pensioners; 96 000 Old Age Pensioners; and 181 500 War Pensioners. (Figures 21 and 22). Of War Pensions, those paid to incapacitated soldiers represented more than 50% of the total expenditure. The average fortnightly rate for an Invalid or Old Age Pension was £1/4/-; for a War Pensioner the average was £1/10/-. (Figure 23) In the case of the Old Age or Invalid Pensioner, this amount was the equivalent of around 15% of the basic wage; for the war pensioner it was around 18.75%.[50]

By June of the following year, the average fortnightly cost of a war pension dropped from £1/10/- to £1/6/-, a 13% drop, yet the number of pensions in force increased significantly. The number paid to incapacitated soldiers rose from 71 512 to 90 389, a 26% increase; the total number of war pensions rose from 181 529 to 225 580, a 24% increase. It seems clear that while overall Commonwealth liability was rising, due to sheer numbers of pensions, there were forces at work which drove that cost down.[51] (Figures 23 and 24).

Figure 21. Commonwealth benefits and war pensions: liability June 1919

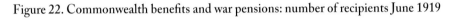

Source: AA(ACT): A571/1, 20/27781, statistics all benefits, June 1919

Figure 22. Commonwealth benefits and war pensions: number of recipients June 1919

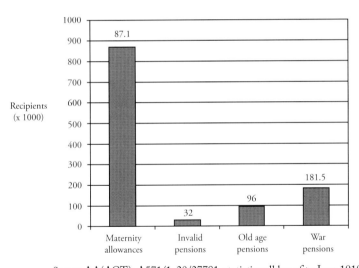

Source: AA(ACT): A571/1, 20/27781, statistics all benefits, June 1919

By 1925, 44% of pensions paid to incapacitated soldiers in New South Wales were at a rate of less than 25% of a full pension, that is to say, less than 10/6 per week. A further 30% received between 25% and 50%, or less than £1/1/0 per week.[52] It has been shown previously that a 50% pension in 1920 for a man, his wife and three children was equivalent to less than half the cost of living estimated by the 1920 Royal Commission. The principal means of cost-cutting was control of the pension assessment system. This was the largest item of expenditure and therefore attracted most attention. These measures

Figure 23. Average fortnightly pension rates for incapacitated soldiers, 1919 and 1920

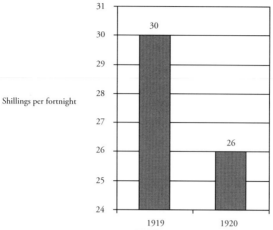

Source: AA(ACT): A571/1, 20/27781, statistics all pensions for year ended June 1919; A2491/1, W3838, War Pensions, Statement for Twelve Months ended June 1920.

Figure 24. Number of pensions paid for incapacitated soldiers, 1919 and 1920

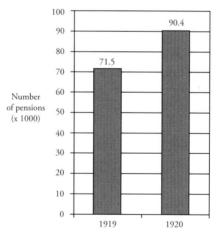

Source: AA(ACT): A571/1, 20/27781, statistics all pensions for year ended June 1919; A2491/1, W3838, War Pensions, Statement for Twelve Months ended June 1920.

have been outlined in previous chapters and in the discussion above, but there were other cost-control techniques available to the Department, some of interest because of their social dimension, others for their disclosure of power relationships within the system. These are examined in the following sections.

Feeding by class and by gender
One of the more fascinating investigations into cost-cutting undertaken during the 1920s was one into the cost of feeding staff and patients in Departmental institutions. In

January 1929, Semmens wrote to the DC Sydney directing investigation of the increase in daily per capita cost in the various Departmental institutions in New South Wales. The DC forwarded a copy of the Memorandum to the Medical Superintendent of the Prince of Wales Hospital at Randwick, E. H. Rutledge.[53] Rutledge replied in February, his principal concern being the rise in the cost of 'Provisions' over the period 1925 to 1928. Meat, milk and eggs, which, he argued, were consumed in large quantities, had undergone a significant increase in cost in this period.[54] The DC concurred and put the case forcibly to Semmens.

One particular food item had been singled out for investigation, a commodity which had indeed been banned previously by the Repatriation Commission – tinned asparagus. It would seem from correspondence that catering for the 'Nurses Quarters' normally included this item. The DC argued that the Superintendent's check of institutional eating habits found the nurses' food bill 'not exorbitant' and that it was worth lifting the ban. He continued,

> Women generally are fastidious over foods and drinks and many would rather have a serving of asparagus for a meal than a juicy steak or lamb cutlet; particularly in the summer heat.[55]

Semmens, however, was not moved. Tinned asparagus along with tinned tongues, oysters and Bovril were banned and reductions were ordered in the use of salmon, jam, proprietary sauces and meats. These 'feeding standards', he argued,

> should have no harmful results to patients and if strictly applied will not reduce the standard and quality of feeding of both patients and staff below what they might reasonably expect.[56]

Consumption of poultry and cream were also to be investigated, and if consumption could not be lowered then the DC was instructed to provide a satisfactory explanation.

Correspondence over this rationing continued until mid 1929 because the Hospital feared complaints over the quality of food it provided. In June, however, rigid guidelines were issued from Melbourne. The banned items remained banned, although Bovril was allowed in 'special cases only, and then under the direction of a medical officer'. Cream was allowed one day per week in Hostels only (not in hospitals) and on one day per week for Nurses, Doctors, the Secretary and Supply Officer of the institution. The same instructions were issued in the case of poultry but with the additional clause that it was 'not to be supplied to Domestic or Orderly Staff Messes'. Patients on Light Diets, where the standard menu could not be used, were another problem. Semmens ordered that 'the list of patients on light and special diets is to be closely scanned daily, with a view to ensuring that patients are not retained on the list longer than is absolutely necessary for their proper treatment and care'.

> The Medical Superintendent of each Institution should be requested to give this matter his personal and careful attention.[57]

Finally, he ordered that no imported foodstuffs were to be purchased. His closing paragraph indicates the importance attached to the exercise:

> The Commission proposes to watch very closely the cost of institutional feeding during the current year, and trusts that all officers concerned will give effect to its desire for greater economy, ensuring at the same time, of course, that a reasonable standard is maintained. The objective in view is a reduction in the general costs of feeding of at least 10%; this means that all items in addition to those mentioned … are to be closely checked.[58]

These were institutions established to care for the sick and injured. Clearly, the cost-cutting measures outlined here affected all those who resided within the institution's walls. Yet it is also abundantly clear that the poorest diets were reserved for the patients and those at the bottom of the organisation's hierarchy, the Domestic and Orderly staff. The best food selections were for those on the highest salaries, doctors, nurses and senior administrators, a group who were in a position to buy additional foodstuffs if they so desired and who were presumably healthy. The impact of the deepening recession on state organisations was felt first by those with the least power to resist.

Fraud everywhere

From its inception, the bureaucracy was obsessed with fraud. It has been argued previously that a poor law mentality, one which assumed fraudulent behaviour and imposed workhouse discipline to control it, was integral to the functioning of the Department. On some occasions this assumption was spelt out quite clearly; on others it is apparent in actions taken.

In 1921, for example, the question of repayment of Departmental loans taken out by soldiers to buy furniture or other items during their civil re-establishment was the subject of intense scrutiny.[59] When a Senior Clerk of the Department visited the New South Wales coal mining district of Cessnock, the Secretary of the Local Committee had a novel suggestion as to how to make debtors 'realise their obligations': garnishee the miners' wages.[60] The idea was seized upon by Deputy Commissioner Farr whose letter to Semmens is worth quoting at length:

> It appears that in this District in particular a common practice among the business people in cases of outstanding debts, is to garnishee the debtors wages (if in employment). I am assured that such action is not in any way taken exception to by the miners in general, neither is the debtors employment in any way prejudiced.
>
> The Secretary is of the opinion that such action should be adopted by this Department in regard to outstanding loans only, of course, in those cases where grantee is in employment and deliberately evades his obligations but who guards against recovery of chattels by making small repayments spasmodically.
>
> … When stating that the Union would take no exception I quite realise that to garnishee a man's wages is legal at the same time the miners carry considerably [*sic*] sway in these districts and can cause no end of trouble if they so desire.

It might be mentioned by the way that the Cessnock District is at the present time, enjoying great prosperity, and according to the money in circulation there should be few genuine cases of distress thus preventing repayments being regularly made.[61]

The historian of the New South Wales coalminers, Robin Gollan, presents a somewhat different picture. According to Gollan, the 'industry was in a state of permanent crisis' during the post-war years and work was increasingly intermittent due to loss of trade, technical breakdowns and strikes, the latter apparently responsible for only one-third of the total time lost.[62] Mining did not share the brief boom experienced by some other industries after the war. As well, the miners' union (the Miners Federation) was in serious financial difficulties.[63] Under the circumstances it is easy to understand the 'spasmodic' nature of debt repayments and the union's inability to prevent the garnishee system from operating.

The proposal was passed from one bureaucrat to another for opinion and in the end the Commission decided that if 'the man is endeavouring to evade his liability' (by not making re-payments), and was 'in receipt of wages or salary which in the opinion of the State Board is sufficient to enable the grantee to live and pay his obligations', then 'action should be taken to enforce compliance'.[64]

Assumed fraud was also behind the twenty-five year delay in granting full pensions to soldiers suffering from tuberculosis. The political and administrative history of the debacle is related by Lloyd and Rees.[65] Of more interest here is the source of expert opinion used by government ministers inquiring into the issue. In the last weeks of the Scullin Labor government, at a time when the social welfare cuts of the Financial Emergency Act were about to be implemented, Scullin wrote to Semmens wanting his report on two proposals: one for an attendant's allowance for blind soldiers, the other for a permanent pension at full rate for soldiers suffering from tuberculosis. Both, it was mooted, might be written into the Repatriation Act. Semmens passed the letter to Courtney whose response typifies the Departmental obsession with fraud and at the same time offers a revealing insight into what 'blindness' meant in the medical bureaucracy's discourse. His report, which formed the basis of Semmens's advice to Scullin, bears quoting at length.[66]

… It is common experience within the Department that efforts to prove the existence of Blindness and of Pulmonary Tuberculosis have been productive of many untrue statements by claimants, and of much medical work and financial outlay that otherwise would not have been needed.

Again, the medical difficulty of diagnosing either of these disabilities is in some instances very great, and even with the honest co-operation of the patient, may be impossible. And this co-operation is not always to be expected where the presence of the disability is financially so beneficial.

…The sources of error in granting these benefits are partly inherent in the nature of the disabilities, and partly result from the weakness of human nature that inclines one to turn disease into a commodity.

Blindness when due to 'loss of both eyes' is of course absolute and irrevocable. But when due to 'loss of vision' it may be partial or temporary. What degree of loss is necessary to constitute blindness? and is this loss permanent or curable? are both questions that in many cases are difficult to settle. The several definitions of blindness testify to the difficulties of the problem, e.g., no useful vision; no economic vision; no social vision; and are various labels thus used.

[With regard to tuberculosis,] the phrase 'benefit of doubt' complicates the problem with specially evil results ... for ultimately diagnosis rests on a lay Tribunal ... when failing to weigh medical evidence and its significance this disease was said to be present when there was no doubt in all the medical minds who knew all the clinical and personal evidence, that it was not so. The importance to the patient of sound professional diagnosis is paramount, but it can also be of the utmost importance when dealing with financial benefits embodied in an Act of Parliament. It is so easy for laymen to find differences of opinion in any technical documents that are not different in reality; sometimes the difference is in verbiage only, and sometimes the opinion relates to events of different periods and based on incomplete or slender evidence.

... [If, as is current practice,] a medical certificate based on the slenderest knowledge or written by any practitioner is to be given sufficient weight as to cast doubt on the combined views of especially qualified authoritative medical men, it is fair to say that claimants will make special efforts to become entitled to benefits so easily obtained and so firmly based as in the Act.[67]

Courtney's argument is intriguing. These two conditions, he contends, were extremely difficult to diagnose, that is, medical knowledge was indeterminate in both cases. Consequently diagnostic mistakes were made. His tone is almost apologetic in this instance: doctors made honest mistakes owing to lack of 'evidence'. These misdiagnoses, if that is what they were, were acceptable within the professional discourse of medicine: a diagnosis of tuberculosis by one doctor and of no tuberculosis by another was a legitimate difference of opinion. The only person seriously affected by this difference was the patient: in Courtney's words, 'the importance to the patient ... is paramount'. But the health of the patient was peripheral to the main thrust of his argument. His principal concerns were with the fraudulent inclination of pensioners and the use made of divided medical opinion by lay persons.

When Courtney speaks of the 'specially evil results' that ensued from a lay Tribunal having ultimate authority to decide a pension case, he is not referring to the patient's health. A Tribunal deciding in favour of a diagnosis of TB was hardly disadvantaging the patient. At worst it meant the individual might receive some treatment for a nonexistent disease and in 1930 that treatment was likely to be rest. Courtney's 'evil' is the cost to the state. While a difference of opinion was unproblematic within the profession, where the patient's health was the issue at stake, only one opinion could be correct when the issue was the 'benefits' of a war pension. That determining opinion belonged to the departmental doctors and their experts. All other doctors were susceptible to the fraudulent 'special efforts' soldiers would make to obtain the pension.

Semmens advised Scullin accordingly:

> Experience shows that these specially generous benefits encourage would-be benefi-
> ciaries to go to any length to make it appear that they are suffering much more than
> they are.[68]

The pension for tuberculosis was not written into the Act until 1943.

Concluding comments

The Financial Emergency Act came into effect in July 1931. As a result, pensions of wives, children and other dependants were reduced, payment of pension arrears was banned or severely limited, Assessment Appeals Tribunals were given power to reduce pensions and the various allowances paid to soldiers and dependants were reduced. Some of these cost-cutting measures were never repealed. The Repatriation Commission, in its Annual Report for 1929-30, complained that 'economic necessity' had forced many ex-soldiers and their dependants 'who have never previously applied for aid', to apply to the Depart-ment; staff complained of the additional 'operational and financial burden'.[69] Yet the number of pension claims the Department received dropped from 15 000 in 1930 to 3 400 in 1934. Departmental historian, A.P. Skerman, attempting to find administrative explanations for the dramatic reduction in claims, as well as for the complaints of Depart-mental staff, suggests that there was a 'rationalisation' of 'unofficial, semi-official and ten-tative approaches' to the Department. In other words, while the administrative load for officers was increased by such 'approaches', the real cost to the Department was lowered by systematic rejection: the percentage of pension claims rejected by the Department in this period rose from 9% in 1930 to 18% in 1933. (Figures 25 and 26).[70]

These were crude responses to the financial crisis and many were highly visible, writ-ten into the Act or its Regulations. By concentrating on these miserable years it is easy to lose sight of the many invisible 'economies' that were effected throughout the post-war decades. Systems of surveillance and control were steadily refined while the role of the medical bureaucrats became increasingly important to limiting pension liability. The small but systematic savings made, justified by reference to the public purse, had an immense human cost, a small part of which has been documented in previous chapters, and no individual or organisation, including the RSSILA, succeeded in counteracting this. Arguably, human agency, the ability of individuals to resist the powerful forces at work in particular economic formations, whether capitalism or state capitalism, was simply impossible in this period. The history of individuals confronted by the powerful alliance of the Australian state with bureaucratised medicine goes some way towards confirming such a bleak view.

The structure of the world the AIF returned to was quite different from that which they left. Meliorism, or reformist liberalism, all but disappeared during the crisis of war and was replaced by a political regime and, in the case of repatriation, a bureaucratic organisa-

Figure 25. Total number of war pension claims 1924-1934

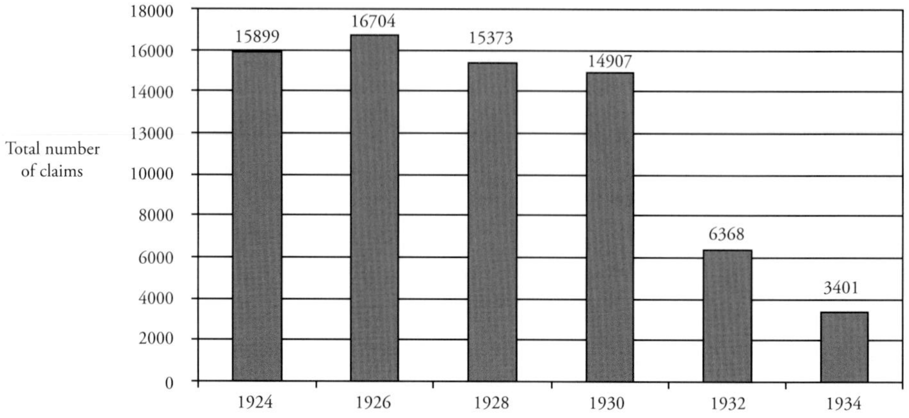

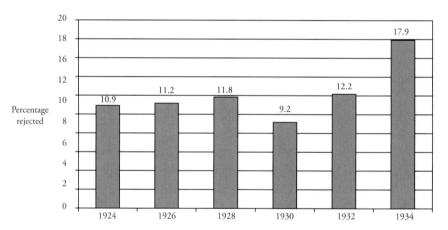

Source: A.P. Skerman, *Repatriation in Australia: a history of development to 1958*,
Repatriation Department, Melbourne 1961, p.63.

Figure 26. Percentage of total war pension claims rejected 1924-1934

Source: A.P. Skerman, *Repatriation in Australia: a history of development to 1958*,
Repatriation Department, Melbourne 1961, p.63.

tion steeped in the values of militarism and classical liberalism. This only becomes apparent after a detailed analysis of vast archival sources. Australian welfare history has tended to look at how much was 'achieved', to look at so-called 'progressive reforms' in the early twentieth century – lists of 'benefits' – but has largely failed to investigate the processes and the procedures that were simultaneously erected to limit state liability. As well, the citizenship discourse has acted to channel investigation into analyses of the make-up of these lists and, within a feminist citizenship discourse, to the gender divisions they contain. This discourse has largely accepted the rhetoric of official documents uncritically in order to construct a picture of 'generous' welfare schemes that supposedly benefited one section of the population at the expense of others.

Yet there is a whole other discourse, an unofficial dialogue always hidden from public view, on the interpretation and application of these public 'benefits', one that systematically and purposefully worked to reject applicants and to contain costs. In repatriation, and in invalid pensions before it, the medical profession, acting as bureaucratic assessors rather than doctors of human ills, were an integral and increasingly important part of this other discourse. War pensions were the most important fiscal component of the repatriation scheme, but they were not welfare benefits: they were compensation payments for human damage which resulted from a labour relationship between an individual and the state. A small group of bureaucrats and doctors, hand-picked for their ideological conformity and working within a carefully constructed system of administration-by-Regulation, during a period of conservative and highly centralised politics, worked diligently to protect the public purse. The social consequences of this process were profound. That it can be described as a 'generous' welfare system simply reveals the immense power of official rhetoric and its strengthening of a hegemonic liberal ideology, one that has characterised Australian welfarism for much of its history.

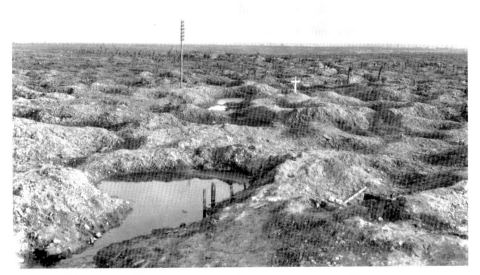

Figure 27. The village of Pozières some months after the battle, April 1917
[Australian War Memorial neg. no. E00532]

Notes to the Chapters

Preface

1. R. Cooter, 'Medicine and the Goodness of War', *Canadian Journal of Medical History*, Vol.7, 1990, p.148.
2. Philippe Dagen, 'The Morality of Horror', *Otto Dix, The War (Der Krieg)*, 5 Continents Editions/ Historial de la Grande Guerre, Milan and Péronne 2003, p.13.
3. Most recently in Australia by Betty Churcher in *The Art of War*, MUP 2004, p.62, where it is juxtaposed with an Albert Tucker image (*Psycho, Heidelberg Military Hospital*) of 'madness'.
4. Otto Dix, *Der Krieg*, Plate XL, Transplantation *Skin Graft*.
5. AWM 41, Butler Papers, item 118, Photographs and diagrams of cosmetic surgery used on facial wounds.
6. The photograph of the Australian soldier with the facial skin graft is different from these images for a number of reasons. To begin with, it is not an image of a dead or decaying soldier. Second, no matter how shocking it may be to the non-professional observer, within the medical profession, and in professional publications of the time, it was evidence of the advances in surgical skills and procedures that allowed some kind of reconstruction of a devastated face; in other words, some kind of face was better than a gaping hole where a nose used to be. Finally, this photograph is the polar opposite of death and decay; it witnesses *life*, beyond the trenches, after the war.
7. The collections of the Australian War Memorial, the National Library of Australia and major state libraries were searched online. The collection of the AWM was also investigated at the Memorial and the assistance of photographic archivists sought. In July 2007 the Veterans' Affairs Minister announced a 'multi-million dollar project' to excavate a site in northern France where it is believed 165 Australians and hundreds of British soldiers might be buried near Fromelles It is believed the German Army buried the dead soldiers. (ABC News, 24 and 26 July 2007)
8. AWM, PR 83/202, Letters of Pte James Agnew, 12th Field Ambulance, AIF. Agnew was the son of James F. Agnew, briefly PDMO of Repatriation and militaristic doctor. His son wished to join the Baptist Ministry after the war but died at the front in September 1917.

Chapter 1

1. David Malouf, *Fly Away Peter*, Penguin, Ringwood 1982, pp.82-87.
2. AWM27, 521.4 [1], letter Gilbert to Secretary RSSILA, December 1919.
3. *CPD*, Vol.91, 24 March 1920, p.657.
4. A.P. Skerman, *Repatriation in Australia*, Repatriation Department, Melbourne 1961, p.327.
5. C. Lloyd and J. Rees, *The Last Shilling*, MUP, Melbourne 1994, p.419; S. Garton, *The Cost of War: Australians Return*, OUP, Melbourne 1996, p.86.
6. *Official Year Book of the Commonwealth of Australia*, Government Printer, Melbourne 1922, pp.659-666.
7. Australian 'welfare' historiography on this subject remains scant and has been contained largely within a traditional liberal historiographical approach. The classic works are T.H. Kewley, *Social Security in Australia 1900-1972*, Sydney 1973; B. Dickey, *No Charity There. A Short History of Social Welfare in Australia*, Nelson, Melbourne 1980; F.G. Castles, *The Working Class and Welfare*, Allen & Unwin, Wellington 1985; M.A. Jones, *The Australian Welfare State*, Allen & Unwin, Sydney 1980. Other more critical works include *Social Policy in Australia: Some Perspectives*, J. Roe (ed), Cassell, Stanmore 1975; *Australian Welfare History*, R. Kennedy (ed), Macmillan, South Melbourne 1982; *Australian Welfare: Historical Sociology*, R. Kennedy (ed), Macmillan, South Melbourne 1989; R.

Beilharz, M. Considine and R. Watts, *Arguing About the Welfare State: the Australian Experience*, Allen & Unwin, North Sydney 1992.

8   On this issue see K. Blackmore, 'Making health policy in Australia: the case of invalid pensions', in V.A. Brown and G. Preston (eds), *Choice and Change: ethics, politics and economics of public health*, Public Health Association, Canberra 1993, pp.82-87.

9   See Chapter 10, 'Economy', p.204ff.

10 S. Macintyre, *The Labour Experiment*, McPhee Gribble, Melbourne 1989, p.10.

11 Broadly, I have assumed the use and meaning of 'ideology' as elaborated by Antonio Gramsci, *Prison Notebooks*, Q.Hoare and G. Nowell Smith (trans and eds), International Publishers, London and New York 1971. C. Ramsay, *The Ideology of the Great Fear*, Johns Hopkins University Press, Baltimore 1992, p.124.

12 Ernest Gellner, *Nations and Nationalism*, Basil Blackwell, Oxford 1983, p.20.

13 C.B. Macpherson, *The Life and Times of Liberal Democracy*, OUP, Oxford 1977, p.43.

14 R. Bendix, *Max Weber. An Intellectual Portrait*, Methuen, London 1966, p.426.

15 Ibid, p.429.

16 Gellner, op cit, p.20.

17 AWM41, Box 61, Hastings Willis to Butler, 9 October 1942.

18 Those works most directly useful here were Alfred Vagts, *A History of Militarism: Civilian and Military*, revised ed, Meridian Books 1959; Samuel P. Huntington, *The Soldier and the State: the theory and politics of civil-military relations*, Vintage Books, New York 1957; Volker R. Berghahn, *Militarism: the History of an International Debate 1861-1979*, CUP, Cambridge 1981; Philip K. Lawrence, *Modernity and War: the Creed of Absolute Violence*, St Martin's Press, New York 1997 and 'Enlightenment, modernity and war', *History of the Human Sciences*, Vol.12, No.1, 1999, pp.3-25; Michael Geyer, 'The Militarization of Europe, 1914-1945', in John R. Gillis (ed), *The Militarization of the Western World*, Rutgers University Press, New Brunswick 1989, pp.65-102; Barton C. Hacker, 'Military Institutions and social order: transformations of western thought since the Enlightenment', *War & Society*, Vol.11, No.2, October 1993, pp.1-23; Charles Townshend, 'Militarism and Modern Society', *Wilson Quarterly*, Winter 1993, pp.71-82; Anne Summers, 'Militarism in Britain before the Great War', *History Workshop Journal*, Vol.2, No.1, pp.104-123; Roger Cooter and Steve Sturdy, 'Of War, Medicine and Modernity: Introduction', in R. Cooter, M. Harrison & S. Sturdy eds, *War, Medicine and Modernity*, Sutton, Stroud 1998.

19 Townshend, op cit, p.75.

20 Vagts, op cit.

21 Vagts, op cit, pp.13 and 17.

22 Townshend, op cit, p.76.

23 J.M. Powell, *An Historical Geography of Modern Australia: the restive fringe*, CUP, Cambridge 1988, p.71.

24 Summers, op cit, outlines the extent of civilian militarism in Britain prior to the war but without defining the word. Nonetheless she seems to imply militarism as ideology. See also Best in Gillis (ed), op cit.

25 On this see also Huntington, op cit, p.93 and passim.

26 Vagts, op cit, p.237.

27 Vagts, op cit, p.34.

28 Cooter, Harrison & Sturdy, op cit.

29 Cooter & Sturdy, op cit, pp.1-2.

30 Lawrence, op cit, p.3.

31 Lawrence, ibid, pp.21-23. He further adds that slaughter with machine guns was common prior to World War One but 'the victims lay outside the domain of European Christendom'.

32 Gellner, op cit, p.42.

33 See Chapter 5 on the 1st Australian Dermatological Hospital and Chapter 7 on the medical boarding process in particular.

34 Michel Foucault, *The Birth of the Clinic*, Vintage, New York 1975 and *Discipline and Punish: the Birth of the Prison*, Penguin 1987.
35 See Chapter 5.
36 P. Weindling, *Health, Race and German politics between national unification and Nazism, 1870-1945*, CUP, Cambridge 1989, pp.283-4.

Chapter 2

1 D.J. Gilbert, 'The Civil Re-Establishment of the A.I.F.', reproduced as an Appendix in A.P. Skerman, *Repatriation in Australia: a history of development to 1958*, p.239.
2 See for example, K.S. Inglis, 'The Anzac Tradition', *Meanjin*, Vol.24, 1965, pp.25-44; Kevin Fewster, 'Allis Ashmead-Bartlett and the Making of the Anzac Legend', *JAS*, Vol.10, June 1982, pp.17-30; Richard White, *Inventing Australia*, George Allen & Unwin, Sydney 1981, Ch.8; Humphrey McQueen, *Gallipoli to Petrov*, George Allen & Unwin, Sydney 1984, Ch.1.
3 *The Argus*, 16 December 1914, p.14.
4 A.G. Butler *Official History of the Australlian Army Medical Services. 1914-1918*, (hereafter Butler), AWM, Canberra 1940, Vol.1, p.178 and n.20.
5 Ibid, pp.249-53.
6 Ibid, pp.262-4.
7 CPD, Vol.LXXVI, p.4671, cited in L.J. Pryor, 'The Origins of Australia's Repatriation policy (1914-1920)', MA, University of Melbourne 1932, p.37.
8 Gilbert, p.240; Pryor, pp.36-41.
9 AWM 27, Item 365[10]; L.L. Robson, *The First A.I.F.*, MUP, Carlton 1982, p.43.
10 Gilbert, p.239. Ernest Scott, 'Australia During the War', *The Official History of Australia in the War of 1914-1918*, Vol.11, UQP and AWM, 1989, p.697, refers to the 'first great impulse'.
11 Scott, pp.697 ff.
12 Pryor, p.35; Scott, p.738; Gilbert, p.239. Robson, p.59 n.40, reports the Australia Day fund in New South Wales as approximately half that mentioned by Gilbert and Scott.
13 Pryor, ibid, cites Bagnall, in the New South Wales parliament, proposing a special taxation to supplement the Commonwealth pension.
14 S.J. Hurwitz, *State Intervention in Great Britain: a study of economic control and social response 1914-1919*, Frank Cass & Co, London 1968 (first edn. 1949), p.244. See also D. Cohen, *The War Come Home: Disabled Veterans in Britain and Germany, 1914-1939*, UCP, Berkeley and London 2001.
15 Robson, pp.59-60; Pryor, p.38. AWM38, 3DRL 7953 [18], letter from Scott to Bean, 3 March 1927, quoting secret cables between Munro-Ferguson and British Secretary of State, 7-17 June 1915.
16 Bill Gammage, *The Broken Years*, Penguin, Ringwood 1974, p.15. On the subscriptions to funds see Scott, p.737.
17 AWM38, 3DRL 8042, item 119D, Notes on Repatriation; *The Argus*, 21 May 1915, p.7.
18 Ian Turner, *Industrial Labour and Politics*, Hale & Iremonger, Sydney 1979, p.72; Stuart Macintyre, *The Oxford History of Australia*, OUP, Melbourne 1986, p.163.
19 G.E. Caiden, *Career Service*, MUP, Carlton 1965, p.122; R.S. Parker, *Public Service Recruitment in Australia*, MUP, Melbourne 1942, p.68.
20 M. Lake, *Limits of Hope: Soldier Settlement in Victoria 1915-1938*, OUP, Melbourne 1987, p.32.
21 Lake, Chapter 2.
22 *The Argus*, 3 September 1914, cited in Pryor, p.13.
23 Cook's scheme proposed £75 for a totally incapacitated soldier plus an additional £30 for his wife; Pearce was proposing £25 for the incapacitated soldier plus £52 for his wife. See Pryor, p.13; Hansard, Thursday 15 October 1914, reproduced in AA(ACT): A571/55, item 15/19194.
24 R.N. Spann, *Public Sector Administration in Australia*, Government Printer, Sydney 1973, p.58.
25 Caiden, p.112. At the same date the staff of Defence was only 29 and spread throughout the states.

26 See Treasury correspondence in AA(ACT): A571/55. *Official Year Book of the Commonwealth of Australia*, Government Printer, Melbourne 1922, No.15, Section XIX.

27 AA(ACT): A571/55, item 15/19194, F.J. Ross to The Secretary, 17 October 1914.

28 On this see K. Blackmore, 'Making health policy in Australia: the case of Invalid Pensions', in *Choice and Change: ethics, politics and economics of Public Health*, PHA, Canberra 1993, pp.15-20.

29 AA(ACT): A571/55, item 15/19194, Collins to Allen, 3 February 1915.

30 AA(ACT): A1317/1, item A6440, War Pension statistics for the year 1915-1916.

31 Scott, pp.842-4; Lake, p.41.

32 AA(ACT): A2, item 19/1163, Memo from Secretary, Prime Minister's Department to Garran, Attorney General, 8 May 1916; Pryor, pp.40-47.

33 Gilbert, p.240.

34 Australian Soldiers' Repatriation Fund, *Report of the Board of Trustees* (henceforth *Board of Trustees*), Schedule 1, Government Printer, Melbourne 1918, p.25.

35 *Board of Trustees*, p.25.

36 AA(ACT): A2, item 16/4018, letter J.C. Watson to G.F. Pearce, 30 March 1916.

37 Ibid, whole file.

38 *Board of Trustees*, p.25.

39 *ADB*, Vol.7, pp.339-341; Helen Bourke, *Worker Education and Social Inquiry in Australia 1913-1929*, PhD thesis, University of Adelaide, 1981, passim; M. Roe, *Nine Australian Progressives*, UQP, St Lucia, 1984, passim. On the increasing number of technical students in Australia in the 1920s see C. Forster, *Industrial Development in Australia 1920-1930*, ANU, Canberra 1964, pp.20, 187-9.

40 Manning Clark, *A History of Australia*, MUP, Melbourne 1987, Vol.6, pp.64-5 and n.36, cites a letter from Bonython to Hughes in October 1917 where Bonython proposes Hughes look into a Barony for Sir John Forrest, a long-time opponent of Hughes. On this see also Gavin Souter, *Lion and Kangaroo*, Fontana, Sydney 1978, p.263; L.F. Fitzhardinge, *William Morris Hughes*, A&R, 1979, Vol.2.

41 *ADB*, Vol.9, pp.86-7; *Labor in Politics*, D.J. Murphy (ed), UQP, St Lucia 1975, p.103; J. Merritt, *The Making of the AWU*, OUP, Melbourne 1986, passim. Watson was a friend of W.S. Robinson according to the latter's edited autobiography: *If I Remember Rightly*, G. Blainey (ed), F.W. Cheshire, Melbourne 1967, pp.80-81; Fitzhardinge, Vol.2, pp.75, 109ff.

42 *Board of Trustees*, Schedule 4; *Minutes of the Repatriation Committee*, 1 July 1918 to 26 March 1920.

43 *ADB*, Vol.7, pp.138-145; W.S. Robinson, op cit. See also F. Carrigan, 'The Imperial struggle for power in the Broken Hill base-metal industry', in E.L. Wheelwright and K.D. Buckley (eds), *Essays in the Political Economy of Australian Capitalism*, Australia & New Zealand Book Company, Frenchs Forest 1983, Vol.5, pp.164-186. Scott, p.567, suggests that the relationship between the Commonwealth government and Collins House was amicably settled by March 1916.

44 Fred Johns, *John's Notable Australians and Who is Who in Australasia*, Second Edition, Adelaide 1908. Williams was General Manager from 1903 to 1920 (*Who's Who in the Commonwealth of Australia*, 1922).

45 *Board of Trustees*, Schedule 4.

46 *Argus*, 5 May 1916, cited in AWM38, 3DRL 8042, item 119D, Notes on Repatriation.

47 *ADB* Vol.9, p.2; *Repatriation*, 26 June 1920, p.9.

48 R.W. Connell & T.H. Irving, *Class Structure in Australian History*, Longman Cheshire, Melbourne 1980, p.287. See also Humphrey McQueen, 'Who were the Conscriptionists?', *Labour History*, Vol.16, May 1969, pp.44-48. Gilbert's description of himself is in Bean's biographical notes, AWM43, item A297, D.J. Gilbert, letter to Bean, 22 January 1937.

49 Gilbert, p.240; *Board of Trustees*, p.5; Scott, p.830; AWM38, 3DRL 8042, item 119D, Notes on Repatriation.

50 *Board of Trustees*, p.6. It also extended to members of the Imperial Reserve Force if they were *bona fide* residents of Australia prior to the war.

51 Ibid.

52 *Board of Trustees*, pp.10-13. Not all the approved Furniture claims were made as gifts. Some were made as loans. See AA(ACT): A2479/1, item 17/3, State War Councils, Notes on Administration.

53 Gilbert, pp.240-41; Scott, p.830; *Board of Trustees*, p.7.

54 *ADB*, Vol.10, p.653.

55 AA(ACT): A2479/1, item 17/3, p.4.

56 Ibid, letter from State War Council Melbourne to Secretary, Board of Trustees, ASR Fund, 5 February 1917.

57 Ibid, letter from Secretary, Board of Trustees, ASR Fund, to Secretary, State War Council, Melbourne, 10 February 1917.

58 Brian Dickey, *No Charity There*, Allen & Unwin, North Sydney 1987, p.90.

59 Dickey, p.89.

60 AWM38, 3DRL 8042, item 119D, Notes on Repatriation; Pryor, p.60; *Board of Trustees*, p.8.

61 *Board of Trustees*, p.11.

62 Pryor, p.57.

63 Scott, pp.737-8.

64 Pryor, p.58; Gilbert, p.240; *Board of Trustees*, pp.6-7.

65 *Board of Trustees*, p.15; Pryor, p.59.

66 AWM38, 3DRL 7953, item 16, Shortage of men and conscription; Robson, Ch.5.

67 Hurwitz, p.104.

68 Fitzgerald, Chapter 5. AA(ACT): old series CP4/1, Prime Minister's Department – Bundles, gives a clear indication of the importance of Australian primary industries in Hughes's negotiations in London.

69 Fitzgerald, pp.71, 78; Scott, p.528. The Round Table was a conservative imperialist organisation which in Australia spawned the Universal Service League: Macintyre, *Oxford*, pp.160-1.

70 Fitzgerald, pp.152-61; Scott, p.763ff; Humphrey McQueen, *Social Sketches of Australia 1888-1975*, Penguin, Ringwood 1978, p.89.

71 Macintyre, *Oxford*, Ch.8. See also Raymond Evans, *Loyalty and Disloyalty*, Allen & Unwin, North Sydney 1987, Ch.5.

72 Scott, p.368; Macintyre, *Oxford*, p.165.

73 Pryor, p.59.

74 In 1927 Scott interviewed Hughes while writing the section on Conscription in *Australia During the War*. While Scott lamented that most of Hughes's comments were 'unpublishable', he came away from the meeting believing that the 'terrible affair at Easter in Dublin absolutely upset our applecart in Australia by complicating the industrial situation by religion': AWM38, 3DRL 7953 [18], letter from Scott to Bean, 23 March 1927.

75 Peter Love, *Labour and the Money Power*, MUP, Melbourne 1984, Chapter 3.

76 G. Sawer, *Australian Federal Politics and Law 1901-1929*, MUP, Melbourne 1972, p.145.

77 Scott, pp.830-31.

78 Fitzhardinge, p.75.

79 Robert D. Cuff, 'Herbert Hoover, the Ideology of Voluntarism and War Organisation during the Great War', *J Am Hist*, Vol.64, No.2, 1977, pp.362-3.

80 James Weinstein, *The Corporate Ideal in the Liberal State: 1900-1918*, Beacon Press, Boston 1968; Robert H. Wiebe, *The Search for Order 1877-1920*, Hill and Wang, New York 1967.

81 Gabriel Kolko, *The Triumph of Conservatism*, Free Press, New York 1963, p.6.

82 *Board of Trustees*, p.16.

83 AWM 25, item 885/2, Secret letter from DMS to DDMS, CCS, 17 November 1916.

84 AWM 25, item 885/2, Adjutant General G.H. Fowke to all Armies, 14 October 1916.

85 AWM 25, item 835/1, D.W. Carmalt Jones, MO in charge Shell Shock, to Officer Commanding No. 4 Stationary Hospital, 29 January 1917.

86 AWM 25, item 885/5, Major Woollard to ADMS 4th Division, 22 August 1916.

87 AWM 25, item 835/5, R.B. Huxtable to ADMS 1st Australian Division, 13 August 1916.

88 Butler, Vol. 3, p.89.
89 Butler, Vol. 3, pp. 102, 156, 180.
90 Fitzhardinge, p.236.
91 Scott, pp.405-9.
92 AWM 25, item 481/28, Report of ADMS, Tidworth, Dispatch No.32, 5 October 1917.
93 AWM 41, Box 60, Letter from Harvey H.S. Blackburn to Treloar, AWM, undated 1925.
94 AA(NSW): SP948/1, item 832, letter K. Smith to Chairman, Repatriation Commission, 3 October 1930.
95 Butler, Vol.2, p.843,
96 Ibid, p.844 and n.101.
97 Evans, Chapter 3.
98 AWM38, 3DRL, item 16, letter Bean to Scott, 16 June 1933 and letter Scott to Bean, 20 June 1933. On Hirschfeld's activities see also Evans, p.49; Scott, pp.156-7.
99 Scott, pp.370-71; Fitzhardinge, p.239.
100 Fitzhardinge, p.249; Gerd Hardach, *The First World War 1914-1918*, Allen Lane, London 1977, p.86.
101 *Board of Trustees*, p.16.
102 Pryor, pp.83-4.
103 Minutes of the Board of Trustees, 11 January 1917, cited in Pryor, pp.86-7.
104 *Board of Trustees*, p.21.
105 Fitzhardinge, pp.241-3.
106 *Board of Trustees*, p.16.
107 *Argus*, 21 January 1917, cited in Pryor, p.88.
108 *Board of Trustees*, p.21.
109 Fitzhardinge, p.249; Sawer, p.134.
110 AA(ACT): A2479, item 17/151, letter from Parkes to Williams, 22 February 1917.
111 AA(ACT): A2479, item 17/148, letter from Williams to Hughes, 26 February 1917.
112 AA(ACT): A2479, item 17/151, letter from Gilbert to Williams, 27 February 1917, annotated by Williams.
113 Sawer, pp.131 and149.
114 Sawer, pp.130-31; Fitzhardinge, pp.256-60,
115 AA(ACT): A2479, item 17/216, Australian Soldiers' Repatriation Fund, March 1917.
116 AA(ACT): A2479, item 17/304.
117 *SMH*, 21 April 1917; *Argus*, 21 April 1917, reproduced in AA(ACT): MP68/2, item 17/350/1.
118 Pryor, p.89.
119 AA(ACT): A2479, item 17/422, Confidential Report to Cabinet, May 1917.
120 AA(ACT): A2479, item 17/148, letter from Williams to Millen, 13 June 1917.
121 Pryor discusses the debates at length, pp.94-7.
122 AWM38, 3DRL 7953, item 16, Bean to Scott, 6 July 1928.

Chapter 3

1 Wilfred Owen, Dulce Et Decorum Est, *The Penguin Book of First World War Poetry*, 2nd ed, 1996.
2 Mark Henshaw, 'War: the prints of Otto Dix', *Artonview* (National Gallery of Australia) No.45, Autumn 2006, p.32.
3 See in particular the works of Cooter, Bourke, Sturdy, Harrison, and Cook in the bibliography.
4 Joanna Bourke is one notable exception.
5 Butler Vol.2, Appendix 1, p.iv. I have grouped 'shell shock (wounded)' with 'woundings' in these figures.
6 Butler, Vol. 3, Table 58, n.162.

7   J.D. Howell, ' "Soldier's Heart": the redefinition of heart disease and speciality formation in early twentieth-century Great Britain', in R. Cooter, M. Harrison & S. Sturdy eds, *War, Medicine and Modernity*, Sutton, Stroud 1998, p.88. For an alternative view that argues for widespread malingering and spurious symptoms amongst soldiers, and for pecuniary motives amongst army doctors, see J.A. Christophers, 'The epidemic of heart disease amongst British soldiers during the First World War', *War and Society*, Vol.15, No.1, May 1997, pp.53-72.

8   Note: these figures are not entirely reliable but the best available. Percentages are approximate only but included for easier appraisal of significance.

9   Butler provides a percentage figure of a total figure of 157,547.

10 Butler, Vol.3, p.97.

11 Butler, Vol.3, Table No.55, p.930.

12 AWM27, 521/4 [1], letter Gilbert (Repatriation Department) to Secretary RSSILA, December 1919. The letter states that there were 2200 amputees in Australia by that date.

13 See Chapter 7. For a recent discussion of this issue see in particular C.E. Rosenberg, 'The Tyranny of Diagnosis: Specific Entities and Individual Experience', *Millbank Quarterly*, Vol.80, No.2, 2002, pp.237-260.

14 See in particular Chapters 7-9.

15 See for example: Lutz D.H. Sauerteig, 'Sex, medicine and morality during the First World War', in Cooter, Harrison & Sturdy eds, 1998, op cit, pp.167-188; M. Harrison, 'The British army and the problem of venereal disease in France and Egypt during the First World War', *Medical History*, Vol.9, 1995, pp.133-158. See also S. Welborn, *Lords of Death*, Fremantle Arts Centre Press, Fremantle 1983.

16 See Lloyd and Rees, passim; AWM41, 526, Pensions – onus of proof; AWM41, 725, Onus of Proof.

17 Wilfred Owen, Dulce Et Decorum Est, *The Penguin Book of First World War Poetry*, 2nd ed, 1996. The latin phrase 'Dulce et decorum est, Pro patria mori' has been used as an inscription on many war memorials (including the Sydney War Memorial) and tombstones. Roughly translated it means 'it is sweet and beautiful to die for one's country'.

18 Butler, Vol.3, p.6, n.4.

19 Butler, ibid, p.9.

20 W.D. Miles, ' The idea of chemical warfare in modern times', *Journal of the History of Ideas*, Vol.31, No.2, 1970, pp.297-304.

21 J.A. Johnson, 'Chemical warfare in the Great War', *Minerva*, Vol.40, 2002, pp.93-106.

22 Miles, op cit; C.E. Heller, 'Chemical Warfare in World War 1: the American experience, 1917-1918', *Leavenworth Papers*, No.10, September 1984, Combat Studies Institute, Fort Leavenworth, p.6, notes 6 and 7.

23 Heller, op cit; Johnson, op cit, p.987, note 15.

24 Butler, Vol. 3, p.11; Heller, op cit, p.15.

25 IPCS INCHEM, ICSC:1225, Benzyl Bromide (accessed March 2006).

26 Ibid.

27 C. Winder, 'The toxicology of chlorine', *Environmental Research*, Vol.85, 2001, pp.105-114; R.B. Evans, 'Chlorine: state of the art', *Lung*, Vol.183, 2004, pp.151-167.

28 Winder, op cit, p.108. Heller, op cit, says this was xylyl bromide: p.7, n.9.

29 Heller, op cit, pp.14-15.

30 Ibid, p.17.

31 Butler, Vol.3, p.15.

32 Winder, ibid.

33 Winder, ibid.

34 Butler, Vol.3, p.36.

35 R. Das, P.D. Blanc, 'Chlorine gas exposure and the lung: a review', *Toxicology and Industrial Health*, Vol.9, No.3, 1993, p.443.

36 Tim Cook, *No Place to Run: the Canadian Corps and gas warfare in the First World War*, UNC Press, Vancouver 1999, p57. Butler dates its introduction to July 1916 based on a 'Very Secret' report by the Physiological Adviser to Gas Services in the BEF, Lt Col Douglas (AWM27, 314/15).

37 AWM27, 314/18: Gas Notes of L/Cpl C.C. Serjeant.

38 Heller, op cit, Table 1, p.15; Butler, Vol.3, p.15.

39 C.R. Warden, 'Respiratory Agents: irritant gases, riot control agents, incapacitants, and caustics', *Critical Care Clinics*, Vol.21, 2005, p.719.

40 D. Evison, D. Hinsley, P. Rice, 'Regular review: Chemical weapons', *BMJ*, Vol.324, 9 February 2002, p.333.

41 Centers for Disease Control, *Fact Sheet: Phosgene* (accessed 14 April 2006).

42 J. Borak, 'Phosgene exposure: mechanisms of injury and treatment strategies', *Journal of Occupational and Emergency Medicine*, Vol.43, No.2, February 2001, p.110; Winder, op cit.

43 Warden, op cit, p.719.

44 Borak, op cit, p.111.

45 Evison, Hinsley & Rice, op cit; IPCS INCHEM, ICSC:0007 (accessed 5 April 2006).

46 Butler, ibid, p15.

47 W.F. Diller 'Late sequelae after phosgene poisoning: a literature review', *Toxicology and Industrial Health*, Vol.1, No.2, 1985, pp.129-136.

48 AWM27, 314/14: Gas casualties, gas defence and notes on various chemicals (Jul-Sep 1918).

49 Heller, op cit, p.23; P.P. Rega, 'Diphosgene', *eMedicine Journal*, Vol.7, No.3, March 4 2006 (accessed 10 April 2006).

50 Heller, op cit, p.15.

51 Heller, ibid; IPCS INCHEM *Chlorodiphenylarsine* ICSC:1526 (accessed 12 April 2006).

52 T. Ochi, T. Suzuki, H. Isono, T. Kaise, 'In vitro cytotoxic and genotoxic effects of diphenylarsinic acid, a degradation product of chemical warfare agents', *Toxicology and Applied Pharmacology*, Vol.200, 2004, pp.64-72.

53 Heller, op cit:23.

54 AWM27, 314/14, op cit.

55 J.C. Prudhomme, R. Bhatia, J.M. Nutik, D.J. Shusterman, 'Chest wall pain and possible rhabdomyolysis after chloropicrin exposure: a case series', *Journal of Occupational and Environmental Medicine*, Vol.41, No.1, January 1999, pp.17-22; IPCS INCHEM *Trichloronitromethane* ICSC:0750 (accessed 12 April 2006); M.A. O'Malley, S. Edmiston, D. Richmond, M. Ibarra, 'Illness associated with drift of chloropicrin soil fumigant into a residential area – Kern County, California, 2003', *Morbidity and Mortality Weekly Report*, Vol.53, No.32, August 20 2004, p.740.

56 Butler Vol.3, p.15.

57 M. Balali-Mood, M. Hefazi, 'The pharmacology, toxicology, and medical treatment of sulphur mustard poisoning', *Fundamental & Clinical Pharmacology*, Vol.19, 2005, pp.297-315; K.J. Smith, C.G. Hurst, R.B. Moeler, H.G. Skelton, F.R. Sidell, 'Sulfur mustard: its continuing threat as a chemical warfare agent, the cutaneous lesions induced, progress in understanding its mechanism of action, its long-term health effects, and new developments for protection and therapy', *Journal of the American Academy of Dermatology*, Vol.32, No.5, May 1995, pp.765-776.

58 Balali-Mood & Hefazi, op cit, p298.

59 Ibid; L. Kelly, D. Dewar, B. Curry, 'Experiencing chemical warfare: two physicians tell their story of Halabja in Northern Iraq', *Canadian Journal of Rural Medicine*, Vol.9, No.3, Summer 2004, pp.178-181.

60 A.B. Thomsen, J. Eriksen, K. Smidt-Nielsen, 'Chronic neuropathic symptoms after exposure to mustard gas: a long-term investigation', *Journal of the American Academy of Dermatology*, Vol.39, No.2, 1998, pp.187-90.

61 A. Blair, N. Kazerouni, 'Reactive chemicals and cancer', *Cancer Causes and Control*, Vol.8, 1997, pp.473-90.

62 Evison, op cit.

63 Balali-Mood & Hefazi, op cit.

64 AWM 27, 314/15: Lt Col Douglas, Note on the Casualties and Deaths caused by gas shells, July 1916 to July 1918, p.1.

65 AWM 27, 314/18, op cit; AWM 27, 314/36: Report of Divisional Gas Officer, 3rd Australian Division, 11 July 1918.

66 AWM 27, 314/21: Lt Col [unidentified] of General Staff, 2nd Australian Division, 28 November 1917.

67 AWM41, 1169: [Withers Narratives] Chemical Warfare (Part I Section II Chapter III).

68 J. McManus, K. Huebner, 'Vesicants', *Critical Care Clinics*, Vol.21, 2005, pp.707-18.

69 J.C. Harris 'Gassed', *Archives of General Psychiatry*, Vol.62, January 2005, pp.15-17; McManus & Huebner op cit; Smith, Hurst, et al op cit; Balali-Mood & Hefazi, op cit; IPCS INCHEM *Sulfur Mustard* ICSC: 0418 (accessed March 2006); Blair & Kazerouni, op cit.

70 Blair & Kazerouni, op cit.

71 Balali-Mood & Hefazi, op cit, p.303.

72 AWM41, 1169, ibid.

73 Ibid.

74 AWM27, 314/18, ibid; Butler, Vol.3, Ch.1.

75 AWM25, 267/44: A Note on Trench Fever, Col AB Soltau, August 1918.

76 Butler, Vol.3, pp.247-8.

77 AWM25, 267/44: Report on cases of an infectious fever, Beard to ADMS 5th Australian Division, April 1917.

78 Ibid, Memo to RMOs from ADMS 5th Australian Division, 17 May 1917.

79 Ibid, Letter from 7th Australian Infantry Brigade to Headquarters, 2nd Australian Division, 29 May 1917.

80 Ibid, Sutton to Battalion Headquarters, 31 May 1917.

81 Butler, Vol.3, pp.251-2.

82 AWM25, 267/44: Third Report on Trench Fever, July 1918.

83 Ibid, Memo ADMS Sutton to Divisional HQ, 30 June 1917.

84 Ibid, Major Brown, No.3 AAH, Dartford, to DMS AIF, 10 December 1917.

85 Ibid, Circular from ADMS 2nd Australian Division 22 March 1918.

86 Ibid, Extract from Third Report on Trench Fever, May 1918.

87 M. Drancourt et al, '*Bartonella Quintana* in a 4000-year-old human tooth', *Journal of Infectious Diseases*, Vol.191, 15 February 2005, pp.607-611; D. Raoult et al, 'Evidence for louse-transmitted diseases in soldiers of Napoleon's Grand Army in Vilnius', *Journal of Infectious Diseases*, Vol.193, 1 January 2005, pp.112-20.

88 D. Raoult, C. Foucault, P. Brouqui, 'Infections in the homeless', *Lancet*, Vol.1, September 2001, pp.77-84; N. Seki et al, 'Epidemiological studies on *Bartonella Quintana* infections among homeless people in Tokyo, Japan', *Japanese Journal of Infectious Diseases*, Vol.59, 2006, pp.31-35.

89 Raoult, Foucault & Brouqui, ibid.

90 V. Jacomo, P.J. Kelly, D. Raoult, 'Natural history of *Bartonella* infections (an exception to Koch's Postulate)', *Clinical and Diagnostic Laboratory Immunology*, Vol.9, No.1, January 2002, pp.8-18; C. Foucault, K. Barrau, P. Brouqui, D. Raoult, '*Bartonella quintana* bacteremia among homeless people', *Clinical Infectious Diseases*, Vol.35, 15 September 2002, pp.684-9.

91 G. Greub, D. Raoult, '*Bartonella*: new explanations for old diseases', *Journal of Medical Microbiology*, Vol.51, 2002, pp.915-923.

92 Greub & Raoult, ibid; P. Mann et al, 'From trench fever to endocarditis', *Postgraduate Medical Journal*, Vol.79, 2003, pp.655-5;

93 M.E. Ohl, D.H. Spach, DH, '*Bartonella quintana* and urban trench fever', *Clinical Infectious Diseases*, Vol.31, 2000, pp.131-5; Jacomo, Kelly & Raoult, op cit.

94 P. Fournier et al, 'Epidemiologic and clinical characteristics of *Bartonella quintana* and *Bartonella henselai* endocarditis', *Medicine*, Vol.80, No.4, 2001, pp.245-51; C. Breitkopf et al, 'Impact of a

molecular approach to improve the microbiological diagnosis of infective heart valve endocarditis', *Circulation*, Vol.111, 2005, pp.1415-1421.

95   AWM 41, 269: Major N. Kirkwood to Butler, 27 May 1935.

96   J.S. Haller, 'Trench Foot – a study in military-medical responsiveness in the Great War, 1914-1918', *Western Journal of Medicine*, Vol.152, No.6, June 1990, pp.729-33.

97   On the condition and its importance in this period generally see AWM 41, 269 and 270. See also Butler, Vol.2, pp.87 and 99, n.39. On the number of amputations see AWM 27, 521/4, op cit.

98   Haller, op cit.

99   Owen to his mother, January 1917, in Jon Stallworthy, *Wilfred Owen*, OUP 1977, pp.156-59.

100   M.G. Miller, 'Of lice and men: trench fever and trench life in the AIF', paper presented at the Second Anzac Medical Society, France, October 1993. http://www.ku.edu/carrie/specoll/medical/liceand.htm, (accessed February 2005).

101   M. Tyquin, *Little by Little: A Centenary History of the Royal Australian Army Medical Corps*, Army History Unit, Department of Defence, Canberra 2003, p.246.

102   AWM25, 481/204: Birdwood to 4th Army Headquarters, 11 December 1916.

103   AWM25, 481/204: Sturdee to Divisional Headquarters, 9 November 1916.

104   Ibid, GOC 2nd Division to GOC 1st Anzac Corps, 13 November 1916.

105   Tyquin, op cit, p248; AWM25, 481/204: DA & QMG 1st Anzac Corps to Headquarters 5th Australian Division, 1 December 1916.

106   AWM 25, 481/204: Manifold to Birdwood, 30 November 1916.

107   Ibid.

108   Ibid, Report on the investigation into the excessive evacuation for Trench foot in the 5th Australian Division, 2 December 1916.

109   AWM41/270, Chapter V-VI, Sundry Notes, 24/9/32.

110   Haller, op cit.

111   A.K. Macdougall (ed), *War Letters of Sir John Monash*, Duffy & Snellgrove, Sydney 2002, pp.129-30.

112   Ibid, 157.

Chapter 4

1   There have been a number of notable exceptions including Hilary Golder's *High and Responsible Office: a history of the New South Wales magistracy*, SUP and OUP, Melbourne 1991 and Paul Ashton, *Waving the Waratah*, New South Wales Bicentennial Council, Sydney 1989. But see also J. Murphy, 'The new official history', *Australian Historical Studies* [Australia], Vol.26, No.102, 1994, pp.119-124.

2   AWM41, Box 61, letter Bean to Butler, 24 July 1942.

3   AA(ACT): A2479, 17/1023, letter Knibbs to Millen, 21 August 1917. See also AA(ACT): MP68/2/1, Box 22, 17/1825 for further evidence of Knibbs's correspondence with Millen.

4   Gilbert, p.242.

5   *ADB*, Vol.10, pp.502-3.

6   See following sections for evidence of Millen's values and approach to repatriation.

7   AA(ACT): A2483, item B18/1296, letter Millen to D. Mackinnon, Chairman State War Council, 28 August 1917; *ADB*, Vol.10, p.130.

8   Desley Deacon, *Managing Gender: the state, the new middle class and women workers 1830-1930*, OUP, Melbourne 1989, pp.51 ff., 123 ff.; Fitzhardinge, p.175.

9   On the factional system see *The Emergence of the Australian party system*, P. Loveday, A.W. Martin & R.S. Parker (eds), Hale & Iremonger, Sydney 1977; D. Jaensch, *Power Politics: Australia's party system*, Allen & Unwin, North Sydney 1983.

10   AA(ACT): A2483, item B18/1296, ibid; B18/3310, letter Lockyer to Jensen, Minister of Trade and Customs, 9 October 1917.

11   AA(ACT): A2479, item 17/933, Gilbert to all State War Councils by telegram, 7 August 1917.

12   AA(ACT): A2479, item 17/1133, contains some of these reports and suggestions. It indicates that the information was requested by the Board of Trustees. However, later sequences of files suggest that the information was for either Lockyer or Millen at a time when there was no Repatriation Department letterhead or filing system and when Gilbert, who probably wrote the letter of inquiry, was both Secretary of the Board *and* acting unofficially as Lockyer's secretary.

13   AA(ACT): A2479, item 17/1133. All subsequent discussion on suggestions from the Councils or Funds derives from this item.

14   Further evidence of under-funding and knowledge that the recipient must fail in the venture can be found in AA(ACT): A2487, item 19/1532, Submission by Victorian State Board to Commission, February 1919.

15   See Chapter 6 for an exposition of the workings of this and other Regulations.

16   For a detailed analysis of War Pensions see Chapter 8.

17   AA(ACT): A2479, item 17/1133, Australia Day Fund Amelioration Committee, Classification of the objects of ameliorative assistance, 6 September 1917, p.3.

18   Ibid, p.4.

19   See AA(ACT): A2479, item 17/1133, note by Lockyer that the officers preparing General Orders should see all the Reports. This is noted as 'done'.

20   AA(ACT): A2479, item 17/1181, extract from letter Secretary to ASR Fund, 28 August 1917. See also A2479, item 17/304, Report of the Disablement and Training Sub-committee in the Report of the New South Wales Council, pp.10-12, on the nature of the sub-committee and its work. Since Gilbert was Secretary to both the ASR Fund and Lockyer, letters were often addressed to the ASR Fund until around October when a Departmental address and stationary were established.

21   AA(ACT): A2479, item 17/58, Minutes of the Disablement and Training Sub-Committee of the State War Council, July to December 1917.

22   AA(ACT): A2483, item B18/1753-B18/1767, letter Gilbert to Lockyer, 15 March 1918.

23   *ADB*, Vol.10, p.314; Scott, pp.399-405; AA(ACT): A2483, item B18/1296, letter Lockyer to Secretary of Victorian Council, D. Barry, 12 October 1917.

24   AA(ACT): A2483, item B18/1296, op cit, Minute from Lewis East to The Comptroller, 26 October 1917.

25   Ibid.

26   Ibid, handwritten annotation on the Minute, 29 October 1917.

27   AA(ACT): A2483, item B18/1296.

28   AA(ACT): A2483, item B18/1968.

29   AA(ACT): A2483, item B18/568, Suggestions, Gilbert to Lockyer, 19 February 1918.

30   AA(ACT): A2483, item B18/568, annotation by Lockyer to Gilbert's memorandum, 20 February 1918; also Minute Paper by Lockyer to Millen, 25 February 1918.

31   AA(ACT): A2483, item B18/1753-1767, letter Lockyer to Gilbert, 4 March 1918.

32   Ibid.

33   See on this issue, AA(ACT): A2483, item B18/1278. On Foll see J. Rydon, *A Biographical Register of the Commonwealth Parliament, 1901-1972*, ANU Press, Canberra 1975. On Givens see *ADB* Vol.9, p.20.

34   AA(ACT): A2483, item B18/1209, letter Gilbert to Lockyer, 23 March 1918.

35   AA(ACT): A2483, item B18/1278, telegram Gilbert to Comptroller, 25 March 1918.

36   Ibid, letter Lockyer to Secretary RSSILA, 2 April 1918.

37   AA(ACT): A2483, item B18/5138, letter Millen to T.J. Hitchman, 19 March 1918; item B18/1416, letter Gilbert to Lockyer, 7 March 1918.

38   AA(ACT): A2483, item B18/5138, ibid.

39   AA(ACT): A2483, item B18/1416, letter Gilbert to Lockyer, 7 March 1918.

40   See, for example, photographs used by the Repatriation Department in both World Wars at AA(ACT): A7342, item M92; the cartoons of George Grosz reproduced in Robert Weldon Whalen, *Bitter Wounds: German Victims of the Great War, 1914-1939*, Cornell University Press, Ithaca 1984;

and for Canada see the posters and illustrations reproduced in Desmond Morton and Glenn Wright, *Winning the Second Battle: Canadian Veterans and the Return to Civilian Life 1915-1930*, University of Toronto Press, Toronto 1987.

41 See for example, AWM Film 139.

42 For the number of amputees see AWM27, 521.4 [1], letter Gilbert to Secretary RSSILA, December 1919. See Butler, Vol.3, p.893ff for a lengthy exposition of the incomplete and misleading nature of AIF medical records. A figure of around 170 000 is commonly cited; see, for example, Stuart Macintyre, *Oxford*, op cit, p.177.

43 G.L. Kristianson, *The Politics of Patriotism: the Pressure Group Activities of the Returned Servicemen's League*, ANU Press, Canberra 1966, pp.10-14; and, 'The Establishment of the RSL', *Stand-to*, March-April 1963, pp.22, 25. See also AA(ACT): A2483, item B18/1277, The Status of the RSSILA, for a clear indication of the negligible status of the organisation in late 1917 and early 1918.

44 Kristianson, *Stand-to*, ibid, pp.25-6.

45 On this see M. Lake, 'The Power of Anzac', in M. McKernan and M. Browne (eds), *Australia Two Centuries of War and Peace*, AWM in association with Allen & Unwin, 1988, p.204.

46 AA(ACT): A2483, item B18/5138, letter from A. Jobson, President of New South Wales Branch, RSSILA, to Millen, 29 June 1918.

47 Ibid, letter Lockyer to Gilbert, 19 March 1918.

48 AA(ACT): A2483, item B18/2037, list of members of State Boards April 1918.

49 AA(ACT): A2483, item B18/1416, official letter Gilbert to Lockyer, 13 March 1918; item B18/5138, letter Maughan to Gilbert, 21 March 1918.

50 Ibid, private letter Gilbert to Lockyer, 13 March 1918.

51 AA(ACT): A2483, item B18/5138, letter Willington to Lockyer, 22 March 1918.

52 On membership of the State Boards see AA(ACT): A2483, item B18/2037, op cit. On the General Labourers' Union see Turner, *Industrial Labour*, op cit, pp.95-6. On the conservatism of the Trades and Labour Council in New South Wales prior to June 1918 and the complex allegiances and groupings within the labour movement in this period see Turner pp.174-181.

53 Pryor, p.97.

54 A letter from Gilbert to the Secretary of the Citizens 'War Chest' Fund, 17 June 1918, quotes Millen as being 'desirous of having all classes represented on the Board': AA(ACT): A2483, item B18/5138.

55 AA(ACT): A2483, item B18/2157, Memorandum from Lockyer to all states, 15 April 1918.

56 AA(ACT): A2487, item 19/215, Minutes of meetings of the State Repatriation Board of NSW, various dates.

57 AA(ACT): A2483, item B18/1753-B18/1767, letter Lockyer to Gilbert, 22 March 1918.

58 Ibid, letter Lockyer to Gilbert, 11 March 1918.

59 Ibid, letter Lockyer to Gilbert, 11 and 12 March 1918.

60 AA(ACT): A2483, item B18/1416, letter Gilbert to Lockyer, 7 March 1918.

61 AA(ACT): A2483, item B181753-B18/1767, letter Lockyer to Gilbert, 11 March 1918.

62 On Farr see *Minutes of the Repatriation Commission*, 2 October 1923; AWM183, Farr, Lieutenant Colonel, A.G.; AWM43, A253, A.G. Farr; *Smith's Weekly*, 1 October 1938. On the hostility between Millen and Repatriation Headquarters and Farr over the period see references in AA(ACT): A2487, items 19/5138, 19/8325, 21/10714 and 22/1863.

63 AA(ACT): A2483, item B18/1416, letter Gilbert to Lockyer, 7 March 1918.

64 *Mufti*, 1 February 1939, p.17; AA(ACT): A3048, Staff position cards, 1919-1951; A2483, item B18/1753-B18/1767; AWM140, Official History, War of 1914-1918, Biographical cards.

65 *Reveille*, 1 August 1939, p.5; *The Queensland Digger*, 1 November 1935, p.6; A3048, op cit.

66 AA(ACT): A2479, item 18/19, Minutes of meeting, Executive Committee, 17 January 1918.

67 *ADB*, Vol.8, pp.654-656; AWM140, Unidentified newspaper clipping, 1 January 1934.

68 *Biographical Register*, Vol.2, p.118.

69 *ADB*, Vol.11, pp.112-3; *Who's Who*, 1919.

70   *ADB*, Vol.11, pp.516-7; *Who's Who in the Commonwealth of Australia*, 1922.

71   Pryor, p.98.

Chapter 5

1   Those most directly useful for the theoretical background of this chapter are: M.S. Larson, *The Rise of Professionalism: a Sociological Analysis*, University of California Press, California 1977; H. Jamous & B. Peloille, 'Changes in the French University-Hospital system', in LA. Jackson (ed), *Professions and Professionalization*, Cambridge 1970; T.J. Johnson, *Professions and Power*, Macmillan 1972; E.T. Layton, *The Revolt of the Engineers*, Case Western University Press, Cleveland 1971; E. Friedson, *Profession of Medicine*, Dodd & Mead, New York 1970; R. Torstendahl & M. Burrage (eds), *The Formation of Professions: Knowledge. State and Strategy*, SAGE, London 1990; John C. Burnham, 'How the idea of profession changed the writing of medical history', *Medical History*, Supplement No.18, Wellcome Institute for the History of Medicine, London 1998.

2   Larson, *The Rise*, p.220. Although retreating somewhat from alleged 'discontinuities' in her original interpretation of the genesis of professionalism, Larson's description of these particular historical characteristics of the professionalization process seem to have withstood later criticisms. See Larson in Torstendahl & Barrage (eds), op cit. See also Johnson, *Professions*, p.84; Layton, *Engineers*, pp.59, 116-7.

3   Jan Goldstein, '"Moral Contagion": a professional ideology of Medicine and Psychiatry in Eighteenth- and Nineteenth-Century France', G.L. Geison (ed), *Professions and the French State, 1700-1900*, University of Pennsylvania Press, Philadelphia 1984, p.196.

4   Goldstein, ibid. See also Jan Goldstein, *Console and Classify: The French Psychiatric Profession in the Nineteenth Century*, CUP, Cambridge 1987.

5   Roger Smith, 'Expertise, procedure and the possibility of a comparative history of forensic psychiatry in the nineteenth century', *Psychological Medicine*, 1989, Vol.19, p.298. See also Roger Smith, *Trial by Medicine: Insanity and Responsibility in Victorian Trials*, Edinburgh University Press, Edinburgh 1981.

6   See for example Torstendahl in R. Torstendahl & M. Burrage (eds), *The Formation*, p.6.

7   These processes have been elaborated by Michel Foucault in his work on eighteenth century France; however, it is suggested here that their application is far broader. A brief account of his numerous lengthy studies, which cover many of these issues, can be found in Michel Foucault, 'The Politics of Health in the Eighteenth Century', Colin Gordon (ed), *Power/Knowledge: selected Interviews and other Writings 1972-1977*, Pantheon, New York 1980, pp.166-182.

8   Kerreen M. Reiger, *The disenchantment of the home: modernizing the Australian family 1880-1940*, OUP, Melbourne 1985; Desley Deacon, 'Taylorism in the Home: the medical profession, the Infant Welfare Movement and the deskilling of women', *A&NZ JS*, Vol.21, No.2, July 1985, pp. 161-173, and *Managing Gender: the State, the New Middle Class and Women Workers 1830-1930*, OUP, Melbourne 1989. See also Patricia Grimshaw, 'Women and the family in Australian history – a reply to The Real Matilda', *HS* Vol.18, No.72, April 1979, pp.412-421; David Tait, 'Respectability, Property and Fertility: the development of official statistics about families in Australia', *LH*, Vol.49, November 1985, pp.83-96; C.L. Bacchi, 'The Nature-Nurture Debate in Australia, 1900-1914' *HS*, Vol. 19, No.75, October 1980, pp.199-212; M. Lewis, 'Milk, Mothers and Infant Welfare', in J. Roe (ed), *Twentieth Century Sydney: Essays in Urban and Social History*, Hale and Iremonger, Sydney 1980.

9   On the importance of these two 'professional' groups in plague control and sanitation generally see A.J.C. Mayne, *Fever, Squalor and Vice: sanitation and social policy in Victorian Sydney*, UQP, St Lucia 1982; Max Kelly, *Plague Sydney 1900*, Doak Press Paddington 1981 and 'Picturesque and Pestilential: the Sydney slum observed 1860-1900' in M. Kelly (ed), *Nineteenth-Century Sydney, essays in urban history*, SUP, Sydney 1978.

10 G.R. Searle, *The Quest for National Efficiency, a study in British politics and political thought, 1899-1914*, Basil Blackwell, Oxford 1971; G. Jones, *Social Hygiene in Twentieth Century Britain*, Croom Helm, Beckenham 1986. See also D. Pick, *Faces of Degeneration, a European Disorder, c.1848-c.1918*, CUP, Cambridge 1989.

11 James W. Barrett, *The Twin Ideals, an educated Commonwealth*, Vol.1, H.K. Lewis & Co, London 1918, pp. 349-50. Barrett was also an enthusiastic follower of Malthus, particularly in his (Barrett's) concern for the falling birthrate in Australia, on which see ibid p.327ff and *ADB*, Vol.7, pp.186-9.

12 AWM27, 370/30.

13 Michael Tyquin, *Neville Howse. Australia's First Victoria Cross Winner*, OUP, Melbourne 1999, p.143.

14 Whilst works on the history of the professionalization of medicine in Australia are few, the mass of empirical data collected by Pensabene is a most valuable source: T.S. Pensabene, *The Rise of the Medical Practitioner in Victoria*, Research Monograph 2 (Health Research Project), ANU, Canberra 1980. See also A.S. McGrath (Cumpston), 'The History of medical organization in Australia', PhD Sydney University 1975; LB. Egan, 'Nobler than missionaries: Australian medical culture c1880-1930', PhD Monash University 1988; Claudia Thame, 'Health and the State: the development of collective responsibility for Health Care in Australia in the First Half of the Twentieth Century', PhD ANU 1974.

15 Pensabene reaches this conclusion on the basis of a somewhat uncritical survey of editorials in *The Argus*

16 Evan Willis, *Medical Dominance: the division of labour in Australian health care*, George Allen & Unwin, Sydney 1983, in particular pp.26ff and 69ff.

17 Ibid, pp.69-81.

18 Major works on the subject are few and can be found in the Bibliography. Significant contributions to date have been by Gillespie, MacLeod, Smith and Lewis.

19 I. Loudon, 'Medical Practitioners 1750-1850 and the period of medical reform in Britain', in A. Wear (ed), *Medicine in Society. Historical essays*, CUP, Cambridge 1992, p.220.

20 Willis, pp.73-5.

21 Pensabene, p.130 and p.132.

22 Ibid, pp.74-5.

23 See the Medical Practitioners Acts Further Amendment Act 1900, especially Sections 1-4.

24 Invalid and Old Age Pensions Act, Sections 27-38. Invalid and Old Age Pensions Act, Pensions Regulations, 1911-1914, Sections 7-16. AA(ACT): A571/1, 11/6133, Dr F.L. Benham – complaint.

25 An earlier draft of this section was published as 'Making health policy in Australia: the case of invalid pensions', in V.A. Brown and G. Preston (eds), *Choice and Change*, pp.82-87.

26 AA(ACT): A2188/1, Commonwealth Treasury, Invalid and Old Age Pensions Rulings and Opinions, Vol.1, p.189.

27 Ibid, p.223.

28 Ibid p.232.

29 Ibid, pp.156, 168.

30 AA(ACT) A571/1, 20127781, Invalid, Old-age Pension and Maternity Allowance.

31 AA ACT): A571/1, 11/7085, Medical examinations.

32 AA(ACT): A2188/1, Vol.2, p.84.

33 Ibid, p.98.

34 Ibid.

35 *ADB*, Vol.7, pp.41-2; Pensabene, pp.54 and 183-4.

36 *ADB*, Vol.8, pp.77-8.

37 AA(ACT): A571/1, 17/2858, Legality of appointing Collins.

38 R. Watts, 'Origins of the Australian Welfare State', in R. Kennedy (ed), *Australian Welfare History: critical essays*, Macmillan, South Melbourne 1982.

39 AA(ACT): A2188/1, Vol.2.

40 AA(ACT): A571/55, 15/17326, Rearrangement of duties and promotion of Commissioner of Old-age Pensions etc.

41 AA(ACT): A2491, W3838, *War Pensions. Statement for the twelve months ended 30th June, 1920*, Government Printer, Melbourne 1920, p.8.

42 Repatriation Department, *Annual Report*, 1921, p.51.

43 Brian Dickey, review, *Journal of the Australian War Memorial*, Issue 30, April 1997, *http://www.awm.gov.au/journal/j30/bkrevs.htm* (accessed 10 July 2006).

44 Dr J.W. Springthorpe after speaking with A.G. Butler, Official Medical Historian, re his history project. AWM 2DRL/0701, Springthorpe Papers, Series 1, Wallet 1 of 2, typed diary, June 17 1918.

45 Michael Tyquin, *Little by Little: a Centenary History of the Royal Australian Army Medical Corps*, Army History Unit, Department of Defence, Canberra 2003; Michael Tyquin, *Gallipoli the Medical War: the Australian Army Medical Services in the Dardanelles campaign of 1915*, NSWUP, Kensington 1993.

46 See also Chapter 8.

47 Tyquin, *Little by Little*, p.100.

48 AWM27, 370/114, Medical Services: Copy of letter from Surgeon General Fetherston DG AAMS to Col Downes ADMS, AIF Egypt – Administration of the AAMC in Egypt and Australia (Nov 1916).

49 Tyquin, ibid, p.215; I.R. Whitehead, 'The British medical officer on the Western Front: the training of doctors for war', *Clio Medica/The Wellcome Series in the History of Medicine*, Vol.55, No.1, p.23.

50 Anne Summers, 'Militarism in Britain before the Great War', *History Workshop Journal*, Vol.2, No.1, p.108.

51 Roger Cooter, *Surgery and Society in Peace and War: orthopaedics and the organization of modern medicine, 1880-1948*, Macmillan, Basingstoke 1993, pp.6-7.

52 The most recent works are S. Braga, *ANZAC Doctor: the life of Sir Neville Howse, VC*, Hale & Iremonger, Alexandria (NSW) 2000; M. Tyquin, *Neville Howse: Australia's first Victoria Cross winner*, Australian Army History Series, OUP 1999. On Butler's relationship with Howse see Brendan O'Keefe, 'Butler's medical histories', *J Aust War Memorial*, Vol.12, 1988, pp.25-34.

53 Geoffrey Serle, *John Monash: a biography*, MUP, 1982, p.43. See also Braga, op cit, p.256.

54 *ADB*, Vol.12, MUP 1990; Melbourne University, *Roll of the Returned*, Government Printer, Melbourne 1926; Guide to the papers of Dr John William Springthorpe, 2DRL/0701, AWM Canberra.

55 After many requests he finally received an answer 'not approved' from Headquarters in London. A colleague informed him that 'some one [is] behind it all, the penalty of trying to play the game and tell the truth'. AWM 2DRL/0701, Series 1, Wallet 1 of 2.

56 AWM2DRL/0701, Series 1, Wallet 1 of 2, Diary entry. Lt Col Arthur Hamilton Tebbutt enlisted on 20 August 1914 having graduated with both a BA and MB from Sydney University and a Diploma in Public Health from Oxford. He was the chief Resident Pathlogist at Royal Prince Alfred Hospital on enlistment aged 29. He served in the AAMC at Gallipoli and was promoted to Senior Bacteriologist. He worked in this capacity at Fromelles, the Somme and later engagements. He was twice mentioned in Despatches and awarded the DSO (NAA B2455).

57 AWM41, 2008, Springthorpe, letter Springthorpe to Butler in reply to a request for assistance in compiling his history re statistics of the war.

58 Service record of James Reiach, NAA B2455.

59 On Consultant Surgeon Ryan see Chapter 7.

60 Butler, Vol.2, pp.834-6. See also ample evidence in the Howse papers (AWM 2DRL, 1351), notably item 12.

61 See multiple references in Braga, Tyquin and Butler.

62 AWM41, 520, Corresondence with Gibson and Wiley concerning venereal disease in the AIF.

63 Ibid.

64 Butler, Vol.3, p.169.

65 AWM41, 520, Butler's handwritten notes.

66 McWhae lost an eye at Gallipoli. After his recuperation he served as the SMO of the Base Depot in England and then as ADMS of all AIF Depots in the UK from January 1917 until the end of the war.

67 AWM war diaries, 1st ADH; NAA B2455, Piero Fiaschi.

68 *ADB – online edition*, Fiaschi, Piero Francis Bruno (1879-1948).

69 Braga, op cit, pp.94-6, 104; see also Tyquin, *Little by Little*, pp.37-8.

70 AWM war diaries, op cit.

71 NAA B2455, Kenneth Smith; AWM28, 2/462, p.6; AWM28, 2/459, p.15; AWM28, 2/459, p.13; AWM183, 183/42, Smith, K. Col.

72 AWM41, 520, including Butler's handwritten notes. One possible explanation for this very odd order is the greater social stigma attached to syphilis.

73 Butler, Vol.3, p.171.

74 AWM183, 183/42, Smith K. Col.

75 On this see Barton C. Hacker, 'Military institutions and social order: transformations of Western Thought since the Enlightenment', *War & Society*, Vol.11, No.2, October 1993, pp.1-23 and 'Military Institutions, Weapons, and social Change: Toward a new history of military technology', *Technology and Culture*, Vol.35, 1994, pp.768-834.

76 AA(ACT): A2483, B18/3360, Pearce to Millen, 11 March 1918.

77 P. Weindling, *Health, race and German politics between national unification and Nazism, 1870-1945*, CUP, Cambridge 1989, pp.283-4.

78 Butler Vol.3, pp.734-37; AA(ACT): A2487, 19/1336, Fetherston to Gilbert, 11 December 1917.

79 Butler, Vol.3, pp.751-57.

80 AA(ACT): A2487, 21/10227, FPWC, Advisory Committees for Military Hospitals and Convalescent Homes, 6 October 1915.

81 Ibid, letter from Semmens to Secretary Department of Defence, 11 July 1921.

82 Gilbert, p.252ff.

83 AA(ACT): A2487, 19/6732, Contagious diseases.

84 PR83/201, Warrant, Capt James F Agnew, AAMC, AIF; Obituary in *Messenger*, 14 July 1922.

85 *Biographical Register*, Vol.1, pp.6-7; AWM [A], Agnew, Captain J.F.; AWM 146, Agnew, Captain J.F.. On the early AAMC see Tyquin, *Little by Little*, op cit; J. Gurner, *The Origins of the Royal Australian Army Medical Corps*, Hawthorn Press, Melbourne 1970.

86 For a similar interest in policing the racial stock in Germany at this date see Weindling, *Health, race*, pp.281-287.

87 AA(ACT): A2487, 19/1336, Report Agnew to Gilbert, 18 September 1918.

88 Ibid, pp.1-2.

89 The functions of doctors in the Department is analysed in greater detail in subsequent chapters. For examples of specific functions in this early period see AA(ACT) A2487, 19/4774, Medical examination of widows, and 22/13425, Medical examination of intending land settlers.

90 AA(ACT): A2487, 19/2912, Minute Agnew to Gilbert, 4 March 1919.

91 AA(ACT): A2487, 19/11257, Departmental Minute Paper and Return, 13 January 1920; Pensabene, Tables 4.5 and 4.6, pp.69 and 72.

92 AA(ACT): A2487, 21/5230, Minute Paper Agnew to Gilbert, 18 November 1919; ibid, list of specific instruments and prices supplied by W. Ramsay, 18 November 1919.

93 AA(ACT): A2487, 19/1336, Report, p.2.

94 P. Weindling, *Health. Race*, pp.281-84.

95 AA(ACT): A2483, B18/485, Minute Paper by Ovington, December 1917.

96 J.S. Gillespie, *The Price of Health, Australian Governments and Medical Politics 1910-1960*, CUP, Sydney 1991, p.8.
97 Pensabene, Appendix 2, p.181 and pp.156-7.
98 Pensabene, p.157. For New South Wales see Gillespie, *Price of Health*, p.9.
99 Willis, p.77.
100 Gillespie, *Price of Health*, p.10.
101 This point is picked up by Wheeler in her thesis, 'Be in it Mate', chapter 10.
102 Gillespie, *Price of Health*, Table 1.2.

Chapter 6

1   Robson, p.197; Imperial War Cabinet *Minutes*, No.22 (28 June 1918), cited in Fitzhardinge, p.324 and n.23.
2   AWM 3DRL, 2222, Bundle 3, item 3, Hughes to Pearce, 7 May 1918.
3   Imperial War Cabinet, *Minutes*, op cit.
4   Gilbert, p.242.
5   Hughes refers to the 'Generals' union' in a cable to Watt, 4 September 1918. See AA(ACT): CP360/8/1, item 1.
6   AA(ACT): A3934/1, SC15/8/Part 1, cables Birdwood to Defence, July 1918, and Defence to Birdwood, 6 August 1918; Scott, p.824.
7   AA(ACT): CP360/8/1, 1, secret cable Hughes to Watt, 1 August 1918; Scott, pp.744-5; Fitzhardinge, pp.338-341.
8   AWM13, 7041/10/1, Repatriation of Australian Troops – General.
9   Compare Appendix A of the discussion paper, ibid, with AA(ACT): A2487, 19/1552, Detailed Return showing occupations of men applying for employment, March 1919.
10 Butler, Vol.3, p.791; Scott, p.827; Fitzhardinge, p.339; *ADB*, Vol.10, pp.134-5; G. Serle, *John Monash*, MUP, Melbourne 1982, p.409.
11 AA(ACT): CP360/8/1, 1, secret cable Hughes to Watt, 4 September 1918; CP360/8/1, 2, secret cable Hughes to Watt, 30 October 1918.
12 AWM25, 245/70, letter Dodds to Birdwood, 24 October 1918.
13 AA(ACT): A3934, SC 15/8/Pt 1, Confidential memo to Cabinet, 28 October 1918.
14 John Monash, *Australian Imperial Force: the history of the Department of Repatriation and Demobilisation from November 1918 to September 1919*, Department of Repatriation, London 1919, p.7 (henceforth cited as Monash); Butler, Vol.3, pp.710-713; A. Gough, 'The Repatriation of the First Australian Imperial Force', *Qld Hist Rev*, Vol.7, No.1, 1978, pp.62-3; Serle, pp.406-7. The official line is accepted by Lloyd and Rees, p.114.
15 See in particular the cables between Hughes and Watt in late 1918 in AA(ACT): CP360/8/1, 2. Garton, *The Cost of War*, p.2, provides a simplistic and triumphal version of events.
16 AA(ACT): A3934/1, SC15/8/part 1, Memorandum for Cabinet, 28 October 1918.
17 AA(ACT): CP360/8/1, 2, secret cable Watt to Hughes, 2 November 1918. See also Lloyd and Rees, p.114.
18 Ibid and AWM 3DRL, 2222/66, bundle 3, secret cable from Hughes to Watt, 21 November 1918. See also Fitzhardinge, pp.351-3; Monash, passim; Serle, p.409.
19 AWM 3DRL 2222, Pearce to Millen, 30 April 1919; AA(ACT): A2487, 19/7763, Ryan to Gilbert, 1 May 1919. See also Butler, Vol. 2, p.798 and n.41.
20 For a description of the scheme, see Lloyd and Rees, pp.124-8.
21 Sources on the propaganda issued to the AIF by both the Departments of Defence and Repatriation are voluminous. See for example AA(ACT): A2487, 19/379, What Australia is doing for Returned Soldiers, and 19/821, Nature and Scope of Assistance Rendered. See also AWM25, 577/4/1, Summary of assistance and benefits, Australian Soldiers' Repatriation Scheme; 245/5, Repatriation Scheme in Australia. What government is doing.; 245/55, Notes on lecture

by Australian Repatriation Officer; 245/70, demobilisation and repatriation – miscellaneous correspondence; and AWM 19, TE 10/310 and TE 10/324 on literature issued by the Repatriation Department late in 1919 through its London office; TE 12/147, AIF Education Scheme; and AWM10, 4334/1/7, Re Lectures on Demobilisation to be delivered to troops; 4332/5/145, Criticisms and Queries regarding Demobilisation appearing in the Press; and AWM13, 7041/10/1, Repatriation of Australian Troops – General.

22　AWM10 [4334/1/7], Gilbert to Owen, 12 March 1919; AA(ACT): A2487, 19/1, Millen to Eller, 15 May 1919.

23　*Who's Who in Australia*; C.D. Coulthard-Clark, *The Citizen General Staff: the Australian Intelligence Corps 1907-1914*, Military Historical Society of Australia, Canberra 1976; *Repatriation*, 26 June 1920, p.8; F. Legg, *The Gordon Bennett Story*, A&R, 1965; *ADB*, Vol. 13, 'Henry Gordon Bennett'; *Listening Post*, 15 July 1937, p.19; AWM 43, A781, Semmens, J.M.; *Reveille*, July 1937; *Age*, 23 December 1915, cited in Lake, *Limits*, p.33; Serle, Ch.2 passim. Semmens, on his forced retirement, applied for a War Pension but it was denied by both the Repatriation Commission and the Entitlement Appeals Tribunal: Lloyd and Rees, p.254.

24　Coulthard-Clark, p.77; AWM19, TE 12/147, AIF Education Service; AWM25, 245/53, Notes on a lecture by an Australian officer; AA(ACT): A2487, 19/7763, Reports by Repatriation officer UK.

25　Lloyd and Rees, p.253.

26　*Kia Ora Coo-ee News*, 6 August 1918, p.4.

27　AWM25, 245/82, Report on Moral [sic], quarter ending 31 December 1918.

28　See, for example, AWM25, 245/65, Memo to all Officers Commanding all units of the AIF from Headquarters, Repatriation and Demobilisation Department, 4 January 1919; and AWM22, 577/4/1, Commanding Officer, Headquarters Egypt to Gilbert, 14 January 1919.

29　AWM 3DRL 2222/7, item 26, Pearce to Millen, 30 April 1919; Serle, p.406; AWM10 [4304/53/86], cutting from the *Sunday Times*, 4 May 1919. The accompanying letter describes this as the first in a series of exposés on 'Brass Hat' bungling. The anonymous 'special correspondent' is clearly hostile towards Monash which invites speculation on Bean's involvement. On this see Serle, pp.397-400.

30　AWM10 [4332/15/145], Report from McCay to Monash, 3 February 1919.

31　AWM25, 245/65, Circular Memo to all AIF units, 1919; AWM13 [7041/10/1], Repatriation and Demobilisation of the AIF, Appendix E. On the Army form and its use see Lloyd and Rees, p.119.

32　AA(ACT): A2483, item B18/3227, Completion of Form 2 on Transport Ships.

33　See Kate Blackmore, War, Health and Welfare, PhD Macquarie University 1994, pp.111-127.

34　C.B. Macpherson, *The Political Theory of Possessive Individualism, Hobbes to Locke*, OUP, Oxford 1962, p.228.

35　Jill Roe, 'Chivalry and social policy in the Antipodes', *HS*, Vol.22, No.88, 1987, p.409, refers to 'an unprecedented array of welfare services'. L. Wheeler, 'War, Women and Welfare', R. Kennedy (ed), *Australian Welfare, historical sociology*, Macmillan, South Melbourne 1989, p.174, uses identical words and also refers to a 'comparatively generous' income security scheme based on a 'new system of citizenship'; Marilyn Lake, 'The Power of Anzac', in M. McKernan and M. Browne (eds), *Australia: Two Centuries of War and Peace*, AWM with Allen & Unwin, 1988, p.222, refers to 'privileged beneficiaries'; Theda Skocpol, writing about the experience in the United States in *Protecting Soldiers and Mothers*, HUP, Cambridge 1992, p.103, refers to 'generous and honorable public aid'. In her thesis, Wheeler provides a superficial and uncritical reading of Millen's and Gilbert's 'success' with finding employment (p.215). Garton's more recent populist history, *Cost of War*, describes a 'welfare apartheid' (p.85), 'generous benefits', a 'privileged class of welfare recipients' (p.86) and a 'pursuit of dependency' (p.109).

36　AA(ACT): A2, item 1920/421, op cit. See also M. Lake, 'The Power of Anzac', pp.218-220.

37　AWM25, 245/70, Memo to all Departments from Public Service Commissioner citing Prime Minister's Department memo, 21 September 1917.

38 On the investigations of staff in the Prime Minister's office see AA(ACT): A3934, SC42 [16], Returned Soldiers miscellaneous; SC42 [13], Returned soldiers in the Prime Minister's Department.

39 For a typical sample of Hughes's response to personal appeals see AA(ACT): A2487, 19/9806; 19/9809; 20/6337.

40 AA(ACT): A2487, 19/124, Enquiry re method of sustenance payments made to discharged soldiers. Analysis of files held by Australian Archives Canberra and of New South Wales files indicates that there were hundreds of appeals to the Department by state and federal ministers and almost all those examined had a similar outcome.

41 See in particular, R. Evans, *Loyalty and Disloyalty*, Ch. 8; A. Moore, *The Secret Army and the Premier*, NSWUP, Kensington 1989, Ch. 1; Ian Turner, *Sydney's Burning*, Alpha Books, Sydney 1969. Reference to 'dinkum diggers' or an equivalent expression was not uncommon. See, for example, letter from the Public Service Commissioner to the Prime Minister's Department, AA(ACT): A664, item 437/401/43, 26 April 1919; and T. King, 'Telling the Sheep from the Goats: "Dinkum diggers" and Others, World War I', in J. Smart and T. Wood (eds), *An Anzac Muster*, Monash Publications in History, No.14, pp.86-99.

42 Lake, 'The Power of Anzac', p.204. But see also F. Cain, *The Origins of Political Surveillance in Australia*, A&R, Sydney 1983, p.39; AA(ACT): A3934, SC42 [16], Returned Soldiers miscellaneous; and *Age*, 9 January 1919.

43 Cain, p.39.

44 Phrase of J.E. Fenton, Labour member for Maribyrnong, *CPD*, Vol.91, p.1699, 30 April 1920.

45 Gibson's description of the political problems of October 1919 in AA(ACT): A1606, D11/1, Minutes of meeting between Prime Minister and Repatriation Commission, 9 October 1919.

46 Fitzhardinge, p.425; Macintyre, *Oxford*, p.191.

47 Lake, 'The Power of Anzac'; Evans, *Loyalty and Disloyalty*, p.151; Kristianson, p.14.

48 AWM27, 521.4[1], letter from Secretary Department of Defence to Acting General Secretary RSSILA, 9 December 1919; Kristianson, ibid. On Hughes's antagonism to the League and Dyett in particular see AA(ACT) references in notes 51 and 52 below.

49 AA(ACT): A461, A394/1/1, Minutes of discussion between Prime Minister and Repatriation Commissioners, 9 October 1919.

50 Fitzhardinge, p.423; AA(ACT): A1606, D11/1, Prime Minister's conferences with soldiers; A461, A394/1/1, Appointment of Repatriation Commission.

51 AA(ACT): A1606, D11/1, Minutes of meeting 16 October, p.2; Lake, 'The Power of Anzac', p.210; *ADB*, Vol.8, p.394.

52 AA(ACT): A1606, D11/1, Meeting 16 October 1919, p.3.

53 Ibid.

54 *CPD*, Vol. 94, 16 November 1920, p.6482, quoting policy speech delivered at Bendigo on 31 October 1919.

55 P.G. Macarthy, 'Wages for unskilled work, and margins for skill, Australia, 1901-21', *AEHR*, Vol.12, No.2, September 1972, p.142.

56 Ibid, p.144.

57 CPP, 1920, Vol.4, *Report of the Royal Commission on the Basic Wage*, 23 November 1920, pp.581 and 586.

58 AA(ACT): A1606, Minutes of meeting 9 October, p.6; Minutes of meeting 16 October, p.10.

59 AA(ACT): A2487, 21/372, Amendments to the Australian Soldiers' Repatriation Act 1917-1918. Hughes had been forwarded a precis of the effects of the increase on 20 October which clearly indicated that the matter needed further investigation before being approved by Treasury.

60 Ibid.

61 Sawer, p.185.

62 AA(ACT): A2487, 21/372, Draft First Schedule submitted to Cabinet 20 February 1920.

63   *Report of the Independent enquiry into the Repatriation System*, Justice P.B. Toose, AGPS, Canberra 1975, (hereafter Toose) pp.276-8; A.P. Skerman, *Repatriation in Australia*, p.68. Wheeler, 'War, Women and Warfare', p.183, is incorrect in this matter.

64   See Treasury précis, AA(ACT): A2487, 21/372, which refers to the maintenance of existing rates. Pryor, p.28, is incorrect.

65   *Report of the Royal Commission on the Basic Wage*, pp.572 and 579. In all instances, figures for Melbourne have been used for consistency.

66   *CPD*, Vol.91, p.657, 24 March 1920.

67   AA(ACT): A1606, D11/1, Minutes of meeting with RSSILA, 10 October 1919, p.10; A2487, 21/372, draft Second Schedule in Commission's proposals, 14 February 1920.

68   *CPD*, Vol.91, 24 March 1920, p.657.

69   AA(ACT): A2487, 21/372, ibid. The special allowance was re-introduced in an amendment to the Act in 1923.

70   AA(ACT): A2487, 21/372, Amendments to the Australian Soldiers' Repatriation Act 1917-1918.

71   Frank Anstey's comment on Gratuities in the House of Representatives in debate on the Supply Bill, 23 October 1919: *CPD*, Vol.90, p.13907.

72   Pryor, pp.160-163.

73   Pryor, p.163.

74   P. Sekules and J. Rees, *Lest We Forget: the history of the Returned Services League 1916-1986*, p.28.

75   AA(ACT): A1606, D11/1, Minutes of meeting 16 October 1919, p.11.

76   Ibid, p.13.

77   The deal came unstuck from Dyett's point of view when Hughes stole the limelight by calling a mass meeting of soldiers in Adelaide. Both sides then engaged in vilification campaigns through the press, Hughes's trump card being the release of the verbatim transcript revealing the Executive's proposals. *Age*, 13 November 1919.

78   *CPD*, Vol.90, pp.13902-13909.

79   *CPD* Vol.90, p.13903, 23 October 1919; *Daily Telegraph*, 2 November 1919.

80   *CPD* Vol.91, p.625.

81   The 'Mining King' is probably a reference to Baillieu and the Collins House group. *CPD*, Vol.91, p.867, 25 March 1920.

82   *CPD*, Vol.91, p.867. See also 1919-20 Budget speech, *CPD*, Vol.90, p.13081; and Anstey in Vol.91, p.13906, 23 October 1919.

83   See also Tudor's breakdown of the increase of revenue due to income tax during the war which, he argued, could cover the cost of the Gratuities. *CPD*, Vol.91, p.692.

84   *CPD*, Vol.91, p.624, 19 March 1920.

85   See War Gratuity Acts 1920, in particular Sections 1-6.

86   *CPD*, Vol.91, pp.1001-1006, 31 March 1920.

87   *CPD*, Vol.90, p.13904, 23 October 1919.

88   AA(ACT): A2421, G181, Part 1, War Gratuity.

89   Ibid, letter from DC Bell to Gilbert, 11 February 1920.

90   See Millen's submission to Cabinet, ibid, 1 March 1920; Gilbert to all DCs, 19 April 1920; War Gratuity Act, 1920, Section 7.

91   Ibid, annotation by Elvins to letter from Tilney to Gilbert, 20 April 1920.

92   Ibid, letter Ryan to Secretary of Repatriation Commission, 15 October 1920.

93   AA(ACT): A2421, G181, Part 2, letter Secretary of Treasury to Semmens, 23 June 1921, with handwritten annotation by Elvins.

94   AA(ACT): A2487, 19/6480, RSL submission.

95   AA(ACT): A1606, D11/1, Minutes of meeting between Prime Minister and Repatriation Commission, 9 October 1919.

96 On the introduction of a quorum of three see AA(ACT): A2483, B18/1561, Reduction of Quorum, April 1918. See *Repatriation Commission, Minutes of Meetings*, for example July 1919. For Gibson acting alone see, for example, 15 July 1919.

97 *Repatriation Commission, Minutes of Meetings*, Meeting of 11 March 1920.

98 According to Turner, over 8 million 'man-days' were lost in industrial disputes in 1919-1920: *In Union is Strength*, 3rd edition, Nelson, Melbourne 1983, p.70.

99 *CPD*, Vol.92, p.2010; AA(ACT): A1606, D11/1, Minutes of meeting with League, 9 October 1919.

100 AA(ACT): A1606, D11/1, cable Millen to Hughes, 18 October 1919.

101 *CPD*, Vol.91, p.658, 24 March 1920.

102 *CPD*, Vol.91, p.809, 25 March 1920.

103 For the repeated reference to the notion of 'suitable men' see the debates on the Bill during March, April and May 1920.

104 *CPD*, Vol.91, p.811, 25 March 1920.

105 *Age*, 14 April 1920.

106 *CPD*, Vol.91, p.1309, 16 April 1920.

107 *Repatriation*, 26 June 1920, p.9.

108 Moorehead was offered the consolation of Chairmanship of the new Victorian State Board.

109 AWM43, A51, J.E. Barrett; *Repatriation*, 26 June 1920, pp.8-9.

110 *Who's Who*; *Repatriation*, 26 June 1920, p.9; AWM43, A863, A. Teece; *Mufti*, 1 February 1939, p.7.

111 *Who's Who*; *ADB*, Vol.8, pp.646-48; Coulthard-Clark, *The Citizen General Staff*, pp.70-71.

112 *ADB*, Vol.12, pp.190-191; *Who's Who*; *Reveille*, December 1935, p.57.

113 F. Legg, *The Gordon Bennett Story*, Angus & Robertson, Sydney 1965, p.144.

Chapter 7

1   Andrew Ure, *The Philosophy of Manufactures or an Exposition of the Scientific, Moral, and Commercial Economy of the Factory System of Great Britain*, Knight 1835, republished Cass 1967, quoted in Bob Young, 'Science *is* social relations', *Radical Science Journal*, Vol.5, 1977, p.78.

2   E.P. Thompson describes the activity of Doctor John Kay, in concert with Edwin Chadwick, as 'perhaps the most sustained attempt to impose an ideological dogma, in defiance of the evidence of human need, in English history': *The Making of the English Working Class*, Penguin, Harmondsworth 1981, p.295. Paupers were also defined as '*sick* paupers' (emphasis added): Meredeth Turshen, 'The Political Ecology of disease', *Review of Radical Political Economics*, Vol.9, No.1, 1977, p.53 and passim.

3   For a survey of these developments in the history of science to 1976 see R. MacLeod, 'Changing perspectives in the social history of science' in I. Spiegel-Rosing & D. de Solla Price (eds), *Science, Technology and Society*, SAGE, London, 1977, pp.149-195; and, more specifically for medicine, see the Introduction to Peter Wright and Andrew Treacher (eds), *The Problem of Medical Knowledge*, Edinburgh University Press 1982, pp.1-22. For recent developments see the *Bulletin* and *Journal* of the *Society for the Social History of Medicine* and A.Wear (ed), *Medicine in Society, historical essays*, CUP, Cambridge 1992.

4   This section draws on the following works, in particular, that of Figlio: Karl Figlio, 'The historiography of Scientific Medicine: an invitation to the human sciences', *Comparative Studies in Society and History*, Vol.19, 1977, pp.262-286; Meredeth Turshen, op cit; Peter Wright, op cit; Bob Young, op cit; Lesley Doyal and Imogen Pennell, *The Political Economy of Health*, Pluto Press, London 1979; S. Kelman, 'The Social Nature of the definition problem in health', *International Journal of Health Services*, Vol.5, No.4, 1975, pp.625-42.

5   Figlio, op cit, p.270. Figlio speaks of polar conceptual influences: one, a mechanistic view of the body, deriving from Descartes; the other, a debate over animism, deriving from Stahl. See also T.S. Hall, *History of General Physiology*, Vol.2, University of Chicago Press, Chicago 1969.

6   Turshen, op cit, p.46; T. McKeown, 'A historical appraisal of the medical task', G. McLachlan and T. McKeown (eds), *Medical History and Medical Care*, OUP, London 1971, cited in Wright, op cit, p.96, n.24. For an enlightening and, for the purposes of this study, contemporary view see also Thorstein Veblen, 'The Place of Science in Modern Civilisation' (1906), in *idem*, B.W. Huebsch, New York 1919, pp.1-31.

7   See Figlio, op cit, pp. 272-3.

8   Claude Bernard, *An Introduction to the Study of Experimental Medicine*, first published Paris 1865, trans. H. Copley Greene, Collier Books, New York 1961. Bernard went on to say that 'Certainly a special force in living beings, not met with elsewhere, presides over their organization; but the existence of this force cannot in any way change our idea of the properties of organic matter – matter which, when once created, is endowed with fixed and determinate, physico-chemical properties' (p.231).

9   Figlio, op cit, p.277 and n.25.

10   Georges Canguilhem, *On the Normal and the Pathological*, trans C.R. Fawcett, D. Reidel Publishing Company, Holland 1978, p.151.

11   Michel Foucault, *The Birth of the Clinic*, Vintage, New York 1975.

12   On which see F. Dagognet, *Le catalogue de la vie*, Paris 1970, cited in Figlio, op cit; I. Waddington, 'The role of the hospital in the development of modern medicine: a sociological analysis', *Sociology*, Vol.7, 1973, pp.211-224.

13   On the philosophical debates over the nature of aetiology see Canguilhem, op cit.

14   There is evidence to suggest that morbidity levels did not seriously change despite a lowering of mortality rates. On this see Doyal and Pennell, op cit, pp.50-51, 55-6 and 62-6.

15   The literature pertaining to this subject is extensive and well represented in bibliographies elsewhere. See particularly Gareth Stedman Jones, *Outcast London*, OUP, Oxford 1971.

16   Workers compensation is a field that has been sorely neglected in historical research until quite recently: an astounding fact when the nexus of legal-medical-state-industry-worker interest that is at stake is considered. Some contributions to the area which grasp the significance are: Anthony Bale, 'Medicine in the industrial battle: early workers compensation', *Social Science and Medicine*, 1989, Vol.28, No.11, pp.1113-1120; P. Weindling (ed), *The Social History of Occupational Health*, Croom Helm, Beckenham 1985; Deborah A. Stone, *The Disabled State*, Temple University Press, Philadelphia 1984; P.W.J. Bartrip and S.B. Burman, *The Wounded Soldiers of Industry. Industrial Compensation Policy 1833-1897*, Clarendon Press, Oxford 1983; Karl Figlio, 'How does illness mediate social relations? Workmen's compensation and medico-legal practices, 1890-1940', in P. Wright and A. Treacher (eds), *The Problem of Medical Knowledge*, Edinburgh University Press, 1982; Janet Schmidt, 'Workers' Compensation: the articulation of class relations in law', *Insurgent Sociologist*, Vol.10, No.1, 1980, pp.46-54. For a legal examination of the background to the first British Act see David G. Hanes, *The First British Workmen's Compensation Act 1897*, Yale University Press, New Haven 1968; for a brief history of workers compensation in New South Wales see Gina Cass, 'Workers' benefit or employers' burden: a history of workers' compensation in New South Wales 1880-1926', *Industrial Relations Monograph Series*, No.8, UNSW 1983.

17   In Britain, the most important pieces of legislation were: the Trades Disputes Acts of 1906, the amendment to the Workmen's Compensation Act in 1906, various factory acts in 1907, the Old Age Pension Act 1908, the coal Miners Regulation Act 1908-11, the Labour Exchanges Act 1911 and the Coal Mines (Minimum Wage) Act 1912. In Australia, Workers Compensation Acts were passed by all state governments between 1902 and 1914. At the federal level: the Old-Age Pensions Act 1909, the Invalid Pensions Act 1910, the Maternity Allowances Act 1912 and the Arbitration Act of 1904 (and Harvester Judgement of 1907). British legislation is listed in Samuel J. Hurwitz, *State Intervention in Great Britain: A study of economic control and social response 1914-1919* (1949),

Frank Cass & Co, London 1968, p.35, n.114. For Australia, see Francis G. Castles, *The Working Class and Welfare*, Allen & Unwin, Wellington 1985; T.H. Kewley, *Australia's Welfare State*, Macmillan, Melbourne 1969.

18 On which see Chapter 5.

19 (Sir) Alfred Keogh in the General Introduction to the English edition of 'Hysteria or Pithiatism' one in the series of medical volumes based on translations of the French *Horizon* Collection, titled in English *Military Medical Manuals*, London 1918, p.v. See also the celebration of this tradition in Rupert Downes, 'What Medicine owes to War and War owes to Medicine', *MJA*, Vol.1, No.3, 1936, pp.73-80.

20 Roger Cooter, 'War and Modern Medicine', in W.F. Bynum & R. Porter (eds), *Companion Encyclopedia of the History of Medicine*, Routledge London, p.1541.

21 R. Cooter & S. Sturdy, 'Of war, medicine and modernity: introduction', in R. Cooter, M. Harrison & S. Sturdy (eds), *War, Medicine and Modernity*, Sutton, Phoenix Mill 1999, pp.6-7.

22 C.B. Macpherson, *The Life and Times of Liberal Democracy, Hobbes to Locke*, OUP, Oxford 1962, pp.74-5. Elsewhere Cooter has suggested the value of this approach: Roger Cooter, 'Essay Review: Discourses on War', *Stud Hist Phil Sci*, Vol.26, No.4, p.643.

23 M. Tyquin, *Neville Howse. Australia's First Victoria Cross* Winner, OUP, Melbourne 1999, p.105.

24 AWM32, 123, AMC Administration, Unofficial letters from Surg Gen Howse in England to Surg Gen Fetherston, Melbourne, letter 15 June 1917.

25 The citation reads: 'valuable services in connection with the war'. NAA: B2455.

26 AWM32, 123, op cit.

27 Butler, Vol.2, p.456.

28 AWM22, 461/14/2020, Downes to CO, No.14 AGH, 7 October 1916.

29 AWM25, 481/190, Instructions to Medical Officers, 2nd Australian Division, July 1917.

30 Butler, ibid, p.458, n.20.

31 Ibid, p.847.

32 On this see the masses of boarding papers held in the previously unused archive of AWM 23.

33 On this lengthy contest between Pearce and Howse, see Butler, Vol.2, pp.472-75, 842-857.

34 *ADB*, Vol.9, p.385.

35 Fetherston's report on Defence policy cited by Butler, Vol.2, p.848.

36 Butler, Vol.2, p.709.

37 Ibid, p.470.

38 Howse was then assisting in the medical organisation of repatriation: *ADB*, Vol.9, p.385; Butler, Vol.2, p.857.

39 AWM25, 273/2, draft report Butler to Howse, December 1919.

40 AWM25, 481/28, Butler's notes of a conversation with Howse, December 1919.

41 AWM41, 2/7.7, Report by Surgeon General Fetherston DGMS on second visit of Inspection 1918, p.50.

42 Ibid.

43 Ibid, p.51.

44 K. Blackmore, 'Law, medicine and the compensation debate', Part 1, *JOH&S A&NZ*, Vol.9, No.1, 1993 pp.59-64. Butler, Vol.3, pp.787-88.

45 See, for example, L.J. Pryor, 'Back from the Wars, the Ex-Serviceman in history', *Australian Quarterly*, June 1946, pp.43-50.

46 The principal works on the administration of post-war pensioning schemes in countries other than Australia are: D. Cohen, *The War Come Home: disabled Veterans in Britain and Germany, 1914-1939*, University of California Press, Berkeley 2001; D. Morton and G. Wright, *Winning the Second Battle: Canadian Veterans and the Return to Civilian Life 1915-1930*, University of Toronto Press, Toronto 1987; R.W. Whalen, *Bitter Wounds: German Victims of the Great War, 1914-1939*, Cornell University Press, Ithaca 1984; A. Prost, *Les Anciens Combattants et la Société Francaise*, Presses de la Foundation Nationale des Sciences politique, Paris 1977; Graham Wootton, *The Politics of*

Influence: British Ex-Servicemen, Cabinet Decisions and Cultural Change 1917-1957, London 1963. See also Robert Bodenger, 'Soldiers' Bonuses: a history of veterans' benefits in the United States, 1776-1967', PhD Dissertation, Pennsylvania State University, 1971. Of these, Whalen and Prost stand out. For accounts of the Australian experience see a populist version in S. Garton, *The Cost of War: Australians Return*, OUP, Melbourne 1996; or a semi-official (commissioned) administrative history of the Repatriation Department in C. Lloyd and J. Rees, *The Last Shilling: a history of repatriation in Australia*, MUP, Carlton 1994.

47   Army Form D1, *Medical History*, p.l.
48   Army Form B178, *Medical History*, Table II, 1917.
49   Army Form D2 (Revised 1.11.1915), *Detailed Medical History of an Invalid*, p.1.
50   Butler, Vol.3, pp.631-2.
51   AWM25, 273/11, DGAMS to GO Commanding-in-Chief, 20 November 1915.
52   *ADB*, Vol.10, p.45; Butler, Vol.3, pp.632-3.
53   AWM27, 370.5[67], Maudsley's reports to Howse 1918 and 1919.
54   Roger Smith, 'Expertise, procedure and the possibility of a comparative history of forensic psychiatry in the nineteenth century', *Psychological Medicine*, Vol.19, 1989, p.291.
55   Smith, ibid, p.296; *ADB*, ibid.
56   On this issue see chapters 8 and 9. Garton, in *Medicine and Madness*, UNSW Press, Kensington 1988, is one of very few Australian historians to examine mental health or illness, but treats the knowledge content of the diagnosis 'neurosis' as unproblematic (see his Chapter 4 and pp.75-6 in particular). On contemporary medical understanding and classification of malingering see R.J. Collie, *Malingering and Feigned Sickness*, Edward Arnold, London 1913 and A. Bassett Jones and L. Llewellyn, *Malingering or the Simulation of Disease*, William Heinemann, London 1917, both works, according to Figlio, ('The Historiography of Scientific Medicine', p.282, n.36), appearing as a direct result of the 1911 British Workmen's Compensation Act.
57   Butler, Vol.3, p.633.
58   AWM 2DRL/0701, Series 1, Wallet 1 of 2, Diary entries.
59   On the problem of lice generally, see Butler, Vol.2, p.32. On the nature and length of leave from the front and the nature of 'recuperation' see, for example, pp.137, 155 and 613.
60   Butler, Vol.2, pp.573-79.
61   AWM23, [BoxAl3], Proceedings of a Medical Board, 28 December 1917. See also AWM23, 12/493/1, Proceedings of a Medical Board, Captain Carey, 30 April 1917
62   Ibid, Proceedings of Medical Board, 20 April 1918.
63   AWM23, 12/411/3, 15 April 1917; 12/411/8, 11 May 1917; 12/411/21, 31 March 1917; 12/411/18, 14 July 1917.
64   AWM25, 371/105, Report to 5th Army HQ by Wilson, 17 October 1918.
65   See AWM25, 371/105 in its entirety.
66   Ibid, Butler to General Tivey, 4 October 1932.
67   M. Foucault, *Discipline and Punish: the Birth of the Prison*, Penguin, Harmondsworth 1987, p.164.
68   AWM25, 885/2, Circular letter from DDMS XVth Corps to Divisional ADMS, 8 September 1916.
69   AWM25, 885/2, Extract from Secret HQ letter to all Armies, 14 October 1916.
70   AWM25, 885/1, Precis of paper on "Shell Shock" 21 January 1917.
71   AA(ACT): A2483, item B18/1000, Pensions Appeal Tribunal, decisions August 21 and 30 1917, p.5.
72   Ibid, p.6.
73   Ibid, p.4.
74   Pers comm., Professor Geoffrey Bolton, January 1995.
75   On aspects of the complex history of medico-legal discourse in Britain see, for example, Roger Smith, *Trial by Medicine*, Edinburgh University Press, Edinburgh 1981 and Karl Figlio, 'How does illness mediate social relations? Workmen's Compensation and Medico-legal Practices', in Wright

and Treacher (eds), ibid. On this issue in relation to workers compensation in Australia see K. Blackmore, 'Law, medicine and the compensation debate', op cit. On medical professionalisation in Australia and the power of the profession see Chapter 5.

76 The treatment in this instance was nine injections of Novarsenobillon and nine grams of mercury: AA(NSW): ST 2817, Box 1380.

77 Karl Figlio, 'Chlorosis and chronic disease in nineteenth-century Britain: the social constitution of somatic illness in a capitalist society', *Social History*, Vol.3, No.2, 1978, p.193, note 92.

78 Venereal disease attracted various penalties including return to Australia, stoppage of pay, stoppage of leave, loss of commissioned rank and incarceration in a penal camp. See Butler, Vol.3, Ch.3

79 See chapters 8 and 9.

80 'Heredity' and 'Constitution' as causative agents in disease are concepts rooted in a late nineteenth century reactionary approach to public health and to the link between social conditions and health. On 'Constitution' see Figlio, ibid, pp.187-194; on the role of hereditarian notions see E.J. Yoxen, 'Constructing Genetic Diseases', in Wright and Treacher (eds), op cit, pp.144-161; Stephen Gould, *The Mismeasure of Man*, Penguin, Harmondsworth 1984; Daniel Kevles, *In the Name of Eugenics*, Penguin, Harmondsworth 1986.

81 AWM25, 371/105, secret report on Blue Cross gassing, August 1918.

82 AA(NSW): ST 2817, Box 1165.

83 AA(NSW): ST 2817, Box 1378.

84 Ibid.

85 On this see the Preface.

86 Lorraine Wheeler, 'War, Women and Welfare', in R. Kennedy (ed), *Australian Welfare: historical sociology*, Macmillan, South Melbourne 1989, p.183.

87 See for example, Wheeler, op cit; and Jill Roe, 'Chivalry and Social Policy in the Antipodes', *Historical Studies*, Vol.22, 1987, pp.395-410.

88 Peter Bartrip, 'The rise and decline of workmen's compensation' in P. Weindling (ed), *The Social History of Occupational Health*, p.163.

89 Garton, *The Cost of War*, pp.85 and 86.

Chapter 8

1 The 'clinical toss-up' is Butler's description of medical assessment for certain disabilities while the 'national purse' is a recurring theme. See his notes on war pensions for draft chapter 16 of Volume 3, AWM27, 521.4[4], part 1.

2 E. Farquhar Buzzard (ed), *Military Medical Manuals*, pp.227-29.

3 Butler is only critical of the poor treatment of doctors in the process. Other accounts are in Gilbert, pp.251-56, and in Lloyd and Rees, Chapter 7, which is largely based on Butler.

4 On Treasury attitude, see Commonwealth Treasury, War Pensions, *Rulings. Opinions and Precedents*, Vols.1 and 2, 1915-1920.

5 AA(ACT): A2487, 19/1336, Minute Paper, Cuscaden to Gilbert, 3 October 1918.

6 AA(ACT): A2483, B18/2429, Lockyer to all Deputy Comptrollers, 11 April 1918.

7 Ibid, Minute Paper, Lockyer to Millen, 18 April 1918.

8 AA(ACT): A2487, 20/6803, letter DC Barrett to Gilbert, 4 January 1919.

9 AA(ACT): A2487, 19/1336, Cameron to DC Brisbane, 8 January 1919.

10 Pryor, pp.129-131; Skerman, p.17.

11 On Departmental salaries see AA(ACT): A3048, [staff cards]. On doctors' salaries see Gillespie, Chapter 1 and p.59; Pensabene passim.

12 On Agnew's relationship with the SMO Sydney, Vivian Benjafield, see AA(ACT): A2483, B18/6918, Re medical Work Sydney, in particular Minute Paper, Agnew to Gilbert, 15 November 1918 and annotation by Gilbert, 18 November 1918. On Agnew's attitude to payment of LMOs as being similar to that of the specialists, see AA(ACT): A2487, 19/1336, Minute Paper, Agnew to

Gilbert, 18 September 1918; AA(NSW): SP948, G509, Part 7, letter Honorary Secretary of BMA to DC Sydney, 6 September 1918; AA(ACT): A2487, 19/2682, letter DC Sydney to Gilbert, 13 September 1918. On specialists' attitudes to payment of LMOs see AA(ACT): A2483, B18/3360, Report Craig to Millen, July 1918, p.5. On Agnew see Chapter 5.

13 See Minutes of the MAC.

14 AA(ACT): A3048, [staff cards]; AA(NSW): SP1037, Box 1, Personal History Dossiers, Henry Hastings Willis; *Report of the Repatriation Commission for Year 1954-1955,* p 47

15 AWM41, Box 59, Butler to Courtney citing (anonymously) Willis's letter, 30 September 1942. Wheeler, 'Be in it Mate!', p.274, suggests the opposite: the MAC 'played a leading role in policy developments'.

16 AA(NSW): SP948/1, G203, letter Drs Scot Skirving and Davidson to DC Sydney, April 1921.

17 Ibid, Semmens to DC Sydney, 22 September 1921.

18 AA(ACT): A2487, 19/5063, Appointment of medical officers by Pensions Department.

19 Ibid, copy of Read's Report, March 1919.

20 Ibid, Agnew to Sinclair, 28 July 1919.

21 Ibid, Memo, Gilbert to PMO Perth, 3 November 1919.

22 Ibid.

23 AWM41, Box 61, Willis to Butler, 9 October 1942.

24 Lloyd and Rees, Ch.7.

25 The idea of this second 'war' is not new: Butler refers to another 'war' in Vol.3, p.73, and Desmond Morton uses the theme as the title of his work on the Canadian system: D. Morton and G. Wright, *Winning the Second Battle.*

26 Commonwealth Treasury, *War Pensions, Rulings. Opinions,* Vol.1 Memo from Secretary of Treasury to Secretary of Department of Defence, 10 January 1916.

27 Ibid, Memo Collins to Higgs, 4 April 1916.

28 Ibid, Collins to Deputy Commissioner, Melbourne, 13 February 1917.

29 Ibid, Opinion on 'Weakness existing prior to enlistment aggravated by military employment', 31 October 1916; AA(ACT): A2421, G249, Part 1, handwritten annotation to Memo from Repatriation DC Farr to Comptroller, 17 July 1918.

30 Commonwealth Treasury, ibid, Memo Collins to all states, 19 April 1917. Butler, Vol.3, p.792, suggests the date of establishment was 1916.

31 *ADB*, Vol.8, p.77.

32 For the tensions in this transfer see AA(ACT): A571/1, 20/44147, Transfer of staff to Repatriation.

33 Ibid. This file indicates transferral of 11 temporary staff from 'Central' branch but gives no figures for the states. Industrial problems with the Public Service Board in New South Wales are also evident.

34 Ibid, letter Gilbert to Commissioner of Pensions, 24 June 1920.

35 On Reiach, see Chapter 5.

36 The volume, complexity and inaccessability of personal medical files of soldiers who served in the war restricted research to soldiers resident in New South Wales. Thus the biographies of DMOs has been similarly restricted to those who had relationships with these soldiers. Given that New South Wales and Victoria had the largest populations, the largest number of pensioners, and the largest War Pensions administrations, it is hoped that this sample is relatively representative. Further research is desperately required to fill out this profile.

37 NAA, B2455.

38 NAA B2455; Newsletter, Australian Society of Indexers, Vol.28, No.3, October 2004; Surgical News (RACS), Vol.3, No.7, 2002 Cowlishaw Symposium, http://www.cursoins.org/surgical_news/vol3_no7/cowlishaw.html (accessed July 2005).

39 NAA, B2455, George Lawson Kerr.

40 AWM140, Parkinson, C.K.; AWM[A], Parkinson, Major C.K.

41 AWM41 [54], copy of letter Parkinson to Butler, 5 November 1935.

42 AWM41 [320], 'Note by Doctor Parkinson' with annotation by Butler.

43 No evidence for Benjafield's appointment could be uncovered, however, it is possible he was appointed by Treasury prior to Agnew's interference in the process and his appointment may have been 'Permanent' within the Public Service.

44 AA(ACT): A2487, 19/4809, letter Roth to Farr, 10 April 1919; AWM25, 273/17, extracts from Reports of PMRB 2nd MD, 1917-18; *SMH*, 4 September 1924; AWM43, A752, Roth, R.E.; AWM[A], Roth, Col. R.E.; Butler, Vol.3, p.594, n.6.

45 See Chapter 10, 'Feeding by class and by gender'.

46 AWM25, 273/17, ibid; AWM140, Benjafield, Major Vivian AAMC; AWM [A], Benjafield Major V..

47 See note 12.

48 NAA B2455; http://www.australiansatwar.gov.au/stories/ (accessed July 2005).

49 NAA B2455; AWM Honours & Awards Database; University of Sydney *Book of Remembrance*.

50 *Annual Report of the Repatriation Commission for the Year ended 30th June, 1950*, p.35. A letter from the Minister for Repatriation to Smith on his retirement commended his 'vigour' and 'ability' but that was all.

51 AWM41, 4/12.11, Smith; AWM140, Smith, Col. K.; AWM43, A812, K. Smith; AWM41, Box 59, various; *Reveille*, April 1935, p.40; AA(ACT): A2421, G408, Pt.2, biographical note on Dr Kenneth Smith.

52 AA(ACT): A2421, G408, Pt.2, retirement of Courtney in 1935.

53 *Medical Directory of Australia*, 1948, p.102; AA(ACT): A2487, 19/8185, letter Courtney to DC Melbourne, 1919; AWM140, Courtney, Lt. Col. C.A.; AWM41, 1/5.21, Dr C. A. Courtney, correspondence; AWM41, Box 59, various.

54 AWM41, Box 59, letters between Butler and Courtney. See in particular letter Courtney to Butler, 26 December 1930.

55 *Duckboard* (organ of the Melbourne branch of the RSSILA) May 1935, pp.3-5.

56 Aside from the educational qualifications and earnings of these doctors, the suburbs of Double Bay, Potts Point, Killara and parts of Stanmore were, in 1920, and still are 'exclusive' middle class Sydney suburbs similar to Toorak, East Melbourne or Malvern in Melbourne.

57 Accurate figures on medical practitioners' incomes are notoriously difficult to obtain. Neither Pensabene nor Gillespie provide specific figures but the specialists' fees demanded of the Department indicate a minimum fee of £2/2/0 per consultation in 1920.

58 AA(ACT): A2487, 22/13802, War pensions payable as compensation for death or incapacity.

59 See file AA(ACT): A1317, A5406, Pensions – cases relating to soldiers employed on home service.

60 *War Pensions Act*, 1914, Regulations, form Z, Claim for War Pension.

61 This period, when pension applications reached their peak, witnessed the most protracted press attacks and returned soldier organisations' campaigns against the pensioning process and saw the birth of the label the 'Cyanide Gang' for the Commission. Toose Report, p.222; *Royal Commission*, 1924; see also *Smith's Weekly* during 1920.

62 K. Blackmore, 'Law, medicine and the compensation debate', Pt.1, pp.59-64.

63 K. Blackmore, 'Law, medicine and the compensation debate', Pts.1 & 2. See also debate over the assessment issue in 'Letters', in two subsequent issues of the Journal; P. Mulvaney and N. Horner, 'The use and abuse of the American Medical Association Guides in Accident Compensation schemes', *Journal of Law and Medicine*, Vol.6, No.2, November 1998, pp.136-146; R. Guthrie, 'Compensation: problems with the concept of disability and the use of American Medical Association Guides', *Journal of Law and Medicine*, Vol.9, No.2, November 2001, pp.185-199; E.M. Shanahan and L.A. Leu, 'The AMA's "Guides to the Evaluation of Permanent Impairment"', *JOH&S A&NZ*, Vol.10, No.4, 1994, pp.323-332.

64 AWM27, 521.4[41], Part 1, letter Butler to Polmeer, 14 September 1937.

65   AWM41, Box 61, letter Butler to Cowen, 16 May 1940.

66   AWM27, 376.31 [10], Butler to Cowen, 16 May 1940.

67   AWM41, Box 59, letter Withers to Butler, 23 October 1931; See also AA(ACT): A2421, G33, AIF medical and other records.

68   AWM27, 521.4 [41, Part 1, draft chapter 16 for Vol.3.]

69   AA(ACT); A2421, G249, Part 1, Minute McPhee to Commission, 19 September 1918; Memorandum, to DCs all states from Comptroller, 8 November 1918.

70   Act No.58 of 1935, Division 4, Section 45W.

71   AA(ACT): A2421, G653, Semmens to D.C. Cameron, MP, 17 October 1924.

72   Ibid, Memorandum, Cornell to Minister, 18 November 1927.

73   AWM41, Box 59, Extracts from evidence given to the Royal Commission, p.6.

74   Repatriation Ruling No.105, 6 February 1920.

75   Skerman, p.28.

76   On this issue see, for example, AA(NSW): SP948/1, G509 Part 7, Medical Treatment; G200/1, Handbook Instructions to Local Medical Officers; G568, Travelling Boards. See also AA(ACT): A2487, 19/1336, After Discharge Medical Treatment Part 1; 19/2997, Local Medical Officers NSW Part 1.

77   AA(ACT): A2487, 21/6493, PDMO Agnew to Secretary of Commission, 19 April 1921.

78   Skerman, p.29.

79   Australian Soldiers' Repatriation Act, 1921, Part III, Section 23, Clause 1.

80   Skerman p.29.

Chapter 9

1   Paraphrase of Philip Adams in *The Weekend Australian*, 1991, May 11-12, p.2.

2   See Note on Sources.

3   On the latter theme see P.W.G. Wright, 'Some recent developments in the sociology of knowledge and their relevance to the sociology of medicine', *Ethics in Science and Medicine*, Vol.6, 1979, pp.93-104.

4   See Chapter 6.

5   Macintyre, *Oxford*, pp.191-97.

6   On this issue see, for example, T.S. Szasz, *The Manufacture of Madness*, Routledge & Kegan Paul, London 1973 and *The Myth of Mental Illness*, Paladin, London 1972; Roger Smith, *Trial by Medicine. Insanity and Responsibility in Victorian Trials*, Edinburgh University Press, Edinburgh 1981.

7   AA(NSW): SP948/1, G514, Medical library file; AA(ACT): A2421, G307, Parts 1 and 2, Medical library. A. Bassett Jones & L. Llewellyn, *Malingering or the simulation of disease*, William Heinemann, London 1917. See also AA(NSW): SP948/1, G188, Unmarried members affected with Lunacy; and G1022, Neurasthenia.

8   Figlio, 'The Historiography of Scientific Medicine', *Comparative Studies in Society and History*, Vol.19, 1977, p.282, n.36.

9   Jones and Llewellyn, ibid, p.v. See also Sir John Collie, *Malingering and Feigned Sickness*, Edward Arnold, London 1913.

10   Collie, ibid, p.vi.

11   Jones & Llewellyn, ibid, p.15.

12   AWM41, Box 59, annotated copy of Gibb's article 'Wounded Souls. A plea for nerve-strained victims of the war', *Overseas*, January 1927.

13   Ibid.

14   AA(NSW): ST2817, Box 2084.

15   AA(NSW): ST2817/1, Box 864.

16   AWM41, 1/5.21, letter Butler to Courtney, 25 June 1934; *ADB*, Vol.9, p.309.

17   See AWM41, 1/5.21, ibid, Interview with Sir Richard Stawell, p.6.

18   Copies of letters Butler to Hirshfeld and Hirshfeld to Butler, in ibid. See also Stawell's critique of radiography in Butler's 'Interview'.

19   Ibid, Courtney to Butler, 28 June 1934.

20   AA(NSW): ST3264/1/0, Box 5490.

21   AA(NSW): ST2817/1, Box 1895.

22   Lloyd and Rees, p.230.

23   Ibid.

24   Skerman, pp.42-3.

25   Ibid.

26   See in particular, Claus Offe, *Contradictions of the Welfare State*, MIT Press, Cambridge Massachusetts 1984, Chapter 6.

27   AA(NSW): ST2817/1, Box 888.

28   AA(NSW): ST2817/1, Box 824.

29   Report of the Royal Commission on the Basic Wage, 1923, p.44.

30   On which see Kristianson, *The Politics of Patriotism*.

Chapter 10

1   Professor Robert MacLennan, commenting on the findings of the report, *Veterans and Agent Orange Health Effects of Herbicides Used in Vietnam*, of which he was a joint author. *SMH*, 8 October 1994.

2   Vietnam Veteran, Mike Boland, reported in *SMH*, ibid.

3   Allan Watson, Vietnam Veteran suffering from leukemia, cited in *SMH*, ibid.

4   The report, *Veterans and Agent Orange, Health Effects of Herbicides Used in Vietnam*, was a review of the US National Academy of Sciences report in 1993 which found exposure to herbicide caused cancers.

5   MacLennan op cit.

6   On this see B. Smith, 'Agent Orange: whose values?', in V.A. Brown and G. Preston (eds), *Choice and Change: ethics. politics and economics of public health*, PHA, Canberra 1993, pp.25-35. Smith comments that 'a minority of veterans ... seized on the allegations as an explanation of their personal discontents, the disabilities of their children and as a likely source of additional repatriation benefits'.

7   Lloyd and Rees, p.361 and passim.

8   See for example, I.B. Campbell, 'Thresholds – fact or fiction', *JOH&S A&NZ* Vol.4, No.4, 1988, pp.319-323; B.J. Castleman and G.E. Ziem, 'Corporate influence on threshold limit values', *American Journal of Industrial Medicine*, Vol. 13, 1988, pp.531-59.

9   Lloyd and Rees, pp.368-9.

10   Ibid, pp.360-379; B. Smith, ibid.

11   Lloyd and Rees, p.360.

12   *Smith's Weekly*, 3 December 1921; 20 August 1921; 21 January 1922.

13   *SMH* 3 March 1922; see also letters in March and April 1922.

14   AA(ACT): A2487, 22/9833, letter Acting Deputy Commissioner to Secretary, 8 June 1922. In the same series, see also 21/18531, Press criticisms – *Smith's Weekly*; 21/10884, Criticism of Department by newspaper 'Smith's Weekly'.

15   See Chapter 6.

16   *Daily Guardian*, 2 September 1924. See correspondence in AA(NSW): SP948/1, G544 and AA(ACT): A458, E382/2.

17   AA(ACT): A458, E382/2, letter Bruce to the Premier [October 1924].

18   See, for example, the entire edition of *Revue D'Histoire*, No.167, July 1992, on Monuments to the dead in the First World War; Annette Becker, *La guerre et la foi. De la mort à la mémoire*

1914-1930, Armand Colin, Paris 1994; Ken Inglis, 'Men, Women and War Memorials: Anzac Australia', *Daedalus*, Vol.116, 1987, pp.48-9.

19 Lloyd and Rees, Chapter 9, 'The Silent Cities'.

20 In New South Wales alone there were 944 official war-related deaths between July 1927 and June 1932: AA(NSW): SP948/1, G1194, Memorandum DC Sydney to Secretary Commission, 26 September 1932.

21 Ibid, Semmens to DC Sydney, May 1928.

22 Ibid, various.

23 See, for example, the Royal Commission on National Insurance (1923 and 1924 and 1925) (1925 and 1927); Royal Commission on Finances of Western Australia, as affected by Federation (1924) (1925); Royal Commission on Health (1925) (1926); Royal Commission on Moving Picture Industry in Australia (1927) (1929); Royal Commission on the Constitution (1927) (1929); Royal Commission on Child Endowment or Family Allowance (1927) (1929); and Macintyre, *Oxford History*, p.226 and n.10.

24 *Medical Journal of Australia*, 30 May 1925, pp.569-70; *Government Gazette*, No.65, 18 September 1924, p.1792. On Blackburn, see *ADB*, Vol.7, pp.308-319.

25 *ADB*, Vol.11, p.118.

26 AA(ACT): A460/1, A5/17, confidential letter Semmens to Page, 30 June 1924; and hostile letter Semmens to Secretary Prime Minister's Department, 19 August 1924.

27 *CPD*, Vol.107, pp.1889-1890, 3 July 1924 and p.2593, 30 July 1924.

28 AA(ACT): A460/1, A5/17, ibid.

29 Ibid. For each member, the four guineas *per day* represented exactly twice the *weekly* war pension paid to a totally incapacitated soldier.

30 See published Commission Report for full details.

31 AWM41, Box 59, letter Withers to Butler, 23 October 1931. [The evidence of the Royal Commission was not published in parliamentary papers. This source represents the only sample of evidence found.]

32 AA(ACT): A460/1, D5/17, Royal Commission – Report. *ADB*, Vol.9, pp.384-6.

33 Skerman, pp.41-48; Lloyd and Rees, p.234, following Skerman.

34 AA(NSW): SP948/1, G873 (Box 315), Circular Letter 459, March 1923.

35 Ibid.

36 For this entire saga see AA(NSW): SP948/1, G1315, (Box 315), Registrar General's Department – check of Marriageable Females 1923-1952.

37 Ibid.

38 Ibid, Memo DC NSW to Secretary, 28 April 1927.

39 Lloyd and Rees, p.379.

40 Pryor, pp.132-3.

41 AA(NSW): SP948/1, G545, Memo Semmens to DC Sydney, 25 March 1926.

42 Ibid, letter DC NSW to Superintendent Red Cross, contained in Memo DC to Semmens, 11 May 1926.

43 Ibid, Minute Paper by SMO Smith, 5 April 1927.

44 Ibid, Barrett to Superintendent, 6 April 1927.

45 On the semantic and medical difference between drunkenness and alcoholism see Bertrand Taithe, *Defeated flesh: welfare, warfare and the making of modern France*, Manchester University Press, Manchester 1999, Ch.7 and passim.

46 AA(NSW): ST817, Box 1115.

47 AA(ACT): CRS13713, Box A, 372, 331, 365, 318.

48 Ibid, letter Blackburn to DC NSW, 28 May 1932.

49 Ibid, Courtney's report of 15 March 1932.

50 AA(ACT): A571/1, 20/27781, statistics on all pensions for year ending June 1919; *Report of the Royal Commission on the Basic Wage*, 23 November 1920, p.90.

51 Ibid; A2491/1, W3838, War Pensions, Statement for the Twelve Months ended June 1920.
52 AA(NSW): SP948/1, G986, 'Table of Rates of Pensions', 1 August 1925.
53 See Chapter 8.
54 AA(NSW): SP948/1, G697, Rutledge to DC NSW, 13 February 1929.
55 Ibid, Memo DC to Secretary, 2 April 1929.
56 Ibid, Semmens to DC NSW, 18 May 1929.
57 Ibid, Semmens to DC NSW, 13 June 1920.
58 Ibid.
59 See Chapter 2.
60 AA(ACT): A2487, 21/9070, Memo DC Farr to Semmens 7 June 1921.
61 Ibid.
62 Robin Gollan, *The Coalminers of New South Wales. A History of the Union 1860-1960*, MUP in association with ANU, Parkville 1963, p.157.
63 Ibid, pp.174-5.
64 Ibid, see annotations to original Memorandum and letter Semmens to Farr, 16 June 1921.
65 Lloyd and Rees, Chapters 12 and 13.
66 AA(ACT): A2421, T1, G277 Part 1, letter Semmens to Scullin, 11 December 1931 in response to Scullin's of 28 October 1931.
67 Ibid, Memorandum Courtney to Secretary of Commission, 2 December 1931.
68 Ibid, letter to Scullin.
69 Skerman, p.63.
70 Ibid, pp.63-71.

Appendix 1

Fortnightly differential rates (£/s/d) of war pensions paid 1920 for 100% incapacity (including wives' pension rates) relative to widows' pension rates and daily AIF rates of pay *

AIF rates of pay per day	Widows' pension	Soldiers' pension	Wives' pension
6/0	£2/7/0	£4/4/0	£1/16/0
7/0	£2/7/0	£4/4/0	£1/16/0
9/0	£2/9/0	£4/4/0	£1/16/0
10/0	£2/12/3	£4/4/0	£1/16/0
10/6	£2/13/9	£4/4/0	£1/16/0
11/6	£2/16/0	£4/4/0	£1/16/0
12/0	£2/17/0	£4/4/0	£1/16/0
13/0	£2/19/6	£4/4/0	£1/16/0
17/6	£3/10/0	£4/4/0	£2/0/0
	£3/17/6	£4/5/0	£2/2/6
	£4/9/0	£4/15/0	£2/7/6
	£5/0/9	£5/0/0	£2/12/6
	£5/12/3	£5/15/0	£2/17/6
	£6/0/0	£6/0/0	£3/0/0

* 'General Pensions Rates', First Schedule, *Australian Soldiers' Repatriation Act* 1920

Appendix 2

Categories of invalids used by the AAMC in 1918 *

A	Fit for general service.
A3	Physically fit, but in need of hardening.
B1a1 4	Temporarily unfit for general service for less than six months, but fit for training. The degree of fitness for training varies and is least in "B1a1" As a rule men in these categories should be fit in at most two or three months.
B1b	Temporarily unfit for general service for less than six months; temporarily unfit for training.
B2a	Temporarily unfit for general service for more than six months; fit for home service.
B2b	Temporarily unfit for general service for more than six months; temporarily unfit for home service.
C1	Permanently unfit for general service; fit for home service.
C1 Aust.	Permanently unfit for general service; fit for home service in Australia. (This classification was adopted in October, 1917, but discarded early in 1918)
C2	Permanently unfit for general service; temporarily unfit for home service.
C3	Permanently unfit for general service permanently unfit for home service.

* Butler, Vol.2, p.458 and n.20, quoting 'Medical work in a Command Depot', Lt Col H. H. Woollard. Comments in parentheses are those of Woollard.

Bibliography

OFFICIAL MATERIAL, UNPUBLISHED

Australian War Memorial Series

AWM [A]	Index Cards and Biographical Index Cards ['Subject Classification']
AWM	Files of Research
AWM 4	AIF unit war diaries, 1914-1918 War
AWM 10	Australian Imperial Force Administrative Headquarters registry, 'A' (Adjutant-General's Branch) files
AWM 11	Australian Imperial Force Administrative Headquarters registry, 'A' (Adjutant-General's Branch) medical (subject) files
AWM 13	Australian Imperial Force Administrative Headquarters registry, 'Q' (Quartermaster-General's Branch) files
AWM 19	Australian Imperial Force Depots in the United Kingdom, Assistant Director of Education files, 1914-1918 War
AWM 22	Australian Imperial Force Headquarters (Egypt), Central registry files
AWM 23	Australian Records Section, General Headquarters 3rd Echelon and British Expeditionary Force (France) files
AWM 24	Anzac Section, General Headquarters 3rd Echelon and British Expeditionary Force (France) index cards
AWM 25	Written records, 1914-1918 War
AWM 27	Records arranged according to AWM Library subject classification [Series of files and miscellaneous official papers from former donated records (DRL) accessions and other series.]
AWM 32	Australian Army Medical Corps files (Tait files)
AWM 38	Official History, 1914-18 War: Records of C.E.W. Bean, Official Historian
AWM 41	Official History, 1914-18 War: Records of A.G. Butler, Historian of Australian Army Medical Services
AWM 43	Official History, 1914-18 War, biographical and other research files
AWM 54	Written records, 1939-45 War
AWM 93	AWM Registry Files, first series
AWM183	Australian War Records Section biographical forms

2DRL 701	Lieutenant Colonel J.W. Springthorpe, reports and correspondence on AAMC in Egypt and England. 1914-1922
2DRL 2351	Major General Sir Neville Reginald Howse
3DRL 251	Major General R.H. Fetherston, reports and administrative papers concerned with his duties as DGMS. 1914-1919
3DRL 2222	G.F. Pearce, Department of Defence papers covering a wide range of military subjects. 1914-1918
3DRL 2574	R.M. Ferguson (later Lord Novar), correspondence as Governor General with the King and General Birdwood. 1914-1920
3DRL 3216	General J. Monash, operations orders and reports from Gallipoli and France. 1915-1919
PR83/201	Agnew, James F. (Captain, AAMC)
PR83/202	Letters of Pte James Agnew, 12th Field Ambulance, AIF
AWM	Films

Australian Archives ACT and NSW series

ACT

AA 1970/559/1	Folders of papers maintained by S.M. Bruce while Australian Minister in London, c1923-c1945
A2	Prime Minister's Department, Correspondence files, annual single number series, c1904-c1920
A457	Prime Minister's Department, Correspondence files, multiple number series, first system, c1900-c1928
A458	Prime Minister's Department, Correspondence files, multiple number series, second system, c1923-c1934
A460	Prime Minister's Department, Correspondence files, Class 5 (Royal Commissions), c1921-c1950
A571	Department of the Treasury [I], Central Office, Correspondence files, annual single number series, c1901-December 1976
A664	Department of Defence [II] (Central Administration), Correspondence files, multiple number series (Class 401), c1912-c1942
A1317	Pensions and Maternity Allowances Office Central, Correspondence files, single number series with alphabetical prefixes, 1913-c1947
A1492	The Rt Hon Viscount Stanley Melbourne Bruce, Correspondence with Rt Hon W.M. Hughes, MP (Prime Minister), c1921-c1923

A1606	Prime Minister's Department, Correspondence files, two-number system with letter prefix, secret and confidential series (Third system), c1926-c1939
A2188	Department of the Treasury [I] and Pensions and Maternity Allowances Office Central, Invalid and Old-Age Pensions – Volumes of Rulings, Opinions, Instructions and Precedents, c1909-c1944
A2189	Department of the Treasury [I] and Pensions and Maternity Allowances Office Central, Invalid and Old-Age Pensions – Index to Volumes of Rulings, Opinions Instructions and Precedents, c1909-c1944
A2421	Repatriation Department [I], correspondence files, 'G' single number series, c1918-c1974
A2479	Repatriation Department [I], correspondence files, annual single number series, 1917-1918
A2481	Repatriation Department [I], correspondence files, 'A' series, 1918-1919
A2483	Repatriation Department [I], correspondence files, 'B' series, 1917-1919
A2487	Repatriation Department [I], correspondence files, annual single number series, 1919-1929
A2489	Repatriation Department [I], correspondence files, 'Red' Series, 1920
A2491	Repatriation Department [I], correspondence files, single number series with 'W' prefix (Australian War Pensions), 1919-1921
A2497	Repatriation Department [I], series title: Subject Index Cards and Booklets for correspondence files A2479, A2481, A248A2487, A2421
A2835	Repatriation Department [I], correspondence files (Staff), 'S' single number series
A3047	Repatriation Department [I], Staff position cards for Repatriation medical institutions, all Mainland States, with reference to 'S' (Staff) single number series
A3048	Repatriation Department [I], Staff position cards by section for headquarters and all states, with references to 'S' (Staff) single number series, 1919-1951
A3934	Prime Minister's Department, Correspondence files, SC secret and confidential series, (old files), c1906-c1931
A6006	Folders of copies of Cabinet papers, 1901
A7342	Repatriation Department [I], Photographs illustrating the history and functions of the Repatriation commission and the Repatriation Department since the end of the First World War, 1920-
B2455	1st AIF Personal Dossiers, 1914-1920
M104	The Rt Hon Viscount Stanley Melbourne Bruce, Folders of annual Correspondence, c1926-c1964

MP68/2	Australian Soldiers' Repatriation Fund and Repatriation Department, General Correspondence of the Australian Soldiers' Repatriation Fund, 1917-1918
MP68/3	Repatriation Department [I], General Correspondence ('A' Series), 1918-1919

NSW

SP948	Deputy Commissioner for Repatriation, NSW, Correspondence – Policy and General (G Files - Old Series), c1921-c1968
SP998	Australian Soldiers' Repatriation Fund and Deputy Comptroller of Repatriation, NSW, and Deputy Commissioner for Repatriation, NSW, Staff establishment registers, 1916-c1960
SP1037	Deputy Commissioner for Repatriation, NSW, Personal History Dossiers, 1914
SP1370	Deputy Commissioner for Repatriation, NSW, Personal Case Files for High Ranked and/or Decorated Veterans of World War I, World War II, the Korean-Malayan War, and the Vietnam War, c1914-c1972
SP1599	Deputy Comptroller and Deputy Commissioner for Repatriation, NSW, Personal case files, parts 'R' and 'H', Australian 1914-1918 War (Deceased) 1955-1978
SP1735	Deputy Comptroller and Deputy Commissioner for Repatriation, NSW, Personal case files, parts 'M' South African, 1914-1918 War (Deceased)
ST2817	Deputy Comptroller and Deputy Commissioner for Repatriation, NSW, Personal Dossiers, Medical Histories and Pensions (Pension Files) 'R', 'M', 'C' & 'H' Groups relating to Deceased ex-Servicemen of 1914-1918 War, c1914-c1964
ST3153	Deputy Comptroller and Deputy Commissioner for Repatriation, NSW, Personal Dossiers, Medical Histories and Pensions (Pension Files) 'R', 'M', 'C' & 'H' Groups relating to Deceased ex-Servicemen of 1914-1918 War, c1914-c1964
ST3264	Deputy Comptroller and Deputy Commissioner for Repatriation, NSW, Personal Dossiers, Medical Histories and Pensions (Pension Files) 'R', 'M', 'C' & 'H' Groups relating to Deceased ex-Servicemen of 1914-1918 War, c1914-c1964
ST3284	Deputy Comptroller and Deputy Commissioner for Repatriation, NSW, Personal Dossiers, Medical Histories and Pensions (Pension Files) 'R', 'M', 'C' & 'H' Groups relating to Deceased ex-Servicemen of 1914-1918 War, c1914-c1964

ST3452   Deputy Comptroller and Deputy Commissioner for Repatriation, NSW, Personal Dossiers, Medical Histories and Pensions (Pension Files) 'R', 'M', 'C' & 'H' Groups relating to Deceased ex-Servicemen of 1914-1918 War, c1914-c1918

ST3584   Deputy Comptroller and Deputy Commissioner for Repatriation and Department of Veterans' Affairs, Branch Office, NSW, Personal Dossiers, Medical Histories and Pensions (Pension Files) relating to deceased Ex-Servicemen for [all wars], c1918

OFFICIAL MATERIAL, PUBLISHED

Australian Soldiers' Repatriation Fund, *Report of the Board of Trustees*, Government Printer, Melbourne, 1918

Commonwealth Treasury, *Invalid & Old Age Pensions Act - Rulings and Opinions*, Vols. 1-3, 1911-1930

Commonwealth Treasury, *War Pensions. Rulings. Opinions and Precedents*, Vols. 1 and 2, 1915-1926

Commonwealth of Australia Parliamentary Papers 1910-30

Commonwealth of Australia Parliamentary Debates 1910-1930

Department of Repatriation, *Repatriation*, 1919-1920

Department of Repatriation, *The Australian Repatriation System*, Canberra, 1975

Government Gazette

Independent Enquiry into the Repatriation System (Justice P.B. Toose), *Report*, AGPS, Canberra, 1975

Repatriation Commission, Medical Advisory Committee, *Minutes of Meetings*, Vol.1, 1919-1926

Repatriation Commission [1], *Minutes of Meetings*, 1918-1920

Repatriation Commission [2], *Minutes of Meetings*, 1920-1930

Royal Commission on the Assessment of War Service Disabilities, *Report*, Government Printer, 1924

Royal Commission on the Basic Wage, *Report*, Government Printer, 1920

War Pensions Entitlement Appeal Tribunal, *Report*, Government Printer, 1929

Commonwealth Acts and Regulations

Australian Soldiers' Repatriation Act 1920

Australian Soldiers' Repatriation Act 1917

Australian Soldiers' Repatriation Regulations 1918

Financial Emergency Acts 1931

Invalid and Old-age Pensions Act 1908-1935

Pensions Regulations 1911-1914

Seamen's Compensation Act 1909

War Gratuity Acts 1920

War Pensions Act 1914

War Pensions Regulations 1915

New South Wales

Anatomy Act 1901

Child Welfare Act 1923

Coroners Act 1898

Friendly Societies Act 1912-1935

Inebriates Act 1900-1912

Invalidity and Accidents Pensions Act 1907

Lunacy Act 1898

Medical Practitioners Act 1898-1912

Noxious Microbes Act 1900

Old-age Pensions Act 1900

Prince Alfred Hospital Act 1902

Public Health Act 1902-1937

Quarantine Act 1897

Registration of Births, Deaths and Marriages Act 1899-1934

Superannuation Act 1916-1935

Venereal Diseases Act 1918

Workmen's Compensation Act 1910-1926

Workmen's Compensation Act Regulations 1910

Victoria

Old-age Pensions Act 1901

Western Australia

Workers' Compensation Act 1902-1912

Tasmania

Workers' Compensation Act 1910

New Zealand

Workers Compensation Act 1908

United Kingdom

Workmen's Compensation Act 1897

NEWSPAPERS AND PERIODICALS

Age

Daily Telegraph

Daily Guardian

Duckboard

Kia Ora Coo-ee News

Listening Post

Mufti

Overseas

Queensland Digger

Reveille

Smith's Weekly

Stand-To

Sunday Times

Sydney Morning Herald

OTHER SOURCES

Australian Dictionary of Biography.

Bacchi, C.L., 'The nature-nurture debate in Australia, 1900-1914', *HS*, Vol.19, No.75, October 1980, pp.199-212.

Balali-Mood, M. Hefazi, M., 'The pharmacology, toxicology, and medical treatment of sulphur mustard poisoning', *Fundamental & Clinical Pharmacology*, Vol.19, 2005, pp.297-315.

Bale, A., 'Medicine in the industrial battle: early workers' compensation', *Social Science and Medicine*, 1989, Vol.28, No.11, pp.1113-1120.

Bale, A., 'The American compensation phenomenon', *IJHS*, Vol.20, No.2, 1990, pp.253-275.

Barnes, B., *Scientific Knowledge and Sociological Theory*, Routledge & Kegan Paul, London 1974.

Barrett, J., *Falling In*, Hale & Iremonger, Sydney 1979.

Barrett, J.W., *The Twin Ideals: an educated Commonwealth*, Vol.1, H.K. Lewis & Co, London 1918.

Bartrip P.W.J. and Burman, S.B., *The Wounded Soldiers of Industry. Industrial Compensation Policy 1833-1897*, Clarendon Press, Oxford 1983.

Bartrip, P., 'The rise and decline of workmen's compensation' in P. Weindling (ed), *The Social History of Occupational Health*, Croom Helm, Beckenham 1985, pp.157-79.

Baruch, G. and Treacher, A., *Psychiatry Observed*, Routledge & Kegan Paul, London 1978.

Bassett, J., *Guns and Brooches: Australian Army Nursing from the Boer War to the Gulf War*, OUP, Melbourne 1992.

Bassett Jones A. and Llewellyn, L., *Malingering, or, the Simulation of Disease*, William Heinemann, London 1917.

Becker, A., *La Geurre et la Foi. De la Mort à la Mémoire 1914-1930*, Armand Colin, Paris 1994.

Beilharz, P. Considine, M. and Watts, R., *Arguing about the Welfare State*, Allen & Unwin, North Sydney 1992.

Below, C., *The Vedgymight History of Australia*, 2nd ed., Hudson, Hawthorn 1984.

Bendix, R., *Max Weber. An Intellectual Portrait*, Methuen, London 1966.

Bennett, L., 'The Federal Conciliation and Arbitration Court in the late 1920s', *LH*, Vol.57, November 1989, pp.44-60.

Berger, P. and Luckman T., *The Social Construction of Reality*, Penguin, Harmondsworth 1984.

Berghahn, V.R., *Militarism: the History of an International Debate 1861-1979*, CUP, Cambridge 1981.

Berkowitz, E.D. and McQuaid, K., 'Bureaucrats as "Social Engineers": federal welfare programs in Herbert Hoover's America', *American Journal of Economics and Sociology*, Vol.39, No.4, 1980, pp.321-335.

Bernard, C., *An Introduction to the Study of Experimental Medicine*, first published Paris 1865, trans. H. Copley Greene, Collier Books, New York 1961.

Berreen, R. and Wearing, M., 'The network of surveillance: the power of official inquiries into poor relief provision in New South Wales, 1898 and 1984' in R. Kennedy (ed), *Australian Welfare: Historical Sociology*, Macmillan, South Melbourne 1989, pp.74-101.

Berridge, V., 'Review Article. Health, Medicine and Social Policy: the Rise of the Longer Twentieth Century', *Journal of Contemporary History*, Vol.35, No. 4, 2000, pp.667-77.

Blackmore, K., 'Aspects of the Australian repatriation process: war, health and responsibility for illness', in J. Smart and T. Wood (eds) *An ANZAC Muster: War and Society in Australia and New Zealand 1914-18 and 1939-45*, Monash Publications in History, No.14, Monash University, Clayton 1992, pp.100-113.

Blackmore, K., 'Law, medicine and the compensation debate', Pt.1, *JOH&S A&NZ*, Vol.9, No.1, 1993, pp.59-64.

Blackmore, K., 'Law, medicine and the compensation debate', Pt.2, *JOH&S A&NZ*, Vol.9, No.2, 1993, pp.147-152.

Blackmore, K., 'Making health policy in Australia: the case of Invalid Pensions', in V.A. Brown and G. Preston (eds), *Choice and Change: ethics. politics and economics of Public Health*, Public Health Association, Canberra 1993, pp.82-87.

Blackmore, K., 'War Health and Welfare: the Great War and its aftermath', PhD thesis, Macquarie University 1994.

Blair, A. Kazerouni, N., 'Reactive chemicals and cancer', *Cancer Causes and Control*, Vol.8, 1997, pp.473-90.

Bodenger, R., 'Soldiers' Bonuses: a history of veterans' benefits in the United States, 1776-1967', PhD Dissertation, Pennsylvania State University 1971.

Borak, J., 'Phosgene exposure: mechanisms of injury and treatment strategies', *Journal of Occupational and Emergency Medicine*, Vol.43, No.2, February 2001.

Bourke, J., *Dismembering the Male: Men's Bodies, Britain and the Great War*, Reaktion Books, London 1996.

Bourke, J., 'The Battle of the Limbs: Amputation, Artificial Limbs and the Great War in Australia', *Australian Historical Studies*, Vol. 110, 1998, pp.49-67.

Bourke, J., 'Effeminacy, Ethnicity and the End of Trauma: the Sufferings of "Shell-shocked" Men in Great Britain and Ireland, 1914-1939', *Journal of Contemporary History*, Vol. 35, No. 1, 2000, pp.57-69.

Braga, S., *ANZAC Doctor: the life of Sir Neville Howse, VC*, Hale & Iremonger, Alexandria 2000.

Breitkopf, C. et al, 'Impact of a molecular approach to improve the microbiological diagnosis of infective heart valve endocarditis', *Circulation*, Vol.111, 2005, pp.1415-1421.

Breul F.R. and Diner, S.J. (eds), *Compassion and Responsibility: Readings in the History of Social Welfare Policy in the United States*, University of Chicago Press, Chicago 1980.

Brooks, A., 'The concepts of "injury" and "disease" in workers' compensation law – a re-examination in the light of recent reforms', *UNSW Law Journal*, Vol.10, No.2, 1987, pp.38-66.

Brumwell, S., 'Home from the wars', *History Today*, Vol. 52, No.1, 1997, pp.53-72.

Buckley, S. and Dickin, J., 'Venereal disease and public reform in Canada', *Can Hist Rev*, Vol.63, No.3, 1982, pp.337-354.

Burgmann, V., 'The Iron Heel: the suppression of the IWW during World War I' in Sydney Labour History Group, *What Rough Beast?*, George Allen & Unwin, Sydney 1982, pp.171-191.

Burnham, J.C., 'How the idea of profession changed the writing of medical history', *Medical History*, Supplement No.18, Wellcome Institute for the History of Medicine, London 1998.

Burry, H. C., 'Accident compensation: gates and gatekeepers', *MJA*, Vol.152, May 1990, pp.450-451.

Butler, A.G., *Official History of the Australian Army Medical Services. 1914-1918*, Vols. 1-3, AWM, Canberra 1940.

Caiden, R.N., *Career Service*, MUP, Carlton 1965.

Cain, F., *The Origins of Political Surveillance in Australia*, A&R, Sydney 1983.

Campbell, C., 'Liberalism in Australian History: 1880-1920', in J. Roe (ed), *Social Policy in Australia*, Cassell, Stanmore 1976.

Campbell, E.W., *The 60 rich families who own Australia*, Current Books, Sydney 1963.

Cane, P., *Atiyah's Accidents. Compensation and the Law*, 4th ed., Weidenfeld & Nicolson, London 1987.

Canguilhem, G., *On the Normal and the Pathological*, trans. C.R. Fawcett, D. Reidel Publishing Company, Holland 1978.

Cass, G., 'Workers' benefit or employers' burden: a history of workers' compensation in New South Wales 1880-1926', *Industrial Relations Monograph Series*, No.8, UNSW, 1983.

Castles, F.G., *The Working Class and Welfare*, Allen & Unwin, Wellington 1985.

Centers for Disease Control, *Fact Sheet: Phosgene*, http://www.bt.cdc.gov/agent/phosgene/basics/pdf/phosgene-facts.pdf (accessed 14 April 2006).

Chalmers, A., 'The sociology of knowledge and the epistemological status of science', *Thesis Eleven*, Vol.21, 1988, pp.82-102.

Chambers, J.W., 'Conscripting for Colossus', in P. Karsten (ed), *The Military in America*, Free Press, New York 1980, pp.275-296.

Churcher, Betty, *The Art of War*, Miegunyah Press/MUP, Carlton 2004.

Childe, V.G., *How Labour Governs*, MUP, Parkville 1964.

Christophers, J.A., 'The epidemic of heart disease amongst British soldiers during the First World War', *War and Society*, Vol.15, No.1, May 1997, pp.53-72.

Clarke, P., *Liberals and Social Democrats*, CUP, Cambridge 1981.

Cohen, D., *The War Come Home: Disabled Veterans in Britain and Germany, 1914-1939*, UCP, Berkeley and London 2001.

Collie, J., *Malingering and Feigned Sickness*, Edward Arnold, London 1913.

Connell R.W. & Irving T.H., *Class Structure in Australian History*, Longman Cheshire, Melbourne 1980.

Connell, R.W., *Ruling Class Ruling Culture*, CUP, Melbourne 1977.

Cook, T., *No Place to Run: the Canadian Corps and gas warfare in the First World War*, UNC Press, Vancouver 1999.

Cooter, R., 'Medicine and the Goodness of War', *Canadian Bulletin of Medical History*, Vol.7, 1990, pp.147-59.

Cooter, R., *Surgery and society in Peace and War: Orthopaedics and the Organization of Modern Medicine, 1880-1948*, Macmillan, Basingstoke 1993.

Cooter, R., 'War and Modern Medicine', in W.F. Bynum & R. Porter (eds), *Companion Encyclopedia of the History of Medicine*, Routledge, London 1994, pp.1536-1573.

Cooter, R., 'Essay Review: Discourses on War', *Stud Hist Phil Sci*, Vol.26, No.4, 1995, pp.637-647.

Cooter, R., 'Review Article: the Resistible Rise of Medical Ethics', *Social History of Medicine*, Vol.8, No.2, 1995, pp.257-270.

Cooter, R. and Sturdy, S., 'Of War, Medicine and Modernity: Introduction', in R. Cooter, M. Harrison & S. Sturdy (eds), *War, Medicine and Modernity*, Sutton, Stroud 1998.

Coulthard-Clark, C.D., *The Citizen General Staff: the Australian Intelligence Corps 1907-1914*, Military Historical Society of Australia, Canberra 1976.

Coward, D., 'Crime and punishment: the great strike in New South Wales, August to October 1917', in J. Iremonger, J. Merritt and G. Osborne (eds), *Strikes: Studies in Twentieth Century Australian Social History*, A&R, Sydney 1973, pp.51-80.

Coward, D., 'The impact of war on New South Wales: some aspects of social and political history, 1914-1917', PhD ANU 1974.

Crouthamel, J., 'War Neurosis versus Savings Psychosis: working-class politics and psychological trauma in Weimar Germany', *Journal of Contemporary History*, Vol.37, No.2, 2002, pp.163-182.

Cuff, R.D., 'Herbert Hoover, the ideology of voluntarism and war organisation during the Great War', *J Am Hist*, Vol.64, No.2, 1977, pp.358-372.

Cuff, R.D., 'Organising for war: Canada and the United States during World War I', Canadian Historical Association, *Historical Papers*, 1969, pp.141-156.

Cuff, R.D., *The War Industries Board: business-government relations during World War 1*, Johns Hopkins University Press, 1973.

Cuff, R.D., 'We band of brothers - Woodrow Wilson's war managers', *Canadian Review of American Studies*, Vol.2, 1974, pp.135-148.

Dagen, Philippe, 'The Morality of Horror', *Otto Dix, The War/Der Krieg*, 5 Continents Editions/Historial de la Grande Guerre, Milan and Péronne 2003, pp.9-23.

Daniel, A., *Medicine and the State*, Allen & Unwin, North Sydney 1990.

Das, R. Blanc, P.D., 'Chlorine gas exposure and the lung: a review', *Toxicology and Industrial Health*, Vol.9, No.3, 1993.

Dawes, J.N.I. and Robson, L.L., *Citizen to Soldier*, MUP, Carlton 1977.

Deacon, D., *Managing Gender, the State, the New Middle Class and Women Workers 1830-1930*, OUP, Melbourne 1989.

Deacon, D., 'Taylorism in the home: the medical profession, the infant welfare movement and the deskilling of women', *A&NZ JS*, Vol.21, No.2, July 1985, pp. 161-173.

Denholm, B., 'Some aspects of the transition period from war to peace 1918-1921', *AQ*, March 1944, pp.39-50.

Dickey B, review, *Journal of the Australian War Memorial*, Issue 30, April 1997, http://www.awm.gov.au/journal/j30/bkrevs.htm (accessed 10 July 2006).

Dickey, B., *No Charity There*, Allen & Unwin, North Sydney 1987.

Dickson, D., *Alternative Technology and the Politics of Technical Change*, Fontana, 1974.

Diehl, J. M., 'Victors or victims? Disabled veterans in the Third Reich', *J Mod Hist*, Vol.59, December 1987, pp.705-736.

Diller, W.F., 'Late sequelae after phosgene poisoning: a literature review', *Toxicology and Industrial Health*, Vol.1, No.2, 1985, pp.129-136.

Otto Dix, The War/Der Krieg, 5 Continents Editions/Historial de la Grande Guerre, Milan and Péronne 2003.

Downes, R., 'What medicine owes to war and war owes to medicine', *MJA*, Vol. 1, No.3, 1936, pp.73-80.

Drancourt, M. et al, '*Bartonella Quintana* in a 4000-year-old human tooth', *Journal of Infectious Diseases*, Vol.191, 15 February 2005, pp.607-611.

Eder, N.R., *National Health Insurance and the Medical Profession in Britain*, Garland Publishing Inc., London 1982.

Edwards, C., *Bruce of Melbourne*, William Heinemann, Melbourne 1965.

Egan, L.B., 'Nobler than missionaries: Australian medical culture c1880-1930', PhD Monash University 1988.

Ellis, U., *A History of the Australian Country Party*, MUP, Melbourne 1963.

Englander, D. and Osborne, J., 'Jack, Tommy, and Henry Dubb: the armed forces and the working class', *The Historical Journal*, Vol.21, No.3, 1978, pp.593-621.

Englander, D., (Review Article), 'People at war: France, Britain and Germany, 1914-18 and 1939-45', *Euro Hist Quart*, Vol.18, 1988, pp.229-238.

Evans, R., *Loyalty and Disloyalty*, Allen & Unwin, North Sydney 1987.

Evans, R., *The Red Flag Riots*, UQP, St. Lucia 1988.

Evans, R.B., 'Chlorine: state of the art', *Lung*, Vol.183, 2004, pp.151-167.

Evatt, H.V., 'Australia on the home front 1914-1918', *AQ*, March 1937, pp.68-75.

Evatt, H.V., *William Holman. Australian Labour Leader*, A&R, 1979.

Evison, D. Hinsley, D. Rice, P., 'Regular review: Chemical weapons', *BMJ*, Vol.324, 9 February 2002, pp.324; 332-35.

Feldman, G.D., 'Economic and social problems of the German demobilization, 1918-19', *J Mod Hist*, Vol.47, March 1975, pp.1-47.

Ferro, M., *The Great War 1914-1918*, Routledge & Kegan Paul, London 1973.

Fewster, K., 'Allis Ashmead-Bartlett and the making of the Anzac legend', *JAS*, Vol.10, June 1982, pp.17-30.

Figlio, K., 'Chlorosis and chronic disease in nineteenth-century Britain: the social constitution of somatic illness in a capitalist society', *Social History*, Vol.3, No.2, 1978, pp.167-197.

Figlio, K., 'How does illness mediate social relations? Workmen's compensation and medico-legal practices, 1890-1940', in P. Wright and A. Treacher (eds), *The Problem of Medical Knowledge*, Edinburgh University Press, 1982, pp.174-224.

Figlio, K., 'The historiography of scientific medicine: an invitation to the human sciences', *Comparative Studies in Society and History*, Vol.19, 1977, pp.262-286.

Finnane, M., 'The politics of police powers', in M. Finnane (ed), *Policing in Australia, Historical Perspectives*, UNSW Press, Kensington 1987, pp.88-113.

Fischer, G., '"Negative Integration" and an Australian road to Modernity', *Australian Historical Studies*, Vol.26, No.104, 1995, pp.452-476.

Fitzhardinge, L.F., *William Morris Hughes*, A&R, 1979.

Fitzpatrick, B., *The British Empire in Australia: an Economic History 1834-1939*, Macmillan, South Melbourne 1969.

Forster, C., *Industrial Development in Australia 1920-1930*, ANU, Canberra 1964.

Foucault, C. Barrau, K. Brouqui, P. Raoult, D., '*Bartonella quintana* bacteremia among homeless people', *Clinical Infectious Diseases*, Vol.35, 15 September 2002, pp.684-9.

Foucault, M., *Discipline and Punish: the Birth of the Prison*, Penguin, 1987.

Foucault, M., *The Birth of the Clinic*, Vintage, New York 1975.

Foucault, M., 'The politics of health in the eighteenth century', in C. Gordon (ed), *Power/ Knowledge: selected Interviews and other Writings 1972-1977*, Pantheon, New York 1980, pp.166-182.

Fournier, P. et al, 'Epidemiologic and clinical characteristics of *Bartonella Quintana* and *Bartonella henselai* endocarditis', *Medicine*, Vol.80, No.4, 2001, pp.245-51.

Friedson, E., *Profession of Medicine*, Dodd & Mead, New York 1970.

Fry, E. (ed), *Common Cause: essays in Australian and New Zealand Labour History*, Allen & Unwin/Port Nicholson Press, North Sydney 1986.

Fussell, P., *The Great War and Modern Memory*, OUP, London and New York 1975.

Gammage, B., 'Australians and the Great War', *JAS*, Vol.6, 1980, pp.26-35.

Gammage, B., *The Broken Years*, Penguin, Ringwood 1974.

Garton, S., *Medicine and Madness*, UNSW Press, Kensington 1988.

Garton, S., *Out of Luck: Poor Australians and Social Welfare 1788-1988*, Allen & Unwin, Sydney 1990.

Garton, S., *The Cost of War: Australians Return*, OUP, Melbourne 1996.

Garton, S., 'Freud versus the Rat: understanding Shell Shock in World War 1', *Australian Cultural History*, Vol.16, 1997-8, pp.45-59.

Gellner, E., *Nations and Nationalism*, Basil Blackwell, Oxford 1983.

Geyer, M., 'The Militarization of Europe, 1914-1945', in John R. Gillis (ed), *The Militarization of the Western World*, Rutgers University Press, New Brunswick 1989, pp.65-102.

Gibbney, H.J. and Smith, A.G. (eds), *A Biographical Register, 1788-1939*, Vols. 1 & 2, ADB, Canberra 1987.

Gilbert, D.J., 'The civil re-establishment of the A.I.F.', Appendix B, in A.P. Skerman, *Repatriation in Australia: a history of development to 1958*, pp.239-265.

Gillespie, J.S., *The Price of Health, Australian Governments and Medical Politics 1910-1960*, CUP, Sydney 1991.

Golder, H., *High and Responsible Office: a History of the New South Wales Magistracy*, SUP and OUP, Melbourne 1991.

Goldstein, J., '"Moral Contagion": a professional ideology of medicine and psychiatry in eighteenth- and nineteenth-century France', G.L. Geison (ed), *Professions and the French State. 1700-1900*, University of Pennsylvania Press, Philadelphia 1984, pp.181-222.

Goldstein, J., *Console and Classify. The French Psychiatric Profession in the Nineteenth Century*, CUP, Cambridge 1987.

Gollan, R., *Radical and Working Class Politics*, MUP and ANU, Carlton 1976.

Gollan, R., *The Coalminers of New South Wales. A History of the Union 1860-1960*, MUP in association with ANU, Parkville 1963.

Gough, A., 'The Repatriation of the First Australian Imperial Force', *Qld Hist Rev*, Vol.7, No.1, 1978, pp.62-3.

Gould, S.J., *The Mismeasure of Man*, W.W. Norton & Co., New York 1981.

Gramsci, A., *Prison Notebooks*, Q. Hoare and G. Nowell Smith (trans. and eds), International Publishers, London and New York 1971.

Graubard, S.R., 'Military demobilization in Great Britain following the First World War', *J Mod Hist*, Vol.19, 1947, pp.297-311.

Greub, G. Raoult, D., '*Bartonella*: new explanations for old diseases', *Journal of Medical Microbiology*, Vol.51, 2002, pp.915-923.

Grimshaw, P., 'Women and the family in Australian history - a reply to *The Real Matilda*', *HS*, Vol.18, No.72, April 1979, pp.412-421.

Gurner, J., *The Origins of the Royal Australian Army Medical Corps*, Hawthorn Press, Melbourne 1970.

Hacker, B.C., 'Military institutions and social order: transformations of Western Thought since the Enlightenment', *War & Society*, Vol.11, No.2, October 1993, pp.1-23.

Hacker, B.C., 'Military Institutions, Weapons, and Social Change: Toward a new history of military technology', *Technology and Culture*, Vol.35, 1994, pp.768-834.

Hall, T.S., *History of General Physiology*, Vol.2, University of Chicago Press, Chicago 1969.

Heller, C.E., 'Chemical Warfare in World War 1: the American experience, 1917-1918', *Leavenworth Papers*, No.10, September, Combat Studies Institute, Fort Leavenworth 1984.

Haller, J.S., 'Trench Foot – a study in military-medical responsiveness in the Great War, 1914-1918', *Western Journal of Medicine*, Vol.152, No.6, June 1990, pp.729-33.

Hancock, K. (ed), *The National Income and Social Welfare*, F.W. Cheshire, Melbourne 1965.

Hanes, D.J., *The First British Workmen's Compensation Act 1897*, Yale University Press, New Haven 1968.

Hardach, G., *The First World War 1914-1918*, Allen Lane, London 1977.

Harris, J.C., 'Gassed', *Archives of General Psychiatry*, Vol.62, January 2005, pp.15-17.

Harris, R., *Murders and Madness: Medicine, Law and Society in the fin de siècle*, Clarendon Press, Oxford 1989.

Harrison, M., 'The British army and the problem of venereal disease in France and Egypt during the First World War', *Medical History*, Vol.9, 1995, pp.133-158.

Harrison, M., 'Medicine and the Management of Modern Warfare', *History of Science*, Vol.34, 1996, pp.379-410.

Harrison, M., 'The Medicalization of War – the Militarization of Medicine', *Social History of Medicine*, Vol.9, 1996, pp.267-76.

Harrison, M., 'Medicine and the Management of Modern Warfare: an Introduction', *Clio Medica: the Wellcome Series in the History of Medicine*, Vol.55, No.1, 1999, pp.1-27.

Henshaw, M. 'War: the prints of Otto Dix', *Artonview* (National Gallery of Australia) No. 45, Autumn 2006.

Higgs, E., 'Medical Statistics, Patronage and the State: the development of the MRC Statistical Unit, 1911-1948', *Medical History*, Vol.44, No.3, 2000, pp.323-40.

Howell, J.D., '"Soldier's Heart": the redefinition of heart disease and speciality formation in early twentieth-century Great Britain', in R. Cooter, M. Harrison & S. Sturdy (eds), *War, Medicine and Modernity*, Sutton, Stroud 1998.

Huntington, S.P., *The Soldier and the State: the theory and politics of Civil-Military Relations*, Vintage Books, New York 1957.

Huppauf, B., 'War and death', in Mira Crouch and Bernd Huppauf (eds), *Essays on Mortality*, University of New South Wales Press, Kensington 1985, pp.65-87.

Hurwitz, S.J., *State Intervention in Great Britain, a study of economic control and social response 1914-1919*, 1st ed. 1949, Frank Cass & Co, London 1968.

Illich, I., *Limits to Medicine*, Marion Boyars, London 1976.

Illich, I., *Disabling Professions*, Marion Boyars, London 1977.

Ingleby, D., 'The social construction of mental illness', in P. Wright and A. Treacher (eds), *The Problem of Medical Knowledge*, Edinburgh University Press, 1982.

Inglis, K., 'Men, women and war memorials: Anzac Australia', *Daedalus*, Vol.116, 1987, pp.48-9.

Inglis, K.S., 'The Anzac tradition', *Meanjin*, Vol.24, 1965, pp.25-44.

IPCS INCHEM (www.inchem.org), *Phosgene* ICSC:0007 (accessed 5 April 2006).

IPCS INCHEM (www.inchem.org), *Chlorodiphenylarsine* ICSC:1526 (accessed 12 April 2006).

IPCS INCHEM (www.inchem.org), *Sulfur Mustard* ICSC: 0418 (accessed March 2006).

IPCS INCHEM (www.inchem.org), *Trichloronitromethane* ICSC:0750 (accessed 12 April 2006).

IPCS INCHEM, (www.inchem.org), *Benzyl Bromide* ICSC:1225, (accessed March 2006).

Jackson, J.A. (ed), *Professions and Professionalization*, CUP, Cambridge 1970.

Jacomo, V. Kelly, P.J. Raoult, D., 'Natural history of *Bartonella* infections (an exception to Koch's Postulate)', *Clinical and Diagnostic Laboratory Immunology*, Vol.9, No.1, January 2002, pp.8-18.

Jaensch, D., *Power Politics. Australia's Party System*, Allen & Unwin, North Sydney 1983.

Jamous H. and Peloille, B., 'Changes in the French university-hospital system', in L.A. Jackson (ed), *Professions and Professionalization*, CUP, Cambridge 1970, pp.111-152.

Jewson, N.D., 'The disappearance of the sick-man from medical cosmology, 1770-1870', *Sociology*, Vol.10, 1976, pp.225-244.

Johns' Notable Australians and Who is Who in Australasia

Johnson, J.A., 'Chemical warfare in the Great War', *Minerva*, Vol.40, 2002, pp.93-106.

Johnson, R., 'The Professions in the class structure', in R. Scase (ed), *Industrial Society: Class, Cleavage and Control*, St. Martin's Press, New York 1977, pp.93-110.

Johnson, T.J., *Professions and Power*, Macmillan, London 1972.

Johnston, P.W., 'Judges of fact and scientific evidence - problems of decision-making in environmental cases', *Western Australian Law Review*, Vol.15, June 1983, pp.122-147.

Jones, E. and Wessely, S., 'The origins of British Military psychiatry before the First World War', *War and Society*, Vol.19, No.2, 2001, pp.91-108.

Jones, G., *Social Hygiene in Twentieth Century Britain*, Croom Helm, Beckenham 1986.

Jones, M.A., *The Australian Welfare State*, Allen & Unwin, Sydney 1980.

Katz, M.B., *The Undeserving Poor*, Pantheon, New York 1989.

Keegan, J., *The Face of Battle*, Penguin, Harmondsworth 1978.

Kelly, L. Dewar, D. Curry, B., 'Experiencing chemical warfare: two physicians tell their story of Halabja in Northern Iraq', *Canadian Journal of Rural Medicine*, Vol.9, No.3, Summer 2004, pp.178-181.

Kelman, S., 'The social nature of the definition problem in health', *International Journal of Health Services*, Vol.5, No.4, 1975, pp.625-42.

Kemp, C.D., *Big Businessmen, Four Biographical Essays*, Institute of Public Affairs, Melbourne 1964.

Kennedy, D.M., *Over Here: the First World War and American Society*, OUP, New York 1980.

Kennedy, D.M., 'Overview: the Progressive Era', *Historian*, Vol.37, 1975, pp.453-468.

Kennedy, D.M., 'The political economy of World War I', *Reviews of American History*, Vol.2, 1974, pp.102-107.

Kennedy, R., 'Charity and ideology in colonial Victoria', in R. Kennedy (ed), *Australian Welfare History*, Macmillan, South Melbourne 1982, pp.51-83.

Kenny, D., 'The relationship between workers' compensation and occupational rehabilitation', *JOH&S A&NZ*, Vol.10, No.2, 1994, pp.157-164.

Keogh A., 'Hysteria or pithiatism', *Military Medical Manuals,* London 1918.

Kessler, H.H., *Disability - Determination and Evaluation*, Lea & Febiger, Philadelphia 1970.

Kevles, D., *In the Name of Eugenics*, Penguin, Harmondsworth 1986.

Kewley, T.H., *Australia's Welfare State*, Macmillan, Melbourne 1969.

Kewley, T.H., *Social Security in Australia 1900-1972*, SUP, Sydney 1973.

Kewley, T.H., 'Social Services in Australia (1900-1910)', *JRAHS*, Vol.33, Part 4, 1947, pp.189-257.

Kincaid, J.C., *Poverty and Equality in Britain*, Penguin 1973.

King, T., 'Telling the sheep from the goats: "Dinkum diggers" and others, World War I', in J. Smart and T. Wood (eds), *An Anzac Muster,* Monash Publications in History No.14, Monash University, Clayton 1992, pp.86-99.

King, T., 'The tarring and feathering of J.K.McDougall: "Dirty Tricks" in the 1919 Federal election', *LH*, Vol.45, 1983, pp.54-67.

Kirkby, D., 'Arbitration and the fight for economic justice', in S. Macintyre and R. Mitchell (eds), *Foundations of Arbitration*, OUP, Melbourne 1989, pp.334-351.

Koch, A.M., 'Rationality, Romanticism and the Individual: Max Weber's "Modernism" and the confrontation with "Modernity"', *Canadian Journal of Political Science*, Vol.26, No.1, 1993, pp.123-144.

Kolko, G., *The Triumph of Conservatism*, Free Press, New York 1963.

Koven, S., 'Remembering and Dismemberment: crippled children, wounded soldiers, and the Great War in Great Britain', *The American Historical Review*, Vol.99, No.4, 1994, pp.1167-1202.

Kristianson, G.L., 'The establishment of the RSL', *Stand-to*, March-April 1963, pp. 19-26.

Kristianson, G.L., *The Politics of Patriotism: the Pressure Group Activities of the Returned Servicemen's League*, ANU Press, Canberra 1966.

La Nauze, J.A., *Alfred Deakin: A Biography*, Vols. 1 & 2, MUP, Carlton 1965.

Lain Entralgo, P., *Doctor and Patient*, trans. F. Partridge, World University Press, 1969.

Laird, J.T., *Other Banners*, AWM and AGPS, Canberra 1971.

Lake, M., *Limits of Hope: Soldier Settlement in Victoria 1915-1938*, OUP, Melbourne 1987.

Lake, M., 'The power of Anzac', in M. McKernan and M. Browne (eds) *Australia: Two Centuries of War and Peace*, AWM with Allen & Unwin, 1988, pp.194-222.

Larson, M.S., 'In the matter of experts and professionals, or how impossible it is to leave nothing unsaid', in R. Torstendahl and M. Burrage (eds), *The Formation of Professions: Knowledge. State and Strategy*, SAGE, London 1990.

Larson, M.S., *The Rise of Professionalism: a Sociological Analysis*, University of California Press, California 1977.

Lasswell, H.D., *Propaganda Technique in the World War*, Kegan Paul, Trench, Trubner & Co. Ltd., London 1938.

Lawrence, P.K., 'Enlightenment, modernity and war', *History of the Human Sciences*, Vol.12, No.1, 1999, pp.3-25.

Lawrence, P.K., *Modernity and War: the Creed of Absolute Violence*, St Martin's Press, New York 1997.

Layton, E.T., *The Revolt of the Engineers*, Case Western University Press, Cleveland 1971.

Legg, F., *The Gordon Bennett Story*, A&R, 1965.

Lewis, M., 'Milk, mothers and infant welfare', in J. Roe (ed), *Twentieth Century Sydney: Essays in Urban and Social History*, Hale and Iremonger, Sydney 1980, pp.193-207.

Lloyd, C. and Rees, J., *The Last Shilling*, MUP, Melbourne 1994.

Loudon, I., 'Medical practitioners 1750-1850 and the period of medical reform in Britain', in A. Wear (ed), *Medicine in Society, historical essays*, CUP, Cambridge 1992, pp.219-248.

Love, P., *Labour and the Money Power*, MUP, Melbourne 1984.

Loveday, P., Martin, A.W. and Parker, R.S. (eds), *The Emergence of the Australian party system*, Hale & Iremonger, Sydney 1977.

Macarthy, P.G., 'Wages for unskilled work, and margins for skill, Australia, 1901-21', *AEHR*, Vol.12, No.2, September 1972, pp.142-60.

Macdougall, A.K. (ed), *War Letters of Sir John Monash*, Duffy & Snellgrove, Sydney 2002.

Macintyre, S., *A Colonial Liberalism: the lost world of three Victorian Visionaries*, OUP, Melbourne 1991.

Macintyre, S., 'Ernest Scott and the Official History of Australia during the war', *1918 and beyond*, Papers from the Australian War Memorial History Conference, September 1993, pp.21-28.

Macintyre, S., *The Labour Experiment*, McPhee Gribble, Melbourne 1989.

Macintyre, S., *The Oxford History of Australia*, OUP, Melbourne 1986.

Macintyre, S., *Winners and Losers: the pursuit of social justice in Australian history*, Allen & Unwin, Sydney 1985.

MacLeod, R. (ed), *Government and Expertise: specialists. administrators and professionals, 1860-1919*, CUP, Cambridge 1988.

MacLeod, R., 'Changing perspectives in the social history of science' in I. Spiegel-Rosing & D. de Solla Price (eds), *Science, Technology and Society*, SAGE, London 1977, pp.149-195.

Macpherson, C.B., *The Life and Times of Liberal Democracy*, OUP, Oxford 1977.

Macpherson, C.B., *The Political Theory of Possessive Individualism, Hobbes to Locke*, OUP, Oxford 1962.

Maizels, A., *Industrial Growth and World Trade*, CUP, Cambridge 1963.

Malouf, David, *Fly Away Peter*, Penguin, Ringwood 1982.

Mann, P. et al, 'From trench fever to endocarditis', *Postgraduate Medical Journal*, Vol.79, 2003, pp.655-5.

Markey, R., 'The ALP and the emergence of a national social policy, 1880-1910', in R. Kennedy (ed), *Australian Welfare History: critical essays*, Macmillan, South Melbourne 1982, pp.103-137.

Marr, S., 'Workers' compensation: body parts for sale', *Legal Service Bulletin*, Vol.10, No.5, 1985, pp.247-8.

Marwick, A., *The Deluge: British Society and the First World War*, Macmillan, Basingstoke 1965.

Mayne, A.J.C., *Fever. Squalor and Vice: sanitation and social policy in Victorian Sydney*, UQP, St Lucia 1982.

McCulloch, J., *The Politics of Agent Orange, the Australian Experience*, Heinemann, Richmond 1984.

McDonald, D.I., 'The Australian Soldiers' Repatriation Fund, an experiment in social legislation', J. Roe (ed), *Social Policy in Australia*, Cassell Australia, Stanmore 1976.

McGrath (Cumpston), A.S., 'The History of medical organization in Australia', PhD Sydney University 1975.

McLachlan, N., 'Nationalism and the divisive Digger', *Meanjin*, Vol.27, September 1968, pp.302-308.

McManus, J. Huebner, K., 'Vesicants', *Critical Care Clinics*, Vol.21, 2005, pp.707-18.

McQueen, H., *Gallipoli to Petrov*, George Allen & Unwin, Sydney 1984.

McQueen, H., 'Who were the conscriptionists?', *LH*, Vol. 16, May 1969, pp.44-48.

Medical Directory of Australia

Meeran, R., 'Scientific and legal standards of proof in environmental personal injury cases', *Lancet*, Vol.339, March 14, 1992, pp.671-672.

Merritt, J., *The Making of the AWU*, OUP, Melbourne 1986.

Miles, W.D., 'The idea of chemical warfare in modern times', *Journal of the History of Ideas*, Vol.31, No.2 1970, pp.297-304.

Miliband, R., *The State in Capitalist Society*, Quartet, London 1973.

Miller, M.G., 'Of lice and men: trench fever and trench life in the AIF', paper presented at the Second Anzac Medical Society, France, October 1993. http://www.ku.edu/carrie/specoll/medical/liceand.htm (accessed February 2005).

Monash, J., *Australian Imperial Force: the history of the Department of Repatriation and Demobilisation from November 1918 to September 1919*, Department of Repatriation, London 1919.

Moore, A., 'Guns across the Yarra: secret armies and the 1923 Melbourne police strike', in Sydney Labour History Group, *What Rough Beast?*, George Allen & Unwin 1982, pp.220-233.

265

Moore, A., 'Policing enemies of the state: the New South Wales police and the New Guard, 1931-32', in M. Finnane (ed), *Policing in Australia. Historical Perspectives*, NSWUP, Kensington 1987, pp.114-142.

Moore, A., *The Secret Army and the Premier*, NSWUP, Kensington 1989.

Morton D. and Wright, G., *Winning the Second Battle: Canadian Veterans and the Return to Civilian Life 1915-1930*, University of Toronto Press, Toronto 1987.

Mosse, G.L, 'Shell-shock as a social disease', *Journal of Contemporary History*, Vol.35, No.1, 2000, pp.101-8.

Murphy, D.J. (ed), *Labor in Politics*, UQP, St Lucia 1975.

Murphy, J., 'The new official history', *Australian Historical Studies* [Australia], Vol.26, No.102, 1994, pp.119-124.

Murray, R.K., *Red Scare: A Study in National Hysteria, 1919-1920*, University of Minnesota Press, Minneapolis 1955.

Nairn, B., *Civilising Capitalism: the beginnings of the Australian Labor Party*, MUP, Melbourne 1989.

O'Keefe, B., 'Butler's medical histories', *J Aust War Memorial*, Vol.12, 1988, pp.25-34.

O'Malley, M.A. Edmiston, S. Richmond, D. Ibarra, M., 'Illness associated with drift of chloropicrin soil fumigant into a residential area – Kern County, California, 2003', *Morbidity and Mortality Weekly Report*, Vol.53, No.32, August 20 2004.

Ochi, T. Suzuki, T. Isono, H. Kaise, T., 'In vitro cytotoxic and genotoxic effects of diphenylarsinic acid, a degradation product of chemical warfare agents', *Toxicology and Applied Pharmacology*, Vol.200, 2004, pp.64-72.

O'Connor, J., *The Fiscal Crisis of the State*, St. Martin's Press, New York 1973.

Offe, C., *Contradictions of the Welfare State*, MIT Press, Cambridge (Massachusetts) 1984.

Ohl, M.E. Spach, DH, '*Bartonella quintana* and urban trench fever', *Clinical Infectious Diseases*, Vol.31, 2000, pp.131-5.

Owen, Wilfred, , 'Dulce Et Decorum Est', *The Penguin Book of First World War Poetry*, 2nd ed, Penguin, 1996.

Parker, R.S., *Public Service Recruitment in Australia*, MUP, Melbourne 1942.

Pensabene, T.S., *The Rise of the Medical Practitioner in Victoria*, Research Monograph 2 (Health Research Project), ANU, Canberra 1980.

Pick, D., *Faces of Degeneration, a European Disorder, c.1848-c.1918*, CUP, Cambridge 1989.

Porter, R. (ed), *Patients and Practitioners: lay perceptions of medicine in pre-industrial society*, CUP, Cambridge 1985.

Powell, J., *An Historical Geography of Modern Australia*, CUP, Cambridge 1988.

Price, R., *An Imperial War and the British Working Class*, Routledge & Kegan Paul, London 1972.

Prost, A., *Les Anciens Combattants et la Société Française*, Presses de la Foundation Nationale des Sciences politique, Paris 1977.

Prudhomme, J.C. Bhatia, R. Nutik, J.M. Shusterman, D.J., 'Chest wall pain and possible rhabdomyolysis after chloropicrin exposure: a case series', *Journal of Occupational and Environmental Medicine*, Vol.41, No.1, January 1999, pp.17-22.

Pryor, L.J., 'Back from the wars, the ex-serviceman in history', *AQ*, June 1946, pp.43-50.

Pryor, L.J., 'The origins of Australia's Repatriation policy (1914-1920)', MA thesis, University of Melbourne, 1932.

Ramsay, C., *The Ideology of the Great Fear*, Johns Hopkins University Press, Baltimore 1992.

Raoult, D. et al, 'Evidence for louse-transmitted diseases in soldiers of Napoleon's Grand Army in Vilnius', *Journal of Infectious Diseases*, Vol.193, 1 January 2005, pp.112-20.

Raoult, D. Foucault, C. Brouqui, P., 'Infections in the homeless', *Lancet*, Vol.1, September 2001, pp.77-84.

Rega, P.P., 'Diphosgene', *eMedicine Journal* (www.emedicine.com/), Vol.7, No.3, March 4 2006 (accessed 10 April 2006).

Reiger, K.M., *The Disenchantment of the Home: modernizing the Australian family 1880-1940*, OUP, Melbourne 1985.

Remarque, E.M., *All Quiet on the Western Front*, Mayflower-Dell, London 1963.

Revue d'Histoire, No. 167, July 1992.

Richter, M., *The Politics of Conscience. T.H. Green and his Age*, Weidenfeld and Nicholson, London 1964.

Rickard, J., *Australia, a Cultural History*, Longman Cheshire, Melbourne 1988.

Rickard, J., 'The anti-sweating movement in Britain and Victoria: the politics of empire and social reform', *HS*, Vol.73, October 1979, pp.582-597.

Rivett, R., *Australian Citizen, Herbert Brookes 1867-1963*, MUP, Carlton 1965.

Robinson, W.S., *If I Remember Rightly*, G. Blainey (ed), F.W. Cheshire, Melbourne 1967.

Robson, L.L., *The First A.I.F.*, MUP, Carlton 1982.

Robson, L.L., 'The origin and character of the First AIF, 1914-1918: some statistical evidence', *HS*, Vol.61, October 1973, pp.737-749.

Rodgers, D.T., review of Skopcol in *Journal of Economic History*, Vol.53, No.3, 1993, pp.697-8.

Roe, J. (ed), *Social Policy in Australia: Some Perspectives*, Cassell, Stanmore 1975.

Roe, J., 'Chivalry and social policy in the antipodes', *HS*, Vol.22, 1987, pp.395-410.

Roe, J., 'Old age, young country: the first old-age pensions and pensioners in New South Wales', *Teaching History*, July 1981, pp.23-42.

Roe, M., *Nine Australian Progressives*, UQP, St Lucia 1984.

Rosenberg, C.E., 'The Tyranny of Diagnosis: Specific Entities and Individual Experience', *Millbank Quarterly*, Vol.80, No.2, 2002, pp.237-260.

Rydon, J., *A Biographical Register of the Commonwealth Parliament. 1901-1972*, ANU Press, Canberra 1975.

Sauerteig, Lutz D.H., 'Sex, medicine and morality during the First World War', in R. Cooter, M. Harrison & S. Sturdy (eds), *War, Medicine and Modernity*, Sutton, Stroud 1998, pp.167-188

Sawer, G., *Australian Federal Politics and Law 1901-1929*, MUP, Melbourne 1972.

Schacht, R., *Alienation*, George Allen & Unwin, London 1971.

Schaff, A., *Alienation as a Social Phenomenon*, Pergamon Press, Oxford 1980.

Schedvin, C.B., *Australia and the Great Depression*, SUP, 1970.

Schmidt, J., 'Workers' compensation: the articulation of class relations in law', *Insurgent Sociologist*, Vol.10, No.1, 1980, pp.46-54.

Scott, E., 'Australia During the War', *The Official History of Australia in the War of 1914-1918*, Vol.11, UQP and AWM, 1989.

Searle, G.R., *The Quest for National Efficiency, a study in British politics and political thought, 1899-1914*, Basil Blackwell, Oxford 1971.

Seki, N. et al, 'Epidemiological studies on *Bartonella Quintana* infections among homeless people in Tokyo, Japan', *Japanese Journal of Infectious Diseases*, Vol.59, 2006, pp.31-35.

Sekuless P. and Rees J., *Lest We Forget: the history of the Returned Services League 1916-1986*, Rigby, Dee Why West 1981.

Serle, G., *John Monash: a Biography*, MUP, Melbourne 1982.

Shanahan, E.M. and Leu, L.A., 'The AMA's "Guides to the Evaluation of Permanent Impairment"', *JOH&S A&NZ*, Vol.10, No.4, 1994, pp.323-332.

Shute, C., '"Blood Votes" and the "Bestial Boche": a case study in propaganda', *Hecate*, Vol.2, No.2, July 1976, pp.7-22.

Silbey, D., 'Bodies and cultures collide: enlistment, the Medical Exam, and the British working class, 1914-1916', *Social History of Medicine*, Vol.17, No.1, 2004, pp.61-76.

Skerman, A.P., *Repatriation in Australia*, Repatriation Department, Melbourne 1961.

Skocpol, T., *Protecting Soldiers and Mothers*, HUP, Cambridge 1992.

Smith, B., 'Agent Orange: whose values?', in V.A. Brown and G. Preston (eds), *Choice and Change: ethics. politics and economics of public health*, PHA, Canberra 1993, pp.25-35.

Smith, K.J. Hurst, C.G. Moeler, R.B. Skelton, H.G. Sidell, F.R., 'Sulfur mustard: its continuing threat as a chemical warfare agent, the cutaneous lesions induced, progress in understanding its mechanism of action, its long-term health effects, and new developments for protection and therapy', *Journal of the American Academy of Dermatology*, Vol.32, No.5, May 1995, pp.765-776.

Smith, R., 'Expertise, procedure and the possibility of a comparative history of forensic psychiatry in the nineteenth century', *Psychological Medicine*, 1989, Vol.19, pp.289-300.

Smith, R., *Trial by Medicine. Insanity and Responsibility in Victorian Trials*, Edinburgh University Press, 1981.

Souter, G., *Lion and Kangaroo*, Fontana, Sydney 1978.

Spann, R.N., *Public Sector Administration in Australia*, Government Printer, Sydney 1973.

Spartalis, P., *The Diplomatic Battles of Billy Hughes*, Hale & Iremonger, Sydney 1983.

Spaull, A., 'Federal Government policies and the vocational training of World War One Veterans: a comparative study', *History of Education Review*, Vol.26, No.2, 1997, pp.33-48.

Stapleton, J., *Disease and the Compensation Debate*, Clarendon Press, Oxford 1986.

Starr, A., *Neville Howse V.C., Biography of an Authentic Australian Hero*, Les Baddock & Sons, Sydney 1991.

Stone, D.A., *The Disabled State*, Temple University Press, Philadelphia 1984.

Sturdy, S., 'War as experiment. Physiology, innovation and administration in Britain, 1914-1918: the case of chemical warfare', *War, Medicine and Modernity*, R. Cooter, M. Harrison and S. Sturdy (eds), Sutton, Stroud 1998, pp.65-84.

Summers, A., 'Militarism in Britain before the Great War', *History Workshop Journal*, Vol.2, No.1, 1976, pp.104-123.

Szasz, T., *The Manufacture of Madness*, Routledge and Kegan Paul, London 1973.

Szasz, T., *The Myth of Mental Illness*, Paladin, London 1972.

Tait, D., 'Respectability, property and fertility: the development of official statistics about families in Australia', *LH*, Vol.49, November 1985, pp.83-96.

Tanner, T.W., *Compulsory Citizen Soldier*, Alternative Publishing Co-operative Ltd, 1980.

Thame C., 'Health and the state: the development of collective responsibility for health care in Australia in the first half of the twentieth century', PhD ANU 1974.

Thane, P., *The Foundations of the Welfare State*, Longman, Harlow 1982.

Thomsen, A.B. Eriksen, J. Smidt-Nielsen, K., 'Chronic neuropathic symptoms after exposure to mustard gas: a long-term investigation', *Journal of the American Academy of Dermatology*, Vol.39, No.2, 1998, pp.187-90.

Thomson, A., '"Steadfast until death"? C.E.W. Bean and the representation of Australian military manhood', *AHS*, Vol.23, October 1989, pp.462-478.

Tilbury, M., 'Incapacity for work in workers' compensation law', *UNSW Law Journal*, Vol.6, No.2, 1983, pp.224-233.

Torstendahl R. and Burrage M.(eds), *The Formation of Professions: Knowledge, State and Strategy*, SAGE, London 1990.

Townshend, C., 'Militarism and Modern Society', *Wilson Quarterly*, Winter 1993, pp.71-82.

Turner, B.S., *Medical Power and Social Knowledge*, SAGE, London 1987.

Turner, L.C.F., 'Australian historians and the study of war, 1964-74', in J.A. Moses (ed), *Historical Disciplines and Culture in Australasia*, UQP, 1979, pp.173-214,

Turshen, M., 'The political ecology of disease', *Review of Radical Political Economics*, Vol.9, No.1, 1977, pp.45-60.

Tyquin, M., *Gallipoli the Medical War: the Australian Army Medical Services in the Dardanelles campaign of 1915*, NSWUP, Kensington 1993.

Tyquin, M., *Neville Howse. Australia's First Victoria Cross Winner*, OUP, Melbourne 1999.

Tyquin, M., *Little by Little: a Centenary History of the Royal Australian Army Medical Corps*, Army History Unit, Department of Defence, Canberra 2003.

University of Melbourne, *Record of active service of teachers, graduates, undergraduates, officers and servants in the European War, 1914-1918*, Government Printer, Melbourne 1926.

University of Sydney, *Book of Remembrance of the University of Sydney in the Great War, 1914-1918*, University of Sydney 1939.

Vagts, A., *A History of Militarism: Civilian and Military*, revised ed, Meridian Books 1959.

Veblen, T., *The Place of Science in Modern Civilisation*, B.W. Huebsch, New York 1919.

Waddington, I., 'The role of the hospital in the development of modern medicine: a sociological analysis', *Sociology*, Vol.7, 1973, pp.211-224.

Wall, R. and Winter, J. (eds), *The Upheaval of War: Family, Work and Welfare in Europe 1914-1918*, CUP, Cambridge 1988.

Ward, S.R., 'Intelligence surveillance of British ex-servicemen, 1918-1920', *Historical Journal*, Vol.16, No.1, 1973, pp.179-188.

Warden, C.R., 'Respiratory Agents: irritant gases, riot control agents, incapacitants, and caustics', *Critical Care Clinics*, Vol.21, 2005, pp.719-737.

Watson, J.S.K., 'Wars in the wards: the social construction of medical work in First World War Britain', *Journal of British Studies*, Vol.41, No.4, 2002, pp.484-510.

Watts, R., 'Origins of the Australian welfare state', in R. Kennedy (ed), *Australian welfare history critical essays*, Macmillan, South Melbourne 1982, pp.225-255.

Wear, A. (ed), *Medicine in Society, historical essays*, CUP, Cambridge 1992.

Webster, I.W., 'Invalid pension: the medical decision', *New Doctor*, Vol.21, 1981, pp. 9-12.

Weindling, P. (ed), *The Social History of Occupational Health*, Croom Helm, Beckenham 1985.

Weindling, P., *Health, race and German politics between national unification and Nazism 1870-1945*, CUP, Cambridge 1989.

Weinstein, J., 'Big business and the origins of workmen's compensation', *Labor History*, Vol.8, No.2, 1967, pp.156-174.

Weinstein, J., *The Corporate Ideal in the Liberal State: 1900-1918*, Beacon Press, Boston 1968.

Welborn, S., *Lords of Death*, Fremantle Arts Centre Press, Fremantle 1983.

Whalen, R.W., *Bitter Wounds: German Victims of the Great War, 1914-1939*, Cornell University Press, Ithaca 1984.

Wheeler, L., 'Be in it mate: war, women and welfare', PhD UNSW 1985,

Wheeler, L., 'War, women and welfare', in R. Kennedy (ed), *Australian Welfare: historical sociology*, Macmillan, South Melbourne 1989, pp.172-196.

White, R., 'War and Australian society', in M. McKernan and M. Browne (eds), *Australia Two Centuries of War and Peace*, AWM in association with Allen & Unwin, 1988, pp.391-423.

Whitehead, I.R., 'The British medical officer on the Western Front: the training of doctors for war', *Clio Medica/The Wellcome Series in the History of Medicine*, Vol.55, No.1, 1999, pp.163-184.

Who's Who in Australia

Who's Who in the Commonwealth of Australia

Wikely, N.J., 'Social security adjudication and occupational lung diseases', *Industrial Law Journal*, Vol. 17, 1988, p.92-104.

Willis, E., *Medical Dominance: the division of labour in Australian health care*, George Allen & Unwin, Sydney 1983.

Winder, C., 'The toxicology of chlorine', *Environmental Research*, Vol.85, 2001, pp.105-114.

Winter, D., *Death's Men: Soldiers of the Great War*, Allen Lane (Penguin), 1978.

Winter, J., 'Shell-shock and the cultural history of the Great War', *Journal of Contemporary History*, Vol.35, No.1, 2000, pp.7-11.

Withers, G., 'The 1916-1917 conscription referenda: a cliometric re-appraisal', *HS*, Vol.20, 1982-3, pp.36-46.

Wootton, G., *The Politics of Influence: British Ex-Servicemen, Cabinet Decisions and Cultural Change 1917-1957*, London 1963.

Wright, P. and Treacher, A.(eds), *The Problem of Medical Knowledge*, Edinburgh University Press, 1982.

Wright, P.W.G., 'Some recent developments in the sociology of knowledge and their relevance to the sociology of medicine', *Ethics in Science and Medicine*, Vol.6, 1979, pp.93-104.

Wright, P.W.G., 'The radical sociology of medicine', *Social Studies of Science*, Vol.10, No.1, 1980, pp.103-120.

Young, Bob, 'Science *is* social relations', *Radical Science Journal*, Vol.5, 1977, pp.65-129,

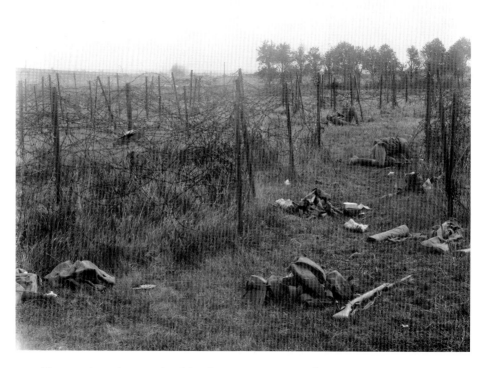

The complete photograph of the illustration appearing (detail) as the frontispiece:
Barbed wire entanglement, Anvil Wood, 2 September 1918
[Australian War Memorial neg. no. E03149]

Index

1st Australian Dermatological Hospital (1st ADH), 91-5, 132, 162

AAMC, 6-9, 21, 46-7, 54-5, 77, 80, 86-9, 127, 133, 137-45, 199

Absent Without Leave (AWL), 144, 147, 182, 185

aetiology, 31, 33, 130-1, 137-40, 143, 145-49, 167-71, 182, 195

Agent Orange, 194-5, 198, 201

'aggravation', 165, 167, 170, 175, 203

Agnew, James, xiv

Agnew, James F, 96-9, 153-5, 159-64, 195

alcohol, 48, 82, 91, 97, 169, 177-9, 186-8, 202-4

Allen, George, 3, 13, 84-5

amputation, 32, 49, 57, 176-80

Appleyard, Sydney V, 159, 191

Australian Intelligence Corps (AIC), 5, 7, 49, 105-6, 126

Australian Soldiers' Repatriation Act, 6, 16, 27, 101, 124-7, 135

Australian Soldiers' Repatriation Fund, 15-18, 21, 27, 136 See also Board of Trustees

Australian War Memorial, xiv-xv, 89, 197, 199

Baillieu, Arthur, 16-17, 19-21, 25-6, 74-5

Barrett, James E, 5, 74, 125-6, 202

Barrett, James W, 79-80

Benjafield, Vivian, 159-62

Bennett, H Gordon, 105, 127, 199

Birdwood, Sir William R, 19, 51-3, 102-3, 134

Board of Trustees, 15-17, 20, 24, 26-7, 72, 74, 76

Bonython, Sir John Langdon, 16-17, 74, 122, 125, 127

British Medical Association (BMA), 80, 85, 95, 100, 153

Bruce, S M, 75, 196, 198-9

Butler, Arthur Graham, 22-3, 30-1, 34, 37-47, 55, 57, 59, 86, 88, 91-5, 132-4, 137-8, 141, 150, 153, 155, 160-3, 167-8, 174, 180-1, 186, 204

censorship, xiv-xv, 59, 126

Cerutty, C J, 85,

chlorine, 34, 36-9, 43

Collins, James, 3, 14, 85, 151, 155-9

Commonwealth loans, 12, 14, 20, 108

compensation, 13, 64, 135-7, 149, 156, 165-6, 183, 188, 193-4, 196, 213 See also workers compensation

conscription, 2, 16-23, 95, 101, 106

conservatism, 4, 7, 20, 24, 27, 61, 70, 73, 86, 95, 124, 127, 151, 156, 165, 173, 213

Cooter, Roger, xiii, 8, 88, 131

Cornell, C J, 3, 85, 158, 165, 169

Courtney, Charles A, 86, 153, 159, 162-4, 174, 181, 184, 195, 203, 209-10

Cowlishaw, Leslie, 159-61, 189

demobilisation, 94, 101-9, 165

diagnosis, 21, 33, 47-8, 52, 134, 137-9, 142, 146-7, 175-87, 210

Dickey, Brian, 86, 94

discipline, 5-9, 21, 47, 53, 55, 57, 74, 87, 92, 94-9, 101, 104, 135-6, 140-2, 144, 150, 155, 158, 164, 173, 177, 202-3, 208

Disordered Action of the Heart (DAH), 47, 141, 147, 186 See also trench fever

Dix, Otto, xiii-xv, 30, 50

Dyett, Gilbert, 110-11, 118-19

Eade, Joseph, 69-71, 73, 126

economy, 2, 4-5, 8, 13, 18, 61, 87-8, 95, 109, 119, 124, 156, 188, 196, 204, 208

Federal Parliamentary War Committee (FPWC), 11, 15-17, 96

Fetherston, R H J, 13, 23, 95, 132-3, 135

Fiaschi, Piero, 93

Fiaschi, Thomas, 93

Figlio, Karl, 129, 145, 173

Financial Emergency Act, 113, 209, 211

Fisher, Andrew, 11-13, 136

Forrest, Sir John, 15-16, 24-5

fraud, 67, 85, 109, 120, 155-6, 173, 179, 199-201, 208-10

funeral benefits, 190, 192, 197-8

furniture, 18, 62-3, 73, 123-4, 208 See also Australian Sodiers Repatriation Fund

Gallipoli, 10, 30, 45, 74-5, 93, 126, 159-63, 182

Garton, Stephen, 149

gas, 32-45, 138, 141, 146-7, 166, 176, 180-4, 194 See also chlorine; phosgene; sulphur mustard

gas mask (respirator), 6, 37-45, 146, 180, 195

Gibson, Robert, 74-5, 109, 121-2, 124-7

Gilbert, David John, 10, 15, 17-18, 20, 25, 59-60, 62, 65-74, 96-8, 105, 107, 109-10, 120, 124-5, 151-2

gonorrhoea, 91-92, 94, 144

Grayndler, Edward, 15-16, 72, 74, 122, 125

Hirschfeld, Eugen, 24, 180

Hirschfeld, O S, 180-2

history of medicine, xiii, 77, 81, 86, 92, 128, 144, 150, 153, 161, 182

Hordern, Sir Samuel, 15-16, 18-19

Howse, Sir Neville, 23, 80, 88, 90-4, 132-4, 138, 199, 201

Hughes, William M (Billy), 2, 12, 16, 18-26, 61, 101-4, 108-10, 112, 116-19, 121, 123-4, 184, 199

ICT See trench foot

ideology, 4, 6-9, 20, 33, 59-60, 75, 77, 85, 99, 124, 126-7, 145-6, 149-50, 153, 165, 173, 187, 194, 213

invalid pension, 3, 82-6, 128, 152, 157-8, 196, 204-5, 213

Kerr, George Lawson, 159-61, 189, 191

Labor, 2, 12, 17, 20, 24-6, 68, 112, 119, 136, 185, 198, 209

labour, 16-18, 20, 80, 87, 101, 104, 108-9, 114, 119, 128, 130, 136, 139, 149, 157, 172, 193, 213

Lake, Marilyn, 12, 109

land settlement, 1, 4, 12, 20-1, 24, 62, 65, 98, 104-5

liberalism, 3-5, 7, 9, 77, 95, 130, 151, 156, 211-12

lice, 46-8 See also trench fever

Lloyd C and Rees J, 187, 209

loans (to returning soldiers), 17, 62-3, 73, 104, 119-20, 123, 208 See also furniture; 'sustenance' payments

Lockyer, Sir Nicholas, 5, 25, 61, 66-74, 99, 107, 125, 151-2, 156

Macpherson, C B, 4, 108, 131

'malingering', 73, 89, 98, 138, 146, 149, 151, 154, 161, 173-80

Manifold, C C, 52-6, 141-2

Maudsley, Henry C, 138-9, 162, 180

Mc Cay, Sir James W, 5, 49, 55-6, 105-6, 160, 196

Mc Whae, Douglas, 92, 94, 163

Medical Advisory Committee (MAC), 96, 152-4, 166, 180-1, 199

medical boarding, 2, 10, 87-90, 132-4, 136-41, 143-8, 159-63, 175, 180, 185 See also Permanent Medical Referee Board

medical bureaucrats, 6, 156, 164, 188, 196, 211

medical history (of individuals), 45, 65, 107, 168, 175, 184-5, 190, 203

medical knowledge, 5, 77, 80, 85, 150-3, 167, 194, 196, 210 See also Chapters 7 and 9 medical statistics, 28, 31, 89, 142, 167

mental health, 173-80 See also malingering; neurasthenia

militarism, 2, 6-9, 86, 94-5, 126, 158, 173, 212

Millen, E D, 12-13, 16, 25-7, 60-3, 66-75, 95, 97, 101-2, 105-9, 112-17, 120-7, 150, 152-3, 158

modernity/modernism, xiii, 6-9, 131

Monash, John, 6, 49, 57, 75, 87-8, 94, 102, 104-6, 164, 180

Moorehead, Harold P, 74-5, 122, 125

mustard gas See sulphur mustard

Nationalist, 2, 24, 107, 110, 112, 119, 124, 196

neurasthenia, 97, 142, 149, 163, 173-9, 189-90, 195

neurosis, 138-9, 173-81

Nurses, 9, 95, 141, 207-8

old age pension, 3, 13, 82-3, 85, 116, 154, 199, 204-5

Owen, Robert H, 74-5, 105-6, 122

Owen, Wilfred, 29, 49-50

Parkinson, Charles K, 159-61, 175-6, 186, 195

Pearce, G F, 13, 15, 23-4, 26, 95, 101, 103, 106, 133-4, 157

Pensabene, T S, 80-1, 99-100

pensions See invalid pension; old age pension; service pension; war pension; widows pension

Permanent Medical Referee Board (PMRB), 136-40, 147-8, 154-5, 158-9, 174-5, 185, 188

phosgene, 37-9, 43-4, 146

police/policing, 3, 14, 63, 65, 82-3, 98, 135, 142, 157, 169, 176, 178, 192, 196, 199-200, 203

Poor Law, 3, 18, 63, 128, 130, 159, 165, 208

Post Traumatic Stress Disorder, 195

professionalisation of medicine, 77-86, 95-100, 131

propaganda, 1, 12, 27, 30, 65, 70, 104-9, 116, 148

Pryor, L J, 11, 19-20, 26, 72, 75, 117

PUO See trench fever

'reconditioning' (of soldiers) See medical boarding

recruiting, 11-12, 22-3, 60, 64, 66, 70, 72, 109, 132, 134, 165

Reiach, James, 90-91, 189

Repatriation Department, establishment of, See Chapter 4

responsibility for health/illness, 135-145, 148, 164, 173

Roth, Reuter Emerich, 159, 161, 175, 186

royal commission, 75, 100, 111, 116, 145, 169, 187, 194, 198, 205

RSSILA/RSL, 1, 69-70, 108-9, 112, 116, 118, 121-2, 126, 169, 178, 193, 211

Rutledge, Edward, 159-62, 207

Ryan, Charles S, 138-9, 148, 162

Ryan, M B, 67-8, 105-6

Sanderson, John, 74-5, 125

Scott, Ernest, 11, 24, 59

Semmens, James, 5, 105-6, 120, 122, 124-7, 153-4, 158, 165, 169, 197, 199-201, 207, 209, 211

service pension, 3, 184

shell shock, 22, 31, 89, 142-3, 163, 174-5, 180

Skerman, A P, 170-1, 187, 211

Smith, Kenneth, 23, 93-4, 132, 159-64, 183, 186, 189-91, 202-3

Smith, Roger, 78, 138

Smith's Weekly, 74, 195-6

'soldier's heart' See Disordered Action of the Heart (DAH)

Springthorpe, John, 88-91, 138-9

State War Council, 11, 15, 17-19, 24-5, 62, 67, 74, 101, 151-2

Sturdy, Steve, 8, 131

sulphur mustard, 40-4

surveillance, 65, 169, 196, 199-201, 204, 211

'sustenance' payments, 1, 17, 62, 67, 98, 104, 108, 112, 123, 185-6

syphilis, 84-5, 136, 144, 190, 203-4

Teece, Ashley, 5, 126, 198

Treasury, 3, 12-14, 61, 74, 76, 82-6, 100, 110-12, 116-20, 151-9, 170, 196, 199, 203-4 See also Collins, James; Allen, George

trench fever, 22, 30-3, 45-8, 65, 144-7, 159

trench foot, 22, 31, 33, 49-57, 134, 141-2, 166

trench warfare, 49-58

tuberculosis, 37, 83-4, 97-8, 180, 183-4, 186-8, 209-11

Tyquin, Michael, 51-2, 86-7, 132

Vagts, Alfred, 7-8

venereal disease, 31-3, 79, 84, 91-7, 136-7, 140, 145, 147, 169, 182-3, 190, 203 See also gonorrhoea; syphilis; 1st Australian Dermatological Hospital

voluntarism, 10-16, 20, 72

war gratuities, 65, 110, 117-20

war loans, 12-13, 20, 101, 108, 118-19 See also Commonwealth loans

war memorials, 197-8

war pensions, 1, 3, 6, 12-14, 17, 33, 58, 62, 64-5, 76, 85-6, 98, 100, 107, 110-16, 124-5, 127, 130, 135, 140, 146, 149, 197-213 See also Chapters 8 and 9

War Pensions Appeal Tribunal (UK), 143

War Pensions Entitlement Appeal Tribunal, 144, 184

war photographs/war images, xiii-xv, 149

war records, 167-170, 172 See also medical statistics

war-relatedness, 145, 147-50, 160, 170

Watson, J C, 15-17

Weber, Max, 5, 7-8, 95, 131

welfare, 2-3, 77-9, 100, 108, 149, 151, 187-8, 196, 204, 209, 212-13

widows pension, 13, 86, 112-14, 193, 199-201

Williams, Oliver Morrice, 16-17, 21, 24-8, 74-5

Willis, Evan, 80-2, 100

Willis, Henry Hastings, 153-6, 159-60, 162-3, 175, 178, 189, 195, 204

workers compensation, 3, 128, 135, 149, 166, 173, 179, 193, 204

Marks of War

War Neurosis and the Legacy of Kokoda

by John Raftery

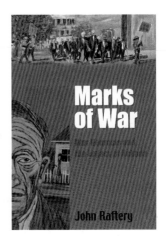

Dr John Raftery spent ten years researching the effects of war on veterans from the infamous Kokoda campaign in 1942, when Australian troops repelled the Japanese in a horrific struggle across the mountains of New Guinea. He found that while many of the men were able to return to a seemingly successful life after the war, they carried the marks of war deep within them. For some, the past has come back to trouble them in their later years. John Raftery paints a very human portrait of the lives of these men, and the difficulties that they and their families have had to cope with.

'This is a graceful and meticulously researched book …'
Allan Young

'… an original, reflective and nuanced analysis of the long-term impact of war'
Joy Damousi

ISBN 978 0 957996 02 1

For more information on this and other Lythrum Press books, visit
www.lythrumpress.com.au

Eyes Right

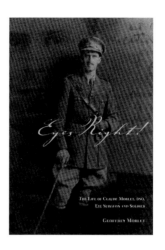

The Life of Claude Morlet, DSO
Eye Surgeon and Soldier

by Geoffrey Morlet

In December 1914 Claude Morlet, a newly qualified doctor, set sail from Melbourne to do his duty for his Country in the First World War. After spending time in Egypt tending the wounded in Australian military hospitals, he got his wish to join the action and arrived in Gallipoli in September 1915, after the initial assault. He recorded his thoughts and observations in diaries and letters back home, many of which have survived, giving a first-hand account of the action. Later in France, caring for the wounded under hazardous conditions, he was Mentioned in Dispatches, and awarded the DSO for his service in action.

Returning from the war, he settled in Perth where he married and established a successful practice as an ophthalmic surgeon. When war again broke out, he enlisted and served in the Middle East before being posted to Tobruk, where he served throughout the siege.

Claude's diaries and letters give a thoughtful and sympathetic view of the lot of the soldier, as well as some acerbic comments on the bureaucratic shortcomings of some of his superior officers. The diaries and letters have been knitted together with further background by his son Geoffrey, and illustrated with photos from Claude's own collection.

Foreword by Major General Digger James

ISBN 978 1 921013 15 7

LYTHRVM

WWW.LYTHRUMPRESS.COM.AU